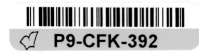
About the Authors

Samir P. Desai, M.D.

Dr. Samir Desai serves on the faculty of the Baylor College of Medicine in the Department of Medicine. He has educated and mentored medical students and residents, work for which he has received teaching awards. He is an author and editor, having written ten books that together have sold over 100,000 copies worldwide.

Dr. Desai is the co-author of the popular *250 Biggest Mistakes 3rd Year Medical Students Make And How To Avoid Them,* a book that shows students how to excel during the third year of medical school. He is also the author of the *Clinician's Guide to Laboratory Medicine: Pocket.* Widely used by students, this book provides a unique step-by-step approach to lab test interpretation while fitting easily in a coat pocket.

He is the founder of www.MD2B.net, a website committed to helping today's medical student become tomorrow's doctor. At the site, a variety of tools and resources are available to help students tackle the challenges of medical school.

With Dr. Rajani Katta, he writes a regular column for www.studentdoctor.net called "The Successful Match." The goal of the column is to provide applicants with a better understanding of the residency selection process. Applicants can then use this information to develop an approach that will lead to a successful residency match.

Recently, he founded www.ImgAssist.com, a website providing guidance to international medical graduates (IMGs) seeking residency positions in the United States. There, IMGs will find key information needed to help them successfully match.

After completing his residency training in Internal Medicine at Northwestern University in Chicago, Illinois, Dr. Desai had the opportunity of serving as chief medical resident. He received his M.D. degree from Wayne State University School of Medicine in Detroit, Michigan, graduating first in his class.

Rajani Katta, M.D.

Dr. Rajani Katta is an Associate Professor in the Department of Dermatology at Baylor College of Medicine. She has authored over 30 articles published in scientific journals, and lectured extensively both nationally and locally on dermatology and contact dermatitis to students, residents, and physicians.

She co-authored *250 Biggest Mistakes 3rd Year Medical Students Make And How To Avoid Them,* the book that shows students how to excel during the third year of medical school. She serves as the course director for dermatology in the basic science years, and has served as the clerkship director for the dermatology rotation. In these capacities, she has seen firsthand the importance of outstanding clinical evaluations in securing a position in a competitive specialty, and her insight in this area has helped students seeking these types of competitive positions.

After graduating with honors from Baylor College of Medicine and completing her internship in internal medicine, she completed her dermatology residency at the Northwestern University School of Medicine.

Contents

Chapter 1

The Application

What does it take to match successfully? What does it take to match into the specialty and program of your choice?

In the 2007 Match, over 40% of all U.S. senior applicants failed to match at the program of their choice. In competitive fields such as dermatology and plastic surgery, over 37% of U.S. senior applicants failed to match at all.

Percentage of U.S. senior applicants who failed to match in 2007	
Specialty	% of U.S. seniors failing to match
Dermatology	38.8%
Plastic surgery	37.5%
Urology	31.3%*
Ophthalmology	30.7%*
Neurological surgery	28.3%*
Orthopedic surgery	19.7%
Otolaryngology	18.4%
Radiation oncology	18.4%
Diagnostic radiology	9.2%
*All applicants (U.S. seniors + other applicants) From www.nrmp.org, www.sfmatch.org, www.auanet.org	

The numbers are significantly worse for osteopathic and international medical graduates:

- 28.4% of the 1,900 osteopathic students and graduates who participated in the 2008 Match failed to match at all.

- 55% of the 10,300 international medical graduates who participated in the 2008 Match failed to match at all.

> **Did you know ...**
>
> Applicants who fail to match may participate in the Scramble. During the Scramble, applicants try to secure a first-year residency position in a program that failed to fill during the Match. In 2008, over 12,000 applicants scrambled for one of only 1,300 positions.

What does it actually take to match successfully? The issue is a hotly debated one, and surveys of students, reviews of student discussion forums, and discussions with academic faculty all find sharp divisions on the topic. In the following 400 plus pages, we answer the question of what it takes to match successfully. We also provide specific evidence-based advice to maximize your chances of a successful match.

Our recommendations are based on data from a full spectrum of sources. We present evidence obtained from scientific study and published in the academic medical literature. The results of these studies can provide a powerful impetus for specific actions. We present anecdotal data and advice that have been published in the literature and obtained from online sources. We also take an insider's look at the entire process of residency selection based on our experiences, the experiences of our colleagues in the world of academic medicine, and the experiences of students and residents with whom we have worked.

Who actually chooses the residents? We review the data on the decision makers. What do these decision makers care about? We review the data on the criteria that matter to them. How can you convince them that you would be the right resident for their program? We provide concrete, practical recommendations based on this data. At every step of the process, our recommendations are meant to maximize the impact of your application.

In Chapter 2, starting on page 21, we present specialty-specific data. Given the high failure to match rates for certain specialties, is there any literature available to applicants to guide them through the residency application process? For each specialty, we present the results of those studies. For example, in radiology, a 2006 survey of residency program directors obtained data from 77 directors on the criteria that programs use to select their residents (Otero). Which criteria did these directors rank as most important in deciding whom to interview? Which selection factors were most important in determining an applicant's place on the program's rank order list? What were the mean United States Medical Licensing Examination (USMLE) Step 1 scores among matched and unmatched U.S. seniors? What percentage of U.S. seniors who matched were members of the Alpha Omega Alpha Honor Medical Society (AOA)? This evidence-based information is critical to developing an application strategy that maximizes your chances of a successful match.

We review each component of the application in comprehensive detail in the following chapters. Each single component of your application can be created, modified, or influenced in order to significantly strengthen your overall candidacy. We devote the next 400 plus pages of this book to showing you, in detail, exactly how to do so.

Letters of Recommendation

Letters of recommendation are a critical component of the residency application. Since you won't be directly writing these letters yourself, it may seem as if you have no control over their content. In reality, you wield more influence than you realize. In our chapter on letters of recommendation, we detail the steps that you can take in order to have the best possible letters written on your behalf. These steps include choosing the correct letter writers and asking in the correct manner. We also discuss the type of information to provide, and the manner in which to provide it, in order to highlight those qualities that you hope your letter writer will emphasize.

The purpose of these letters is to emphasize that you have the professional qualifications needed to excel. The letters should also demonstrate that you have the personal qualities to succeed as a resident and, later, as a practicing physician. Since these letters are written by those who know you and the quality of your work, they offer programs a personalized view. In contrast to your transcript and USMLE scores, they supply programs with qualitative, rather than quantitative, information about your cognitive and non-cognitive characteristics.

What do the faculty members reviewing applications look for in a letter of recommendation? The first item noted is the writer of the letter. In a survey of program directors in four specialties (internal medicine, pediatrics, family medicine, and surgery), it was learned that a candidate's likelihood of being considered was enhanced if there was a connection or relationship between the writer and residency program director (Villanueva). "In cases where there was both a connection between the faculty members and in-depth knowledge of the student (i.e., personal knowledge), the likelihood was that the student's application would be noted." In a survey of 109 program directors of orthopedic surgery residency programs, 54% of directors agreed that the most important aspect of a letter was that it was written by someone they knew (Bernstein).

In another study, the academic rank of the writer was found to be an important factor influencing the reviewer's ranking of the letter, with 48% of the reviewers rating it as important (Greenburg). A survey of physical medicine and rehabilitation (PM&R) program directors asked respondents to rate the importance of letters of recommendation in selecting residents (DeLisa). The study showed that the "most important letters of recommendation were from a PM&R faculty member in the respondent's department, followed by the Dean's letter, and the PM&R chairman's letter." Next in importance were letters from a PM&R faculty member in a department other than the respondents' followed by a clinical faculty member in another specialty. The University of Texas-Houston Medical School Career Counseling Catalog gives this advice: "letters of recommendation from private physicians or part-time faculty, and letters from residents are generally discounted."

For international medical graduates (IMGs), this issue becomes even more important. A survey of 102 directors of internal medicine residency programs sought to determine the most important predictors of performance for IMGs (Gayed). When rating the importance of 22 selection criteria, the lowest rated criterion was letters of recommendation from a foreign country, with 93% of program directors feeling that such letters were useless.

What else do the faculty members reviewing applications look for in a letter of recommendation? They seek evidence of an applicant's strengths and skills. Most applicants assume that their letter writers know what to say and what information to provide in a letter to substantiate their recommendation. However, that is a dangerous assumption. In an analysis of 116 recommendation letters received by the radiology residency program at the University of Iowa Hospitals and Clinics (O'Halloran), reviewers noted the following:

- 10% were missing information about an applicant's cognitive knowledge
- 35% had no information about an applicant's clinical judgment
- 3% did not discuss an applicant's work habits
- 17% did not comment on the applicant's motivation
- 32% were lacking information about interpersonal communication skills

In another review of recommendation letters sent during the 1999 application season to the Department of Surgery at Southern Illinois University, writers infrequently commented on psychomotor skills such as "easily performed minor procedures at the bedside," "good eye-hand coordination in the OR," "could suture well," and so on (Fortune).

Our chapter on letters of recommendation, starting on page 159, reviews strategies to locate letter writers who will be most helpful to your candidacy. We review how to identify these writers and how to approach them. Most importantly, we describe the type of evidence you can provide to the writer and the professional manner in which to provide it. Your letter writers want to write the best letter possible, and you can do much more than you realize to make this a reality.

Personal Statement

For most students the most dreaded aspect of the residency application is the personal statement. It is very frustrating trying to put into words your vision for your medical career. Most students don't understand one basic fact about the personal statement, though. Unlike just about every other aspect of the application, you have complete control over the personal statement. You decide the content, the structure, and the form of the statement. This is a unique opportunity to impress the selection committee. In your statement you can showcase your strengths and those qualities that set you apart from other candidates. You can weave in evidence that confirms your qualities. You can use this opportunity to convince a faculty member that you would be an ideal candidate for their particular program. This is information that is not readily apparent to programs from their review of other application components.

Individual specialties, residency programs, and application reviewers assign varying degrees of importance to the personal statement. In the screening phase, reviewers whittle down a large applicant pool to a select group that is ultimately extended interview invitations. At some programs, the personal statement is used minimally, if at all, during this screening phase. In others, the personal statement is considered very important.

- The website for the University of Washington Family Medicine Residency states that the "personal statement is the primary component that will be used to select applicants who are invited for an interview. Please write a careful and thoughtful document." In fact, a 1993 study of family practice residency program directors found that the personal statement ranked second only to the Dean's letter for making decisions about whom to interview (Taylor). With regard to the ranking of applicants, it was third in importance, following only the interview and the Dean's letter.

- The University of Texas-Houston Department of Orthopedic Surgery states that the "personal statement is read by each of our orthopedic faculty members, and is considered by our faculty to be a very important part of the application process. It is often used as a point of departure for interviewing the student" (http://www.med.uth.tmc.edu/med/administration/student/ms4/2003CCC.htm).

- In a survey of the Association of Program Directors in Radiology, 79% of programs considered the statement to be extremely or somewhat important for selecting an applicant to interview (www.apdr.org).

Adding to the importance of the personal statement is this fact: a poorly conceived and executed personal statement may be detrimental to your application. Otherwise excellent candidates have been ranked lower, or even rejected, because of a poorly written statement. As reinforced by the University of Alabama at Birmingham department of obstetrics and gynecology—"poorly written personal statements may detract from an otherwise excellent application" (http://www.obgyn.uab.edu/medicalstudents/obgyn/uasom/documents/2005ResidencyGuidelines.pdf).

When you create a personal statement, you need to consider your audience. When reading a personal statement, what do faculty members look for? What are they trying to determine? Consider the following:

- In a survey of orthopedic surgery residency program directors, 43% agreed that "the most important aspect of a personal statement is to learn more about the candidate's personal interests and backgrounds," while 32% stated that "the most important aspect of a personal statement was to gain insight into an applicant's ability to write and to communicate effectively" (Bernstein).

- In a study evaluating the content of personal statements, members of the radiology residency selection committee at Wayne State University ranked eleven content areas from least to most important (Smith). Most important was a candidate's explanation as to why they chose to pursue a career in radiology. Personal attributes was second in importance, while perception of radiology defined as the applicant's ability "to explicitly state what he/she feels are the most important characteristics of either radiologists or the practice of radiology" was third.

- At the website for the Wayne State University pathology residency, the program writes that "your personal statement should summarize your particular background and interests and depict you as a person. You should indicate in your personal statement why you are interested in Pathology, what kind of experience you have had with Pathology, and what career path you plan to follow after training." (http://www.med.wayne.edu/Pathology/residencytraining/FAQ.htm)

- The article "Crafting a Great Personal Statement," written by Drs. McGarry and Tammaro, program directors of the internal medicine residency program at Brown Medical School, provides additional insight and recommendations (McGarry). The authors write that "a great personal statement will make the program director eager to meet you and potentially work with you...A poorly written PS can cast doubt on your dedication and focus for a demanding profession like medicine..."

In our chapter on the personal statement starting on page 187, we review in more detail what programs seek in the personal statement. We review different approaches and provide a springboard to brainstorming and developing your own statement. We review in detail how to conceive and execute a personal statement that reflects your individual strengths and skills, while convincingly conveying your excellent fit with the specialty and with the individual program in a convincing manner.

Dean's Letter (MSPE)

Applicants must submit a letter from the Dean as part of their application. Known previously as the Dean's letter, this letter is now termed the Medical Student Performance Evaluation (MSPE). The typical MSPE contains an assessment of both a student's academic performance and professional attributes. The MSPE is particularly helpful when used as a tool to compare your performance in medical school relative to your peers.

Because this component is not written by them, students often don't realize the steps that they can take to influence its content. At many schools, students *are* involved in the development of this letter. In Chapter 9 starting on page 226, we review the steps that applicants can take to maximize the quality of the MSPE, from choosing a letter writer, to providing the correct type of information, to the follow through.

The following table summarizes the studies on the importance of the Dean's letter in the residency selection process.

Importance of the Dean's Letter in the residency selection process	
Study	Findings
Survey of program directors in family medicine and obstetrics and gynecology inquiring about the importance of various application components (Taylor)	In deciding whether to invite an applicant for an interview, obstetrics and gynecology program directors ranked the medical school transcript, Dean's letter, and USMLE score highest (in descending order). The Dean's letter was also among the top three factors used by family practice residency program directors for making decisions about interview invitations.
Survey of family practice residency program directors inquiring about the importance of various application components (Travis)	This study, done as a follow-up to the Taylor study, again showed that the dean's letter continues to be one of the top three criteria used in the residency selection process.

Importance of the Dean's Letter in the residency selection process	
Survey of program directors in internal medicine inquiring about the usefulness of various application components in making decisions about interview invitations and ranking applicants (Adams)	The Dean's letter was rated highly or moderately useful by 87% of respondents, and 82% rated the Dean's letter as highly or moderately useful for making ranking decisions.
Questionnaire sent to PM&R program directors inquiring about the importance of various application components (DeLisa)	Most program directors used multiple criteria to complete their rank list, but the most important were the interview, letters of recommendation, medical school transcript, and the Dean's letter (in descending order of importance).
Questionnaire sent to radiology residency program directors to determine the importance of various application components (Otero)	Respondents were asked to assign a zero to ten score regarding the importance of variables related to extending interview invitations. The USMLE score was ranked highest with a score of 8.65 followed by the Dean's letter at 7.52.
Survey of orthopedic residency program directors to determine what program directors value most highly (Bernstein)	Dean's letter was ranked 10th out of a group of 26 variables used in the resident selection process.
Survey of orthopedic residency program directors to determine the most important attributes to obtaining a residency (Bajaj)	Dean's letter was ranked 7th in importance for resident selection.
Survey of program directors of American Osteopathic Association-approved primary care graduate training programs regarding the importance of 22 variables used in the residency selection process (Bates)	Dean's letter was ranked 18th out of a group of 22 variables.
Study to learn about characteristics of an applicant that might predict future success in an emergency medicine residency (Hayden)	It was found that the Dean's letter correlated fairly well with overall success in the residency. In particular, the letter's categorical rating was found to be a strong predictor of performance during residency training.
Study comparing the Dean's letter categorical ranking (outstanding, excellent, very good, good) of University of Rochester students with program director ratings of these students nine months into their internship (Lurie)	The Dean's letter ranking was found to be a significant predictor of performance in internship.

Curriculum Vitae (CV)

Curriculum vitae is a Latin expression meaning the "course of one's life." Known as CV for short, this document provides an overview of a candidate's academic and professional background. While similar to a resume, a CV includes additional information such as research experience, publications, and presentations.

Programs within most specialties require applications to be submitted through the Electronic Residency Application System (ERAS). Using ERAS, applicants take information on the CV and enter it into the ERAS common application form (CAF). While this process limits what you can do with the look of your CV, the presentation of the information retains the same importance.

Applicants also need to generate a formal CV, as this will be used by letter writers and may be needed by faculty when interviewing.

From the standpoint of a residency selection committee member, reviewing a vast number of CVs from applicants is a difficult process. Therefore, in many cases, your CV will be skimmed. Since you have a limited opportunity to impress the residency selection committee, every line, word, and number on your CV becomes important. We review how to describe and position experiences and achievements in order to maximize their impact. We review techniques such as the utilization of numbers and action verbs to highlight your accomplishments. We review how to create a professional CV, how to utilize the correct structure and format, and how to maximize the impact of every word, line, and number.

Audition Elective

An "audition" elective essentially serves as an extended interview and should be regarded as such. For students applying to competitive specialties or programs, audition electives are considered a must by some programs. These four- or eight- week rotations offer students the chance to highlight skills and qualities that aren't easily judged by the typical application materials. Students can showcase their clinical acumen, their skills in patient interaction, their abilities to work with colleagues and faculty, and their enthusiasm for the particular program and specialty. These electives also offer additional opportunities to highlight a student's qualifications for the program. Opportunities include deeper investigation of difficult cases, performing thorough literature searches, volunteering to give presentations, or seeking opportunities to publish in their chosen field.

In some specialties, particularly those that are more competitive, audition electives become very important:

- In a survey of program directors representing multiple specialties, Wagoner and Suriano found that 86% of program directors would give preference to students who had performed at a high level in an audition elective (Wagoner).
- In a survey of orthopedic surgery residency program directors, *the most important criterion in the resident selection process* was considered to be an applicant's performance during a rotation at the director's program (Bernstein). Of note, applicants were also asked about their impressions regarding

the importance of these factors, and this factor was not cited among their top three.

- In another survey of orthopedic surgery residency program directors, performance on a local rotation was considered *the most important attribute in obtaining a residency.* This was followed by class rank and the interview (Bajaj).
- In a survey of 2003 dermatology applicants, the audition elective was similarly important. A total of 53% of applicants matched at a program in which they had some prior experience. Of these, 29% matched at an institution affiliated with their own medical school, 18% matched with an institution where they had done an audition elective, and 6% matched with a program where they had done a research elective/ fellowship (Clarke).

In other specialties, by contrast, the audition elective may not have much of an effect. Following is a summary of the literature on the importance of this criterion to different specialties.

Importance of audition electives by specialty	
Survey	**Results**
Survey of orthopedic residency program directors inquiring about those factors considered most important in the resident selection process (Bernstein). Applicants were also asked about their impressions regarding the importance of these factors.	Most important criterion was an applicant's performance during a rotation at the director's program. Of note, applicants did not cite this factor among their top three.
Survey of 2003 dermatology applicants (Clarke)	53% of applicants matched at a program where they had some prior experience, highlighting the importance of audition electives: • 29% matched at an institution affiliated with their medical school • 18% matched with an institution where they had done an audition elective • 6% matched with a program where they had done a research elective/fellowship
Survey of orthopedic residency program directors (Bajaj)	Performance on a local rotation was the most important attribute to obtaining a residency.
Survey of 41 PM&R program directors inquiring about the residency selection process (Garden)	While the interview was the most important overall factor, of the academic variables presented, an elective performed at the program director's hospital and the Dean's letter were rated highest.

Importance of audition electives by specialty	
Survey of 94 emergency medicine residency program directors inquiring about the criteria directors use to select residents (Crane)	Respondents were asked to rate each item on a scale of 1 (least important) to 5 (most important). Performance at an elective at the program director's institution received a mean score of 3.76, making it a moderately important factor. Of note, it did have the largest standard deviation of all responses, suggesting that programs vary in the degree of importance attached to these electives.
Study reviewing the outcome of 99 students who completed audition electives in surgery (Fabri)	Results showed that while audition electives increase the probability of receiving an interview, these electives had no effect on the probability of matching with general surgery residency programs. However, authors noted that surgical specialties viewed audition electives differently, with some placing high priority on these electives.
Survey of 89 radiology residency program directors from 2005 (www.apdr.org)	31% rated an audition elective in their department as an extremely important criterion for selecting an applicant for interview; 23% rated an elective as an extremely important criterion for ranking.

Our chapter on the audition elective, starting on page 237, describes each advantage of the audition elective, and details how to derive the maximum benefit from each. We review what factors to consider when choosing an elective and describe how to deliver an outstanding performance.

The Competitive Edge

If you're planning on applying to a competitive program or a competitive specialty, you'll need to bring into play all of the recommendations throughout this book. In Chapter 11, we review in detail how to add an extra competitive edge to your application. For competitive programs, publications may boost the strength of your application. The possibility of being published in the medical literature is available to all students. We tell you how to locate such opportunities and walk you through the steps needed to submit an outstanding product.

We also discuss research. Many applicants who apply to competitive programs will have participated in research. *Those applicants are your competition.*

In 2007 the NRMP published data on how applicant qualifications affect match success. Included among the data were the percentage of U.S. seniors who had participated in research projects and the percentage with publications. In each of the fields shown in the following table, over 75% of U.S. seniors applying to the field had participated in research projects. In highly competitive fields such as dermatology, orthopedic surgery, plastic surgery, and radiation oncology, over 90%

of U.S. seniors had participated in research projects. Even in the fields that are not the most competitive, including the fields of anesthesiology, pathology, and general surgery, over 80% of U.S. seniors had participated in research projects.

Percentage of U.S. seniors in the 2007 Match participating in research and reporting publications			
Specialty	% of U.S. seniors having participated in research projects	% of U.S. seniors with publications*	Of note ...
Anesthesiology	80%	51%	82/84 applicants with > 5 publications matched. Over 90% of applicants with no publications or research experience matched
Dermatology	93%	86%	Most applicants participate in research. Only 26 applicants had no research experience. Of this group, 16 did not match. Of the 136 applicants with > 5 publications, 35 did not match. 35 of 59 with no publications did not match.
Emergency medicine	77%	50%	All applicants with > 5 pubs matched. Nearly 90% of applicants with no publications or research experience matched
Obstetrics and gynecology	77%	46%	7/59 with > 5 pubs did not match 59/509 with no pubs did not match 196/220 with no research experience matched
Orthopedic surgery	93%	65%	19/117 with > 5 pubs did not match 62/244 with no pubs did not match 34/53 with no research participation matched
Otolaryngology	95%	88%	6/65 with > 5 pubs did not match 17/68 with no pubs did not match 10/14 with no research participation matched

Percentage of U.S. seniors in the 2007 Match participating in research and reporting publications			
Pathology	80%	54%	Only 2/56 with > 5 pubs did not match 12/143 with no pubs did not match 58/64 with no research participation matched
Physical medicine and rehabilitation	75%	46%	All applicants with > 5 pubs matched
Plastic surgery	93%	76%	7/40 with > 5 pubs did not match 28/63 with 1-5 pubs did not match 16 of 33 with no pubs did not match 5/10 with no research participation matched
Radiology	88%	63%	11/136 with > 5 pubs did not match 38/336 with no pubs did not match 101/114 with no research participation matched
Radiation oncology	97%	89%	4/62 with > 5 pubs did not match 7/16 with no pubs did not match 3/4 with no research participation matched
General surgery	84%	57%	9/100 with > 5 pubs did not match 48/385 with no pubs did not match 129/147 with no research experience matched
*Includes abstracts, publications, and presentations Data from http://www.nrmp.org/data/chartingoutcomes2007.pdf			

The Interview

Contrary to common belief, the purpose of the interview is *not* to determine if you have the qualifications needed to be a resident at the institution. By granting you an interview, the program has already made that determination. Rather, the purpose of the interview is to assess fit. Are you the right fit for the program? Is the program the right fit for you?

Although the CV, personal statement, letters of recommendation, and other aspects of the application are all of great importance, there is no disputing the fact that the interview is possibly the most critical step of the residency application process. While the other elements of the application will help you get an interview, your interview performance will strongly influence your ranking.

- In a survey of directors of orthopedic surgery residency programs, 22% of programs stated that once invited for an interview, they placed candidates on equal footing, with ranking decisions based solely on interview performance (Bernstein).
- A survey of 205 directors of obstetrics and gynecology programs found that the medical school transcript, Dean's letter, and USMLE scores ranked highest when deciding whom to interview. However, when it came to ranking decisions, the interview was considered most important (Taylor).
- A survey of program directors in internal medicine found that the interview was most useful for ranking decisions, with 96% of respondents reporting that they found the interview to be highly or moderately useful (Adams).

Surveys of program directors over the years have consistently found the interview to be a major factor used to rank applicants. In fact, the results of multiple studies indicate that the interview is *the most* valuable factor used in the ranking of applicants.

Surveys of residency program directors regarding the importance of the interview	
Study	Findings
Survey of program directors of family practice and obstetrics/gynecology investigating the value directors place on various selection criteria (Taylor)	Directors in both specialties ranked the interview as most valuable in the ranking of applicants.
Survey of 24 faculty members at a University of Minnesota primary care internal medicine residency program to determine the importance of various selection criteria (Leonard)	Personal and interpersonal qualities were given the greatest weight and were considered to be more important than academic success.
Survey of 96 residency program directors in Ontario, inquiring about the importance of various selection factors (Provan)	84% of the program directors considered the personal interview to be the most important selection criterion.
Study done at The Children's Hospital of Philadelphia to better understand the impact of interview on the ranking of applicants (Swanson)	Interview scores were found to be the most important tool for the ranking of applicants.

Surveys of residency program directors regarding the importance of the interview	
Survey of 282 family practice residency program directors to determine the strategies used by programs to select residents (Galazka)	The interview was the most important element in the resident selection process.
Survey of program directors of osteopathic rotating internships and residency programs in internal medicine, obstetrics-gynecology, general surgery, orthopedic surgery, and pediatrics to determine the relative importance of academic and nonacademic variables in the selection process (Bates)	The interview was most highly valued in the resident selection process.
Survey of 94 emergency medicine residency program directors to determine the importance of various residency selection criteria (Crane)	The interview was the second most important selection criterion, following the emergency medicine rotation grade.
Survey of orthopedic residency program directors and applicants (Bajaj)	According to faculty, the interview was the third most important attribute to obtaining a residency, following performance on a local rotation and class rank. Of note, applicants did not give interviews the same level of importance, citing performance on a local rotation, USMLE Step 1 score, and recommendation letters as the three most important criteria.

Unfortunately, many otherwise qualified applicants lose any chance of matching into the residency program of their choice because of a poor interview. In a study of internal medicine residency applicants, one third of applicants were ranked less favorably following an interview (Gong). In a study of emergency medicine residency programs, with data obtained from 3,800 individual interviews, a total of 14% of interviews resulted in unranked applicants (Martin-Lee). The conclusion here is that the interview has the potential to destroy your chances. Preparation is critical.

Unfortunately, we find that most applicants don't give interview preparation the priority that it deserves. Applicants spend months of intense study in preparing for the USMLE exam. They then turn around and spend a few casual hours preparing for interviews. This one critical mistake can ruin your chances of matching successfully.

We devote a full four chapters to the interview process. In these chapters, we review the type of research that must be done before each interview. We review what to expect from the typical interview day and the different types of interviews you may encounter. We discuss what to say and how to say it. We review the common interview questions and delve into the intent behind the questions so that you can prepare your responses. We prepare you for what to say when you don't know the answer. These chapters will prepare you for what to do before, during, and after the interview.

Before the Interview

A significant degree of advance planning is necessary to excel during an interview. You need to understand what interviewers are looking for when they speak to applicants. What are they trying to determine? What qualities are they seeking in their future residents? How can you project these qualities? How can you guide the interview to a discussion of your achievements that emphasize these qualities?

A survey of directors of plastic surgery residency programs asked them to rank 20 items that were used in the evaluation of applicants during the interview process (LaGrasso). The survey showed that the highest ranked criteria were leadership qualities, apparent maturity, answers to questions, candidate's interest in teaching/academics, and attitude toward questions. Sixth in importance were questions posed by applicants.

A study of program directors in physical medicine and rehabilitation asked program directors about the importance of different applicant characteristics assessed during the interview (DeLisa). Ranked highest were compatibility with the program, ability to articulate thoughts, ability to work with the team, ability to listen, and commitment to hard work.

We will show you how to take this knowledge and use it when preparing your interview responses. Have you held leadership positions? Does your prior employment or volunteer experience demonstrate a commitment to hard work? A review of your strengths and advance preparation are necessary to guide the interview in a direction that emphasizes these strengths. We also review the advance prep work that you'll need to perform for each program and each interviewer. As emphasized in the *Pritzker Residency Process Guide,* "If granted an interview, run a Medline search of the faculty's publications. Get some notion of who your interviewers are likely to be, and what their program emphasizes" (http://pritzker.uchicago.edu/current/ students/ResidencyProcessGuide.pdf). We review effective ways to research each program as well as each interviewer. Gaining this knowledge well in advance of the interview can help you create rapport and allow you to ask the specific, customized types of questions that are most likely to create a favorable impression.

Chapter 12 also tells you what to expect in an interview. We tell you what to expect from the standard traditional one-on-one interview. We also prepare you for the increasingly used behavioral interview, as well as the panel interview and the conversational interview.

Interview Questions

In Chapter 13 we review common interview questions and delve into the intent behind the questions. Does the faculty member really care about your flight into town? Why do they want to know where you see yourself in 10 years? How can you best respond to the intent behind the question?

We also prepare you for specific areas of caution. Were you ready to talk about perfectionism as your greatest weakness? That response joins the other trite, overused responses that leave faculty with a negative impression. Many interviewers end their questioning with "do you have any questions for me?" "Questions asked by applicant" is actually a criterion used by some programs in evaluating applicants. This question can be used as an opportunity to emphasize your interest in the program, and your fit with the program. It's also the type of question that can sink your chances. We provide a full table of potential questions, and specifically review the ones that should never be asked of a faculty member.

During the Interview

A successful interview involves much more than anticipating interview questions and preparing the content of your answers. While most applicants focus their attention on content, nonverbal communication skills are just as important. It is estimated that 65% to 90% of every conversation is interpreted through body language (Cole). Of concern for applicants, high levels of anxiety have been shown to adversely affect a variety of nonverbal communication factors, including eye contact, body language, voice level, and projected confidence (Freeman). Even small details can alter perceptions. In the *Lancet* article "Getting a grip on handshakes," it was reported that "a strong correlation was found between a firm handshake—as evidenced by strength, vigor, duration, completeness of grip, and eye contact—and a good first impression..." (Larkin).

In Chapter 14, we talk about steps you can take to decrease anxiety, and the steps you need to take to manage the nonverbal messages during an interview. In her article, "Anxiety Patterns in Employment Interviews," Young wrote that "anxious individuals are less likely to be hired...possibly because interviewers perceive highly anxious people to be less trustworthy, less task-oriented...than low anxiety interviewees" (Young).

We also suggest what to say and what to do when you don't know the answer to a question. We review how to handle the situations that you may not be expecting, such as a silent interviewer or inappropriate or illegal questions. These occur more often than you might expect. A survey of urology residency applicants found that "being asked about marital status was recalled by 91% of male and 100% of

female, if they had children by 25% of male and 62% of female, applicants, respectively" (Teichman). We review these types of scenarios,
since advance awareness and preparation is the key to interview performance.

After the Interview

Post-interview communication is a critical component of the interview
process. However, many applicants don't recognize this fact. In one
study, only 39% of applicants sent follow-up communication to every
program with which they interviewed; 55% communicated only with
select programs (Anderson). In Chapter 15, "After the Interview,"
starting on page 344, we review the three cornerstones of post-interview communication and how to correctly thank a program for the
opportunity to interview. We review what to say when a program con-
tacts you. Statistics reveal that this is a common occurrence.

We also help you plan how to communicate and what to say to
the top programs on your list. In Rule #172, we elaborate further on
the fact that your expressed interest in a program can, in some cases,
impact their interest in you. Is there a chance that your communication with a program following the interview can influence your ranking? Absolutely. Not for every faculty member, and not for every
program, but there is a chance that at some programs your
expressed interest in the program may influence your ranking.

How would your interest in a program affect their interest in you?
Your negative interest can provide a negative influence. Negative
interest can be perceived as the lack of any communication from the
applicant following the interview. Some programs don't wish to rank
highly those applicants who have no interest in the program, because
that lack of interest can be an indicator of a poor fit.

A positive interest can be a positive influence. An applicant who
ranks a program highly is likely to feel that the program would be a
good fit for his interests and abilities, which is what a program seeks.
An applicant who plans to rank a program highly would be thrilled to
match there, and that hopefully translates to an enthusiastic, hard-
working resident. It is also a point of pride for many programs to
match those applicants at the top of their own rank list. In a study
examining communication between programs and applicants, the
authors wrote that "some program directors appear to construct their
match lists with the goal of "matching well" i.e., not having to go too
far down their lists. To achieve this, knowing where applicants plan to
rank them is a high priority" (Miller).

However, programs do differ widely in their beliefs on the value of
post-interview communication. For some programs, what you say following the interview will have no effect whatsoever on the program's
decision-making process. In a study looking at recruitment behavior,

the authors wrote that "program directors were very skeptical of student ranking assurances" (Carek).

However, the authors felt that such assurances had an effect on ranking decisions at some programs. They felt that the impact of the rank order list was "limited to one third of programs" (Carek). Such information is clearly important to some programs.

Surveys of applicants support this belief. When Miller and his colleagues surveyed graduating students at ten U.S. medical schools, they found that 23% were asked how they planned to rank the program, and 21.7% were told that their level of interest would have bearing on their ranking (Miller).

Surveys of program directors support this belief as well. In one study, emergency medicine residency program directors were asked to rate the importance of 20 items in the resident selection process. An applicant's expressed interest in the program was found to be a moderately important selection factor. In this study, it ranked of higher importance than the USMLE Step 1 score, although the standard deviation was high, indicating that there were significant differences in how program directors viewed this factor (Crane).

Other surveys noted that programs commonly tell applicants to keep in touch if they have an interest in matching with their program, as outlined in the following table.

Post-interview communication: Does it help?	
Study	Findings
Survey of emergency medicine residency program directors (Crane)	Respondents were asked to rate the importance of 20 items in the resident selection process on a scale of 1 to 5, with five being most important. An applicant's expressed interest in the program was found to be a moderately important selection factor with a mean score of 3.30 and a standard deviation of 1.19. Of note, it was ranked of higher importance than the USMLE Step I score and nearly as high as the USMLE Step 2 score. The authors commented on the large standard deviation, emphasizing considerable differences between programs in the way they viewed post-interview communication.
Survey of fourth-year students at three medical schools (Anderson)	57% were told by a program following the interview to keep in touch if they had an interest in matching there; 21.4% of programs said that confirmatory rank-order statements from applicants had some positive effect; 2% of programs stated that such statements had a significant positive effect.
Survey of family practice program directors (Carek)	82% of programs told at least some of their applicants to keep in touch if they had an interest in matching with their program.
Survey of urology residency program directors (Teichman)	67% of programs told applicants to keep in touch if they had an interest in matching in their program.

Ranking Residency Programs

Even at this late phase of the application process, applicants need to be aware of the dangerous potential pitfalls. Most applicants agonize over the top three programs on their list, but don't spend equivalent time with the bottom three programs on their list. Per the words of the San Francisco Matching Program: "Pay attention to the bottom of your list! Each year some applicants tell us that they omitted a lower choice because they overestimated their chances elsewhere. They ended up unmatched because the omitted program turned out to be their only offer. The only reason not to list a program is that you would rather remain unmatched to explore other options after the match" (www.sfmatch.org).

Applicants sometimes create a rank list that is too short, or don't follow through with all the programs at which they interviewed, in the mistaken belief that they are a "lock" at a specific program. In their Statement on Professionalism, the NRMP writes that each year it is "contacted by applicants who believe that an error has occurred in the Match because they did not match to programs whose directors had promised them positions (i.e., had promised to rank them high enough to ensure a match). In every case, the NRMP has determined that the applicant did not match to the desired program because, contrary to the applicant's expectation, the program did not rank the applicant high enough on the program's rank order list for the applicant to match there" (www.nrmp.org).

Do program directors actually promise positions to applicants? Studies have shown that students often do believe they have received informal commitments from programs. In a survey of fourth-year students at three schools, 43% felt that they had received informal commitments from at least one program (Anderson). In a survey of urology residency applicants, 40% felt that they had received informal commitments (Teichman). In Chapter 16, we review other pitfalls that await applicants at this late yet critical stage of the process.

The Successful Match

There are no shortcuts and no easy answers when it comes to a successful match. The residency application process is prolonged and difficult, and while success is never guaranteed, our evidence-based advice and insiders' perspectives provide the specific, concrete recommendations that will maximize your chances of achieving the ultimate goal: that of a successful match.

Chapter 2

Specialty-Specific Information

In this chapter we present salient points related to residency matches in specialties arranged in alphabetical order from anesthesiology to urology.

Anesthesiology

How competitive is the specialty?

The attractiveness of anesthesiology as a career choice for U.S. senior medical students has fluctuated widely over the years. The number of students pursuing anesthesiology reached a low point in the mid-1990s. Since then, however, there has been growing interest in the field. As of 2008, the specialty can best be described as moderately competitive.

What percentage of available positions is filled by U.S. seniors? What about other applicants?

In recent years over 95% of the available positions (PGY-1 or PGY-2) filled through the NRMP match. As of 2007 there were 4970 total residents training in a total of 131 anesthesiology residency programs (Brotherton). 75.1% were U.S. MDs, 14.8% were IMGs, 10% were osteopathic graduates, and 0.2% were Canadian graduates. As shown in the following tables, categorical positions are available at the PGY-1 and 2 levels.

Anesthesiology: positions filled by U.S. seniors 2004-2008 (for PGY-1 positions)		
Year	Positions offered total	Percentage of positions filled by U.S. seniors
2008	666	78.7%
2007	575	77.9%
2006	552	81.7%
2005	463	70.4%
2004	443	72.7%
Data from www.nrmp.org		

Anesthesiology: positions filled by U.S. seniors 2004-2008 (for PGY-2 positions)

Year	Positions offered total	Percentage of positions filled by U.S. seniors
2008	698	78.2%
2007	763	74.7%
2006	759	77.6%
2005	820	72.0%
2004	846	68.0%
Data from www.nrmp.org		

Is there any literature available to guide applicants through the residency application process for anesthesiology?

In 1999 Wagoner and Suriano surveyed anesthesiology program directors about the residency selection process. Of the 201 surveys sent, responses were received from 31 directors.

Anesthesiology residency program directors' rankings of academic criteria used in the residency selection process

Criteria	Mean	Standard deviation
Grades in required clerkships	3.87	0.76
Class rank	3.74	0.77
Grades in senior electives in specialty	3.74	1.00
USMLE Step 1 score	3.73	1.19
Medical school academic awards	3.68	0.75
USMLE Step 2 score	3.66	0.92
Number of honors grades	3.52	1.09
Grades in other senior electives	3.52	1.03
Membership in AOA	3.29	1.13
Medical school reputation	3.29	0.82
Published medical school research	3.27	0.94
Grades in pre-clinical courses	2.71	1.04

Wagoner NE, Suriano JR. Program directors' responses to a survey on variables used to select residents in a time of change. *Acad Med* 1999; 74(1): 51-58.

Which academic criteria are ranked highest by program directors?

According to Wagoner's survey, grades in required clerkships, class rank, grades in senior electives in the specialty, and USMLE Step 1 score are the top four academic criteria.

How do programs select residents?

As is the case with other specialties, programs will look closely at the entire application for an anesthesiology residency. In 2005 faculty from the Department of Anesthesiology at the University of Pittsburgh offered insight into the residency selection process at their program (Metro). Factors considered important in deciding whom to interview included USMLE scores, medical school performance, the Dean's letter, personal statement, and letters of recommendation.

Following the interview at the University of Pittsburgh, interviewers are asked to rank the applicant on a scale of 1 to 5 (with 5 being the highest score) in the following areas:

- Grades and honors
- USMLE test scores
- Dean's letter
- Letters of recommendation
- Personality aspects
- Enthusiasm, energy, liveliness
- Drive, motivation to excel
- Assertiveness
- Warmth, friendliness, humor
- Poise, composure
- Maturity
- Intellectual aspects
- Intelligence and problem solving skills
- Articulateness, communication skills
- Critical or analytical skills
- Quality of answers
- Quality of questions
- Strength and appropriateness of goals
- Knowledge of anesthesia as a specialty
- Knowledge of Pitt program

Interviewers are also asked to give an overall recommendation using terms such as outstanding, very desirable, acceptable, marginal, and undesirable. At the end of the interview season the selection committee meets as a group. Following a discussion of each applicant, members are asked to rank the applicant on a scale from 1 (undesirable) to 5 (outstanding). These scores are averaged to yield a final score which is used to form the program's rank list.

How important are letters of recommendation?

Dr. McDade of the University of Chicago recommends applicants obtain letters of recommendation from anesthesiologists who are well-known in the field (www.ama-assn.org). For applicants who do not have this option, he recommends selecting anesthesiologists "who know you well and think highly of you." Surgeons and internists who know you well should also be considered as potential letter writers. Dr. Gimenez, program director at the University of California-Irvine, feels that letters should ideally be written by faculty members in the departments of anesthesiology, critical care, and surgery (www.ucihs.uci.edu).

How important is AOA?

Being a member of AOA was eighth in importance. The NRMP reports that 7.5% of U.S. seniors who matched to anesthesiology in 2007 were members of AOA.

How important is the USMLE?

The mean USMLE Step 1 score for 2007 U.S. senior applicants who matched was 220. Of note, 142 of the 184 applicants with Step 1 scores < 200 matched. Applicants with low USMLE Step 1 scores can strengthen their application by showing improvement on the Step 2 CK exam. Dr. Moore, chair and program director at the University of California-Davis, states that "Step 1 is important as basic sciences particularly physiology, biochemistry, and pharmacology are the foundations of anesthesiology practice."

Is it necessary to do an audition elective?

While it is not necessary to do an audition elective, Dr. Gimenez writes that "if the program has direct knowledge of the student they have a better chance of being accepted into the program." This assumes that the applicant performs at a high level.

How important is research experience?

Among 12 academic criteria, Wagoner found that published medical school research was next to last in importance. Among 2007 applicants, 200 of the 214 applicants reporting no prior research experience matched. Dr. Luehr, program director at the University of Texas-Houston, writes that "although not necessary, research experience is viewed very positively and encouraged for those applying to our specialty."

How important is the interview?

Dr. Moore feels that an applicant's performance during the interview "is the deal breaker/maker."

References

American Board of Anesthesiology. Available at www.abanes.org.
American Society of Anesthesiologists. Available at www.asahq.org.
Brotherton SE, Etzel SI. Graduate medical education, 2006-2007. *JAMA 2007;* 298 (9): 1081-1096.
Gimenez, K. Residency selection handbook: anesthesiology. From www.ucihs.uci.edu.
Leuhr S. Career counseling: anesthesiology. Available at http://www.uth.tmc.edu/ med/administration/student/ms4/2003CCC.htm
McDade W. Residency programs: an inside look. From www.ama-assn.org.
Metro DG, Talarico JF, Patel RM, Wetmore AL. The Resident Application Process and its correlation to future performance as a resident. *Anesth Analg 2005;* 100: 502-505.
Moore P. A guide to the perplexed: residency guide. From www.ucdmc.ucdavis.edu.
Wagoner NE, Suriano JR. Program directors' responses to a survey on variables used to select residents in a time of change. *Acad Med* 1999; 74(1): 51-58.

Dermatology

How competitive is the specialty?

Dermatology is tremendously competitive, with many more applicants than available positions. In 2007, out of 407 U.S. seniors applying to dermatology, 158 failed to match. In other words, 39% of U.S. seniors applying to dermatology failed to match. Dr. Shea, section chief and program director at the University of Chicago, writes that their program "is extremely competitive. This year we had 530 applications for 4 slots, and interviewed about 36 candidates."

What is the percentage of available positions filled by U.S. seniors? What about other applicants?

As of 2007, there were 1,069 total residents training in a total of 112 dermatology residency programs (Brotherton). 94.9% were U.S. MDs, 3.0% were IMGs, 1.6% were osteopathic graduates, and 0.5% were Canadian graduates.

Dermatology: positions filled by U.S. seniors 2004-2008 (for PGY-2)		
Year	Positions offered, total	Percentage of positions filled by U.S. seniors
2008	297	77.4%
2007	288	78.5%
2006	276	78.3%
2005	288	75.0%
2004	263	79.1%
From www.nrmp.org		

Note in the previous table that the percentage of "positions filled by U.S. seniors" does not take into account applicants who are applying for a second time or applying following completion of another residency. Also, the data presented in this table does not include programs that incorporate PGY-1 years into their total residency.

How important are audition electives?

In 2003 Dr. Clarke of Penn State University reported the results of a survey sent to 278 applicants who had matched that year (Clarke). 108 responses were received. This survey found the following:

- The mean number of applications submitted was 46.7 per student.
- The average number of interviews granted was 10.4.
- Those with both MD and PhD degrees had significantly more interviews.
- 53% matched at a program where they had had prior experience.

Clearly, audition electives are important in this highly competitive specialty. However, Dr. Miller, program director at Penn State University, cautions applicants not to take this to an extreme (Miller). "We realize that you need to get your 'foot in the door' by doing an elective and possibly spending an elective month completing a dermatology-focused project. But do not go overboard! What impresses us is a medical school experience that takes it all in, not just dermatology."

Who should be asked to write letters of recommendation?

Academic dermatology is a small community. As such, faculty members tend to know one another quite well. Strong letters of recommendation from senior faculty who are well known to the program carry great weight.

Miller encourages applicants to "think carefully about letters of recommendation. These letters usually come from colleagues we know in the field. Most of us also know your chairperson or residency program director. One of your letters should come from one of them. That letter should be strong and personal. Letters of recommendation can separate you from other applicants."

Dr. Hebert, Professor of Dermatology at the University of Texas-Houston, states that "we also look for letters from the chairman of the dermatology program in which the student trained."

What is the importance of the personal statement?

With so many highly qualified applicants from an academic standpoint, dermatology programs take a close look at the personal statement. Several dermatology faculty members offer their advice to applicants, as shown in the following table.

Advice for dermatology applicant	
Heymann	Heymann feels that the personal statement takes on "immense importance" assuming that applicants are equally qualified. Particularly appealing to him are statements that give him insight into the applicant as a person. Is this "someone I want to meet face-to-face?"
Shea	Shea "looks for statements that reveal personality, are articulate and engaging, and tell a compelling story, rather than giving a boring recital of the obvious...However, avoid eccentric projections that could create a negative impression."
Miller	Miller makes note of some common personal statement themes: • Being a visual person • Dermatology offering opportunity to care for a wide range of patients, including those of all ages • Ability to do procedures Miller encourages applicants to think beyond these reasons to make the statement unique. "The bottom line is to balance why you are interested in the field with you are, weighing more heavily on 'who you are.'"

How important is AOA?

The NRMP reports that 47% of U.S. seniors who matched to dermatology in 2007 were members of AOA. Being an AOA member does not guarantee acceptance; 28 of the 145 AOA applicants did not match.

How important is the USMLE?

The mean USMLE Step 1 score for 2007 U.S. senior applicants who matched was 238. Dr. Ellis, the program director of the dermatology program at the University of Michigan, wrote that "last year, more than 100 of our applicants had achieved the top percentile on the United States Medical Licensing Examination" (Kia).

Of note, the mean score among U.S. senior applicants who did not match was 226. Only 2 of 19 applicants with scores < 200 successfully matched.

Is research experience required?

Among 2007 applicants, nearly 95% had participated in at least one research project, with over 80% claiming at least one abstract, publication, or presentation. The Southern Illinois department of dermatology states that "exposure to research and participating in research are preferable. More importantly is attempt at publication and experience in scientific writing." Dr. Shea, chief of the section of dermatology at the University of Chicago, encourages applicants to "publish something (ideally in dermatology, but any publication is valuable, showing your ability to think, write, act independently, and follow through on projects).

A study that surveyed dermatology programs across the country found that of 36 programs responding, students participated in some type of research activity in nearly all of the programs (Wagner). In 35 programs, students were involved in case reports and case series, while in 31 programs they participated in clinical research projects and in 25 programs they participated in laboratory benchwork. Of these programs, 33 offered at least one elective in dermatology research, with 29 of those programs permitting visiting medical student participation. However, 19 of the programs had no specific method to inform students about their research opportunities.

Of note, being published is no guarantee of a residency position. Among 2007 applicants, 35 of the 136 applicants claiming > 5 abstracts, publications, or presentations failed to match.

What recommendations do you have regarding the interview?

The interview is a major factor used by programs to rank applicants. We present advice offered by several academic dermatologists in the following table.

Advice for the dermatology interview	
Heymann	Heymann encourages applicants to be themselves. "Honesty and integrity are of paramount importance; insincerity easily shines through. I am trying to learn if you will be a good 'fit' for our program." He stresses the importance of asking stimulating questions to learn as much as possible about the program. "There is a tremendous difference between the applicant who takes the time and effort to learn about our program and faculty's expertise compared with the person who only applies to be near his girlfriend in Philadelphia. After the interview is done, spend a few minutes to write us a note."
Miller	Miller offers similar advice. "We tell them to answer every question from their heart – not give the answer they think the interviewer expects or wants. If you earned an interview, you made the final cut and that is the time to find out if you are a 'fit' for the program. The only way that can be determined is by being yourself."
Twede	Twede relates a story from his interview days. "The interviewer … cautioned me about using the phrase 'I'm a visual person' during future interviews. He commented that some academic dermatologists find the phrase trite, vague, and overused and therefore might not enhance my application."

Shea	Shea states that, "If granted an interview, run a Medline search of the faculty's publications. Get some notion of who your interviewers are likely to be, and what their program emphasizes... If asked why you are interested in a particular program, do not say that it is for geographic reasons (your home town, pleasant climate, etc.). Give a thoughtful, professional interview."

Applicants are often asked about their future plans. "Are you thinking private practice or academics?" is a commonly asked question that you should be prepared to answer.

In the article, "Academia is the life for me, I'm sure," Robert Gielczyk, a third-year dermatology resident at the University of Michigan, wrote that his goal was to "match into a position, any position" given that the field is extremely competitive. To him, it seemed that "applicants interested in academics might have an advantage over those interested in private practice. Most of the interviewers worked in academic settings. It would make sense that academic clinicians at academic medical centers would desire residents interested in academics. In fact, I do not remember a single interview in which the topic of entering academics did not arise." (Kia).

Even if you're not interested in becoming a full-time faculty member, you should think about, and be prepared to discuss, your academic goals and interests. Be it teaching, research, writing, volunteering, or in another fashion, how will you contribute to the advancement of the field?

References

American Academy of Dermatology. Available at www.aad.org.
American Board of Dermatology. Available at www.abderm.org.
American Osteopathic College of Dermatology. Available at www.aocd.org.
American Society of Dermatology. Available at www.asd.org.
Brotherton SE, Etzel SI. Graduate medical education, 2006-2007. *JAMA* 2007; 298 (9): 1081-1096.
Clarke JT, Miller JJ, Sceppa J, Goldsmith LA, Long E. Success in the dermatology resident match in 2003: perceptions and importance of home institutions and away rotations. *Arch Dermatol* 2006; 142(7): 930-932.
Hebert A. Career counseling: dermatology. Available at http://www.uth.tmc.edu/med/administration/student/ms4/2003CCC.htm
Heymann WR. Advice to the dermatology residency applicant. *Arch Dermatol* 2000; 136(1): 123-124.
Kia KF, Gielczyk RA, Ellis CN. Academia is the life for me, I'm sure. *Arch Dermatol* 2006; 142: 911-913.
Miller J, Miller OF, Freedbert I. Dear dermatology applicant. *Arch Dermatol* 2004; 140: 884.
Shea CR. Pritzker residency process guide: dermatology. Available at http://pritzker.uchicago.edu/current/students/ResidencyProcessGuide.pdf
Twede JV. Being a visual person. *Arch Dermatol* 2006; 242: 1357-1358.
Wagner, RF, Ioffe B. Medical student dermatology research in the United States. *Dermatol Online J* 2005; 11(1):8.
Wu JJ, Tyring SK. The academic strength of current dermatology residency applicants. *Dermatol Online J* 2003; 9(3): 22.
http://edaff.siumed.edu/Year4/SurveyResults_041102.pdf - 2001 survey of program directors at SIU.

Emergency Medicine

How competitive is the specialty?

Emergency medicine is among the more competitive specialties. Dr. Wilhelm of the University of Texas-Houston states that their program receives approximately 500 applications for 10 resident positions. From this group, interviews are offered to about 80 applicants.

What is the percentage of available positions filled by U.S. seniors? What about other applicants?

As of 2007, there were 4,379 residents training in a total of 140 emergency medicine residency programs (Brotherton). Of the total, 85.4% were U.S. MDs, 5.3% were IMGs, 9.0% were osteopathic graduates, and 0.3% were Canadian graduates.

Emergency medicine residency: positions filled by U.S. seniors 2004-2008 (for PGY-1 positions)

Year	Total positions offered	Percentage of positions filled by U.S. seniors
2008	1,399	77.4%
2007	1,288	79.7%
2006	1,251	75.5%
2005	1,188	80.0%
2004	1,151	77.5%

From www.nrmp.org

Emergency medicine residency: positions filled by U.S. seniors 2004-2008 (for PGY-2 positions)

Year	Positions offered total	Percentage of positions filled by U.S. seniors
2008	76	59.2%
2007	97	79.4%
2006	115	80.9%
2005	144	83.3%
2004	144	82.6%

From www.nrmp.org

Is there any literature available to applicants to guide them through the residency application process?

Two surveys of emergency medicine residency program directors are available to help applicants through the process of securing a residency position:

- In 1999, Dr. Crane of the University of Illinois at Chicago reported the results of a questionnaire sent to emergency medicine program directors. In it, he inquired about the criteria programs use to select their residents. Of the 118 surveys sent, responses were received from 94 directors (79.7%).

Emergency medicine program directors' rankings of academic criteria used in the residency selection process

Criteria	Mean	Standard deviation
Emergency medicine rotation grades	4.79	0.50
Interview	4.62	0.64
Clinical grades	4.35	0.70
Recommendations	4.11	0.85
Grades (overall)	3.95	0.64
Elective at the program director's institution	3.76	1.25
Board scores (overall)	3.35	0.77
USMLE Step 2	3.34	0.93
Interest expressed	3.30	1.19
USMLE Step 1	3.28	0.86
Awards/achievement	3.16	0.88
AOA status	3.01	1.09
Medical school attended	3.00	0.85
Extracurricular activities	2.99	0.87
Basic science grades	2.88	0.92
Publications	2.87	0.99
Personal statement	2.75	0.96

From Crane JT, Ferraro CM. Selection Criteria for Emergency Medicine Residency Applicants. *Acad Emerg Med.* 2000; 7:54-60.

- In 1999, Wagoner and Suriano surveyed program directors about the residency selection process. Of the 132 surveys sent, responses were received from 36 directors. Grades in senior electives in the specialty were the most important academic criterion, followed by grades in required clerkships and number of honors grades.

How important are audition electives?

According to Crane, performance at an elective done at the program director's institution carried some importance. However, the authors noted that the mean rating score had a large standard deviation, suggesting considerable variability in the importance that programs attach to these rotations. Dr. Wilhelm recommends audition electives for applicants with less than stellar grades as well as for those who desire to train at a particular program.

How important are letters of recommendation?

Letters of recommendation were ranked fourth in importance. The Society of Academic Emergency Medicine encourages applicants to obtain one or more letters from academic emergency medicine faculty. Dr. Oman, program director at the University of California-Irvine, states that applicants should obtain letters from faculty members in the departments of emergency medicine, critical care, surgery, and medicine. Dr. Wilhelm states that "letters are probably the most carefully read portion of the application" and emphasizes the importance of obtaining letters from emergency physicians with academic ranks. "The positions of chairman, residency director, and assistant residency director or medical student coordinator are recognizable to other directors even if the names of those individuals are not."

Dr. Loftipour and colleagues in the departments of emergency medicine at the University of California Irvine School of Medicine and the University of California San Diego School of Medicine authored an excellent article entitled "Becoming an emergency medicine resident: A practical guide for medical students." The authors write that "an exceptional letter from a respected faculty member may sway residency program directors to offer an applicant with non-competitive scores and evaluations an interview due to the importance programs place on clinical abilities. Therefore, it is valuable for a student to orchestrate time to work with a well-known EM faculty member, such as program director or assistant program director, clerkship director, research director, or Chief/Chair. Opportunities include tag-alongs, research, or educational and leadership positions in an EMIG [emergency medicine interest group]" (Loftipour).

In contrast to other specialties, emergency medicine has developed a standardized letter of recommendation (SLOR). Generally, departments designate a particular faculty member to write the SLOR. Try to determine who that person is at your institution and then work with that attending as much as possible. If you don't have the opportunity to work directly with him, he will write your letter based on information from other faculty and residents.

The writer of the SLOR is asked to provide a bottom-line match recommendation. The choices available include "guaranteed match," which is the best superlative the applicant can receive. In a review of SLORs, 23% of applicants received this designation (Girzadas). In another study, Girzadas found that the following factors were important in securing the "guaranteed match" rating:

- Having extended contact with the letter writer. Working with the writer for an extended period of time (defined as more than ten hours of contact in the emergency department) increased the chance of receiving the rating twofold over those who had less contact.

- Working with the writer in other capacities. Applicants who worked with the writer in other settings, such as research, increased their chances of receiving the rating.
- Having a staff physician write the letter rather than a senior physician such as the chair or residency director. The authors hypothesized that staff physicians may have more direct contact with applicants, making them feel more comfortable in giving them the rating. Also postulated was the tendency of senior physicians to be more selective in giving applicants the highest rating.
- Doing as well as possible in the rotation. The EM rotation grade was the strongest predictor of the rating.
- Demonstrating an outstanding work ethic and ability for differential diagnosis were also positively associated with the highest rating.

How important is the personal statement?

In Crane's survey, the personal statement ranked last in importance. However, individual programs do attach varying degrees of importance to the statement. Dr. Loftipour states that the statement "should pique the reader's curiosity through a story or personal anecdote, such as a patient encounter, leadership experience, or special accomplishment. Because the readers are emergency physicians well acquainted with the specialty, the statement should not describe what EM is, but rather how the specialty suits the student."

How important is AOA?

According to Wagoner, being a member of AOA was eleventh in importance. The NRMP reports that 12.4% of U.S. seniors who matched to emergency medicine in 2007 were members of AOA.

How important is the USMLE?

The mean USMLE Step 1 score for 2007 U.S. senior applicants who matched was 220. Dr. Fling, program director at University of California-Davis, states that "high board scores certainly help, but most EM programs focus on the 'whole package.' Very low board scores hurt most applicants." Additional recommendations include "for those whose Step 1 score falls below the mean, it is recommended to take Step 2 before submitting the EM application" (Loftipour).

How important is research experience?

Among 12 academic criteria, Wagoner found that published medical school research was next to last in importance. Among 2007 applicants, 245/271 claiming no research experience matched. The Society for Academic Emergency Medicine has the following to say about the importance of research experience: "Research experience helps, but it is not necessary. It will strengthen an applicant's position. The research involved does not necessarily have to be in emergency medicine. Mostly, it denotes a student who goes above and beyond the expected. There may be volunteer work or other ways to show this."

How important is the interview?

The interview is clearly an important selection factor. In Crane's survey, it was ranked second in importance. Dr. Loftipour states that "some common pitfalls include emphasizing geography rather than program strengths, a lack of meaningful questions, and unfamiliarity with previous research projects."

References

American Academy of Emergency Medicine. Available at www.aaem.org.
American Academy of Emergency Medicine Resident and Student Association. Available at www.aaemrsa.org.
American Board of Emergency Medicine. Available at www.abem.org.
American College of Emergency Physicians. Available at www.acep.org.
American College of Osteopathic Emergency Physicians. Available at www.acoep.org.
Balentine J, Gaeta T, Spevack T. Evaluating Applicants to Emergency Medicine Residency Programs. *J Emerg Med.* 1999; 17:131-134.
Blumstein HA, Cone DC. Medical Student Career Advice Related to Emergency Medicine. *Acad Emerg Med.* 1998; 5:69-72.
Brotherton SE, Etzel SI. Graduate medical education, 2006-2007. *JAMA* 2007; 298 (9): 1081-1096.
Council of Emergency Medicine Residency Directors. Available at www.cordem.org.
Counselman FL, Griffey RT. Fourth-year Elective Recommendations for Medical Students Interested in Emergency Medicine. *Am J Emerg Med.* 1999; 17:745-746.
Crane JT, Ferraro CM. Selection Criteria for Emergency Medicine Residency Applicants. *Acad Emerg Med.* 2000; 7:54-60.
DeBlieux P, Keim S, Chisholm C. Taming the Residency Application Process. Medical Student Emergency Medicine Symposium, May 22, 2000. Society for Academic Emergency Medicine Website.
Fling M. A guide to the perplexed: residency guide. From www.ucdmc.ucdavis.edu.
Garmel GM. Letters of Recommendation: What Does 'Good' Really Mean? *Acad Emerg Med.* 1997; 4:833-834.
Girzadas DV, Harwood RC, Dearie J, Garrett S. A comparision of standardized and narrative letters of recommendation. *Acad Emerg Med 2000;* 7(8): 963.
Girzadas DV, Harwood RC, Delis SN, Stevison K, Keng G, Cipparrone N, Carlson A, Tsonis GD. Emergency medicine standardized letter of recommendation: predictors of guaranteed match. *Acad Emerg Med 2001;* 8(6): 648-653.
Harwood RC, Girzadas DV, Carlson A, Delis S, Stevison K, Tsonis G, Keng G. Characteristics of the emergency medicine standardized letter of recommendation. *Acad Emerg Med* 2000; 7(4): 409-410.
Keim SM, Rein JA, Chisholm C, et al. A Standardized Letter of Recommendation for Residency Application. *Acad Emerg Med.* 1999;6:1141-1146.
Koscove EM. An Applicant's Evaluation of an Emergency Medicine Internship and Residency. *Ann Emerg Med.* 1990;19:774-780.
Loftipour S, Luu R, Hayden SR, Vaca F, Hoonpongsimanont W, Langdorf M. Becoming an emergency medicine resident: a practical guide for medical students. *J Emerg Med* 2008; Jun 10 (epub).
Lubavin B, Phelps M. Pearls of Wisdom for Your Emergency Medicine Rotation. *J Emerg Med.* 2001; 20:211-212.

Mahadaven SV, Garmel GM. The Outstanding Medical Student in Emergency
Medicine. *Acad Emerg Med.* 2001; 8(4): 402-403.
Martin-Lee L, Park H, Overton DT. Does Interview Date Affect Match List Position in
the Emergency Medicine National Residency Matching Program Match? *Acad
Emerg Med.* 2000; 7:1022-1026.
Oman J. Residency selection handbook: emergency medicine. From
www.ucihs.uci.edu.
Rosen P, Hamilton GC. Pro vs Con: Four vs Three. Society for Academic
Emergency Medicine Website.
Society for Academic Emergency Medicine. Available at www.saem.org.
Wagoner NE, Suriano JR. Program directors' responses to a survey on variables
used to select residents in a time of change. *Acad Med* 1999; 74(1): 51-58.
Wilhelm G. Career counseling: emergency medicine. Available at http://
www.uth.tmc.edu/med/administration/student/ms4/2003CCC.htm

Family Medicine

How competitive is the specialty?

Family medicine is among the less competitive specialties.

What is the percentage of available positions filled by U.S. seniors? What about other applicants?

As of 2007, there were 9,456 total residents training in a total of 464 family medicine residency programs (Brotherton). 46.5% were U.S. MDs, 39.2% were IMGs, 14.1% were osteopathic graduates, and 0.2% were Canadian graduates.

Family medicine residency: positions filled by U.S. seniors 2004-2008

Year	Positions offered, total	Percentage of positions filled by U.S. seniors
2008	2,636	43.9%
2007	2,603	42.1%
2006	2711	41.4%
2005	2761	40.5%
2004	2864	41.4%

From www.nrmp.org

Is there any literature available to applicants to guide them through the residency application process?

There are two surveys of family medicine residency program directors available to applicants to guide them through the process of securing a residency position:

- In 1995 Taylor and colleagues surveyed family practice residency program directors, inquiring about the importance of various criteria used to make interview and ranking decisions. The three most important factors used to make interview decisions were the Dean's letter, personal statement, and transcript. The interview was found to be most important in ranking an applicant.

- In 1999 Wagoner and Suriano surveyed family practice residency program directors about the residency selection process. Of the 503 surveys sent, responses were received from 105 directors.

Family medicine residency program directors' rankings of academic criteria used in the residency selection process

Criteria	Mean	Standard deviation
Grades in required clerkships	4.03	0.73
Grades in senior electives in specialty	3.86	0.88
Number of honors grades	3.64	0.86
USMLE Step 2 score	3.48	0.94
Grades in other senior electives	3.45	0.77
Class rank	3.37	0.83
Membership in AOA	3.25	0.96
Medical school academic awards	3.24	0.69
USMLE Step 1 score	3.21	0.93
Medical school reputation	3.18	0.96
Grades in pre-clinical courses	2.85	0.77
Published medical school research	2.37	0.87

Wagoner NE, Suriano JR. Program directors' responses to a survey on variables used to select residents in a time of change. *Acad Med* 1999; 74(1): 51-58.

How important is the personal statement?

Among factors used to make interview decisions, Taylor found that the personal statement was second in importance. The Department of Family Medicine at the University of Chicago states that "we weigh these fairly significantly. It is a great opportunity to express your unique strengths and interests. Describe how you developed your interest in the field of family medicine, and why you feel family medicine is the specialty for you."

How important are letters of recommendation?

Applicants are advised to obtain at least one letter from a family medicine physician. Also highly valued are letters from other primary care faculty members, including internists, pediatricians, and obstetrician/gynecologists.

How important are audition electives?

Audition electives are generally not necessary for resident selection. However, you have to consider the strength of your application. For example, if you have a red flag in your application, performing at a high level during an audition elective may alleviate concerns. Audition electives also allow applicants the opportunity to assess their fit for a particular program.

How important is AOA?

According to Wagoner, being a member of AOA was seventh in importance. The NRMP reports that 5.7% of U.S. seniors who matched to family medicine in 2007 were members of AOA.

How important is the USMLE?

The mean USMLE Step 1 score for 2007 U.S. senior applicants who matched was 211. Dr. Nelsen, associate program director at the University of California-Davis, states that their program "gives no systematic weight to USMLE Step 1, but if it's low this could be a red flag to other evidences of academic difficulties which, collectively, might drop a student from contention."

How important is research experience?

Among 12 academic criteria, Wagoner found that published medical school research was last in importance. In general, research experience is not necessary to secure a residency position.

How important is the interview?

Taylor found that the interview was most useful to program directors in ranking an applicant. The Department of Family Medicine at the University of Chicago recommends having "three times as many questions as you think you'll need, and you'll probably end up asking them all."

References

American Academy of Family Physicians. Available at www.aafp.org.
American Board of Family Practice. Available at www.abfp.org.
American College of Osteopathic Family Physicians. Available at www.acofp.org.
Association of Family Practice Residency Directors. Available at www.afprd.org.
Brotherton SE, Etzel SI. Graduate medical education, 2006-2007. *JAMA* 2007; 298 (9): 1081-1096.
Dumas, C. Career counseling: family practice. Available at http://www.uth.tmc.edu/med/administration/student/ms4/2003CCC.htm
Hern T, Hickner J, Ewigman B. Pritzker residency process guide: family medicine. Available at http://pritzker.uchicago.edu/current/students/ResidencyProcessGuide.pdf
Nelsen K. A guide to the perplexed: residency guide. From www.ucdmc.ucdavis.edu.
Taylor CA, Weinstein L, Mayhew HE. The process of resident selection: a view from the residency director's desk. *Obstet Gynecol* 1995; 85(2): 299-303.

Wagoner NE, Suriano JR. Program directors' responses to a survey on variables
    used to select residents in a time of change. *Acad Med* 1999; 74(1): 51-58.
Strolling through the match. Available at www.aafp.org (American Academy of
    Family Physicians).

Internal Medicine

How competitive is the specialty?

Overall, internal medicine is among the less competitive specialties.
The number of positions available far exceeds the number of U.S.
seniors who apply to the field. However, one must take into account
the prestige of the residency program. Programs that are considered
top tier are quite competitive.

What is the percentage of available positions filled by U.S. seniors? What about other applicants?

As of 2007, there were 22,099 total residents training in a total of 386
internal medicine residency programs (Brotherton); 50.3% were U.S.
MDs, 44.1% were IMGs, 5.4% were osteopathic graduates, and 0.3%
were Canadian graduates.

Internal medicine residency: positions filled by U.S. seniors 2004-2008		
Year	Positions offered total	Percentage of positions filled by U.S. seniors
2008	4,858	54.8%
2007	4,798	55.9%
2006	4,735	56.3%
2005	4,768	55.8%
2004	4,751	54.8%
From www.nrmp.org		

Is there any literature available to applicants to guide them through the residency application process?

There are two surveys of internal medicine residency program directors available to applicants to guide them through the process of
securing a residency position:

- In 2000 Dr. Adams of the University of Colorado surveyed 407
  program directors in internal medicine to determine which
  factors are most important in deciding whom to interview and
  how to rank applicants. A total of 332 responses were received
  (81.5%). The results are discussed below.

- In 1999 Wagoner and Suriano surveyed program directors about the residency selection process. Of the 646 surveys sent, responses were received from 96 directors.

Internal medicine residency program directors' rankings of academic criteria used in the residency selection process

Criteria	Mean	Standard deviation
Grades in required clerkships	4.07	0.79
USMLE Step 2 score	3.96	0.85
Number of honors grades	3.84	0.75
Membership in AOA	3.75	0.94
Class rank	3.72	0.89
Grades in senior electives in specialty	3.65	0.84
Medical school academic awards	3.55	0.87
USMLE Step 1 score	3.47	0.91
Medical school reputation	3.37	0.78
Grades in other senior electives	3.17	0.72
Published medical school research	2.95	0.94
Grades in pre-clinical courses	2.77	0.84

Wagoner NE, Suriano JR. Program directors' responses to a survey on variables used to select residents in a time of change. *Acad Med* 1999; 74(1): 51-58.

How important are audition electives?

Audition electives are not essential to match into internal medicine.

How important are the letters of recommendation?

Adams found that 79% of program directors found the chairman's letter to be highly or moderately useful in making interview decisions, and 77% found the chairman's letter to be highly or moderately useful in ranking applicants.

How important is the personal statement?

Adams reported that 61% of program directors found the personal statement to be highly or moderately useful in making interview decisions, and 57% found the statement to be highly or moderately useful in ranking applicants.

How important is AOA?

According to Wagoner, being a member of AOA was fourth in importance. The NRMP reports that 12.6% of U.S. seniors who matched to internal medicine in 2007 were members of AOA.

How important is the USMLE?

The mean USMLE Step 1 score for 2007 U.S. senior applicants who matched was 222. According to Adams, 94% of program directors found USMLE scores to be highly or moderately useful for making interview decisions. Dr. Henderson, program director at University of California-Davis, states that his program doesn't "pay much attention to Step 1 unless it's very low (below 200 or so)...The most competitive programs may use Step 1 scores because they can, having many excellent applicants."

How important is research experience?

Among 12 academic criteria, Wagoner found that published medical school research was next to last in importance. Participation in research is not necessary although research experience, especially if it leads to publication, may enhance competitiveness at the more competitive programs.

How important is the interview?

According to Adams, the interview was found to be most useful for ranking decisions, with 96% of respondents reporting the interview to be highly or moderately useful.

References

American Board of Internal Medicine. Available at www.abim.org.
American College of Osteopathic Internists. Available at www.acoi.org.
American College of Physicians. Available at www.acponline.org.
Association of Program Directors in Internal Medicine. Available at
    www.apdim.med.edu.
Adams LJ, Brandenburg S, Blake M. Factors influencing internal medicine
    program directors decisions about applicants. *Acad Med* 2000; 75: 542-3.
Brotherton SE, Etzel SI. Graduate medical education, 2006-2007. *JAMA* 2007;
    298 (9): 1081-1096.
Farnie, MA. Career counseling: internal medicine. Available at http://
    www.uth.tmc.edu/med/administration/student/ms4/2003CCC.htm
Henderson M. A guide to the perplexed: residency guide. From
    www.ucdmc.ucdavis.edu.
Society of General Internal Medicine. Available at www.sgim.org.
Wagoner NE, Suriano JR. Program directors' responses to a survey on variables
    used to select residents in a time of change. *Acad Med* 1999; 74(1): 51-58.

Neurology

How competitive is the specialty?

As with other specialties, prestigious programs are highly competitive. However, neurology overall is among the less competitive specialties.

What is the percentage of available positions filled by U.S. seniors? What about other applicants?

As of 2007, there were 1,507 total residents training in a total of 122 neurology residency programs (Brotherton). Of these, 57.1% were U.S. MDs, 36.5% were IMGs, 6.1% were osteopathic graduates, and 0.3% were Canadian graduates.

Neurology residency: positions filled by U.S. seniors 2007-2008 (for PGY-1 positions)		
Year	Positions offered total	Percentage of positions filled by U.S. seniors
2008	177	59.3%
2007	160	51.9%
From www.nrmp.org		

Neurology residency: positions filled by U.S. seniors 2007-2008 (for PGY-2 positions)		
Year	Positions offered total	Percentage of positions filled by U.S. seniors
2008	398	56.8%
2007	379	57.8%
From www.nrmp.org		

How important are audition electives?

Audition electives are not necessary for residency selection.

How important are letters of recommendation?

Dr. Scheiss of the University of Texas-Houston states that "test scores assume secondary importance. Far more important are letters from physicians—not necessarily neurologically trained—that speak to the character, intellectual curiosity, diligence and the passion for neurology of the applicant. These letters should be based on direct observation of the applicant."

How important is the personal statement?

Dr. Scheiss feels that it is of "utmost importance" for applicants to communicate their desire to be a neurologist.

How important is AOA?

The NRMP reports that 14.5% of U.S. seniors who matched to neurology in 2007 were members of AOA.

How important is the USMLE?

The mean USMLE Step 1 score for 2007 U.S. senior applicants who matched was 219. Although board scores are not as important in this specialty, if you have a low score, you should consider taking the USMLE Step 2 CK exam.

How important is research experience?

Research experience is not required for acceptance into a neurology residency program. However, it may increase an applicant's chances of matching with the more academic programs, particularly if it leads to publication.

How important is the interview?

As with other specialties, the interview is an important factor in ranking applicants for a neurology residency program.

References

American Academy of Neurology. Available at www.aan.com.
Brotherton SE, Etzel SI. Graduate medical education, 2006-2007. *JAMA* 2007; 298 (9): 1081-1096.
Scheiss M. Career counseling: neurology. Available at http://www.uth.tmc.edu/ med/administration/student/ms4/2003CCC.htm

Neurological Surgery

How competitive is the specialty?

Neurological surgery is a highly competitive specialty. In the 2008 match, 70 applicants, or approximately 20% of the applicant pool (including U.S. seniors and other applicants), were left unmatched.

What is the percentage of available positions filled by U.S. seniors? What about other applicants?

As of 2007, there were 881 total residents training in a total of 97 neurological surgery residency programs (Brotherton). 88.6% were U.S. MDs, 10.4% were IMGs, 0.3% were osteopathic graduates, and 0.6% were Canadian graduates.

In the 2008 match, 173 of 179 positions were filled through the match. Of this group, 88% were U.S. seniors.

Neurological surgery residency: positions filled by U.S. seniors 2003-2008		
Year	Positions filled total	Percentage of positions filled by U.S. seniors
2008	173	89%
2007	170	89%
2006	165	85%
2005	154	87%
2004	149	94%
2003	157	89%
From www.sfmatch.org		

How important are the letters of recommendation?

Letters of recommendation, particularly from neurosurgeons who know you well, are important. The American Association of Neurological Surgeons considers "letters from 'famous' individuals that do not speak of you in a personalized fashion" as less useful. Applicants should have at least two letters written by neurosurgeons. Dr. Shaver of the Medical College of Georgia states that "it is also important to get a letter of recommendation from the chairman of the Neurosurgery department of your medical school."

How important is the personal statement?

Program directors recommend that applicants clearly describe the reasons that led them to choose a career in neurosurgery. Applicants often underestimate the importance of the statement. The American Association of Neurological Surgeons encourages applicants to "take the time to do it well. It is important to your future."

How important is the USMLE?

The average USMLE Step 1 score for 2008 matched applicants was 236. The average score for unmatched applicants was 203. Dr. Muizelaar, program director at University of California-Davis, writes that "grades and numbers must be high."

How important is research experience?

Dr. Muizelaar writes, "Research in medical school is highly desirable, especially in basic or clinical sciences related to neurosurgery."

How important is the interview?

As with other competitive specialties, the interview is of great importance. The Department of Neurological Surgery at the University of Chicago states that "all faculty interview each applicant and questions vary from assessment of medical knowledge to more general aspects of preparedness for residency, knowledge of requirements and commitment, maturity, and prior skills."

References

American Association of Neurological Surgeons. Available at www.neurosurgery.org.
Brotherton SE, Etzel SI. Graduate medical education, 2006-2007. *JAMA* 2007; 298 (9): 1081-1096.
Frim D, Rice H. Pritzker residency process guide: neurological surgery. Available at http://pritzker.uchicago.edu/current/students/ResidencyProcessGuide.pdf
Muizelaar JP. A guide to the perplexed: residency guide. From www.ucdmc.ucdavis.edu.
Shaver EG. Neurosurgery. From www.womensurgeons.org (Association of Women Surgeons).
Society of Neurological Surgeons. Available at www.societyns.org

Obstetrics and Gynecology

How competitive is the specialty?

Obstetrics and gynecology is a moderately competitive specialty.

What is the percentage of available positions filled by U.S. seniors? What about other applicants?

As of 2007, there were 4,739 total residents training in a total of 250 obstetric and gynecology residency programs (Brotherton). Of these, 71.1% were U.S. MDs, 21.2% were IMGs, 7.5% were osteopathic graduates, and 0.3% were Canadian graduates.

Obstetrics and gynecology residency: positions filled by U.S. seniors 2004-2008		
Year	Positions offered total	Percentage of positions filled by U.S. seniors
2008	1,163	72.1%
2007	1,155	72.5%
2006	1,154	72.4%
2005	1,144	67.5%
2004	1,142	65.1%
From www.nrmp.org		

Is there any literature available to applicants to guide them through the residency application process?

There are two surveys of obstetrics and gynecology residency program directors available to applicants to guide them through the process of securing a residency position:

- In 1995 researchers surveyed obstetrics and gynecology program directors to determine which factors are most important in deciding whom to interview and how to rank applicants. The medical school transcript, the Dean's letter, and USMLE scores ranked highest for making decisions about whom to interview. The interview was considered most important for ranking decisions (Taylor).

• In 1999 Wagoner and Suriano surveyed program directors about the residency selection process. Of the 257 surveys sent, responses were received from 69 directors.

Obstetrics and gynecology residency program directors' rankings of academic criteria used in the residency selection process

Criteria	Mean	Standard deviation
Grades in required clerkships	4.19	0.63
Number of honors grades	4.09	0.72
USMLE Step 1 score	4.04	0.70
USMLE Step 2 score	3.96	0.85
Class rank	3.91	0.79
Medical school academic awards	3.81	0.80
Membership in AOA	3.75	0.91
Medical school reputation	3.56	0.90
Grades in senior electives in specialty	3.52	1.02
Published medical school research	3.49	0.98
Grades in other senior electives	3.33	0.90
Grades in pre-clinical courses	3.25	0.79

Wagoner NE, Suriano JR. Program directors' responses to a survey on variables used to select residents in a time of change. *Acad Med* 1999; 74(1): 51-58.

How important are audition electives?

Dr. Tony Ogburn, program director at the University of New Mexico, recommends an audition elective if an applicant is particularly interested in a certain program. The Department of Obstetrics and Gynecology at the University of Chicago states that "completing an elective at a desired program can be very helpful. This is especially applicable for very competitive positions."

How important is AOA?

Being a member of AOA was seventh in importance. The NRMP reports that 11.8% of U.S. seniors who matched to obstetrics and gynecology in 2007 were members of AOA.

How important is the USMLE?

The mean USMLE Step 1 score for 2007 U.S. senior applicants who matched was 214. Of note, 218 of 274 applicants with scores < 200 matched. Dr. Paik, program director at the University of California-Davis, states that "a low USMLE score does not preclude someone from going into obstetrics and gynecology."

How important is research experience?

Among 12 academic criteria, Wagoner found that published medical school research was ninth in importance. Among 2007 applicants, 196 of 220 applicants with no research experience matched.

How important is the interview?

According to Taylor, the interview was found to be most useful for ranking decisions.

References

American Board of Obstetrics and Gynecology. Available at www.abog.org.
American College of Obstetrics and Gynecology. Available at www.acog.org.
American College of Osteopathic Obstetricians and Gynecologists. Available at www.acoog.com.
Association of Professors of Gynecology and Obstetrics. Available at www.apgo.org.
Blanchard A, Gilmore-Bradford E. Pritzker residency process guide: obstetrics and gynecology. Available at http://pritzker.uchicago.edu/current/students/ResidencyProcessGuide.pdf
Brotherton SE, Etzel SI. Graduate medical education, 2006-2007. *JAMA* 2007; 298 (9): 1081-1096.
Espey E, Ogburn T. Guidelines for pursuing a residency in obstetrics and gynecology: 2005-2006. From (http://obgyn.unm.edu/clerkship)
Monga, Yoemans E. Career counseling: obstetrics and gynecology. Available at http://www.uth.tmc.edu/med/administration/student/ms4/2003CCC.htm
Paik C. A guide to the perplexed: residency guide. From www.ucdmc.ucdavis.edu.
Taylor CA, Weinstein L, Mayhew HE. The process of resident selection: a view from the residency director's desk. *Obstet Gynecol* 1995; 85(2): 299-303.
Wagoner NE, Suriano JR. Program directors' responses to a survey on variables used to select residents in a time of change. *Acad Med* 1999; 74(1): 51-58.

Ophthalmology

How competitive is the specialty?

Ophthalmology is highly competitive. Of note, 179 applicants in the 2008 match, or approximately 28% of the applicant pool (including U.S. seniors and other applicants), failed to match.

What is the percentage of available positions filled by U.S. seniors? What about other applicants?

Most positions are filled by U.S. seniors. As of 2007, there were 1,225 residents training in 117 ophthalmology residency programs (Brotherton). Of these, 90.4% were U.S. MDs, 8.0% were IMGs, 1.1% were osteopathic graduates, and 0.4% were Canadian graduates.

Ophthalmology: positions filled by U.S. seniors 2003-2008

Year	Positions filled total	Percentage of positions filled by U.S. seniors
2008	453	86%
2007	449	80%
2006	446	88%
2005	443	86%
2004	438	82%
2003	434	82%
From www.sfmatch.org		

Is there any literature available to applicants to guide them through the residency application process?

In 1999, Wagoner and Suriano surveyed program directors about the residency selection process. Of the 135 surveys sent, responses were received from 46 directors.

Ophthalmology residency rankings of academic criteria used in the residency selection process

Criteria	Mean	Standard deviation
Grades in required clerkships	4.16	0.69
Number of honors grades	4.00	1.03
Class rank	3.87	0.81
Membership in AOA	3.87	1.06
Grades in senior electives in specialty	3.72	0.93
USMLE Step 2 score	3.61	0.99
USMLE Step 1 score	3.60	0.89
Medical school academic awards	3.55	0.96
Medical school reputation	3.42	0.81
Grades in other senior electives	3.39	0.80
Published medical school research	3.36	1.02
Grades in pre-clinical courses	3.07	0.80
Wagoner NE, Suriano JR. Program directors' responses to a survey on variables used to select residents in a time of change. *Acad Med* 1999; 74(1): 51-58.		

How important are audition electives?

If you are interested in doing your residency at a particular program, doing an audition elective there may be advisable. Dr. Ksiazek, program director at the University of Chicago, states that "if you are really interested in a particular program, an on-site rotation is a must."

How important is the personal statement?

Dr. Ksiazek encourages applicants to "place great attention on the personal statement. This is your chance to paint a picture of yourself for the reader and to differentiate yourself from everyone else...Often the personal statement is the deciding factor in granting an interview."

How important are the letters of recommendation?

Dr. Simpson, program director at the University of California-Irvine, feels it is "critical" for applicants to obtain letters from ophthalmology professors who truly "know you. If he/she is famous, or has connections to a particular program, it does help—but a letter from a renowned ophthalmologic academic that states: 'I understand from my residents that this student was good...' would be a real negative."

How important is the USMLE?

Very important. The average USMLE Step 1 score among 2008 matched applicants was 232.

How important is research experience?

While ophthalmology research is not required, it can certainly be helpful. Most applicants have participated in some type of research. For prestigious programs, lack of research experience or even a publication can remove an applicant from further consideration.

How important is the interview?

The interview is an important factor in determining a program's rank list. Dr. Ksiazek urges applicants to "research the program before you get there and ask program-specific questions. You do not want to blend into a sea of other applicants by asking the same old questions."

References

American Academy of Ophthalmology. Available at www.abop.org.
Brotherton SE, Etzel SI. Graduate medical education, 2006-2007. *JAMA* 2007; 298 (9): 1081-1096.
Kellaway J. Career counseling: ophthalmology. Available at http://www.uth.tmc.edu/med/administration/student/ms4/2003CCC.htm
Ksiazek S. Taylor TL. Pritzker residency process guide: ophthalmology. Available at http://pritzker.uchicago.edu/current/students/ResidencyProcessGuide.pdf
Lee AG, Golnik KC, Oetting TA, Beaver HA, Boldt HC, Olson R, Greenlee E. Abramoff MD, Johnson AT, Carter K. Re-engineering the resident applicant selection process in ophthalmology: a literature review and recommendations for improvement. *Surv Ophthalmol* 2008; 53(2): 164-176.
Simpson J. Residency selection handbook: ophthalmology. From www.ucihs.uci.edu.
Wagoner NE, Suriano JR. Program directors' responses to a survey on variables used to select residents in a time of change. *Acad Med* 1999; 74(1): 51-58.

Orthopedic Surgery

How competitive is the specialty?

Orthopedic surgery is a highly competitive field. In recent years, the specialty has attracted tremendous interest, with many more applicants than positions available. In 2007 out of 719 U.S. seniors applying to orthopedic surgery, 142 failed to match. In other words, 19.7% of U.S. seniors applying to orthopedic surgery failed to match.

What is the percentage of available positions filled by U.S. seniors? What about other applicants?

As of 2007 there were 3,187 total residents training in a total of 152 orthopedic surgery residency programs (Brotherton); 96.9% were U.S. MDs, 2.3% were IMGs, and 0.8% were osteopathic graduates.

Orthopedic surgery: positions filled by U.S. seniors 2004-2008		
Year	Positions offered total	Percentage of positions filled by U.S. seniors
2008	636	93.1%
2007	616	93.8%
2006	615	89.6%
2005	610	91.8%
2004	589	93.0%
From www.nrmp.org		

Is there any literature available to applicants to guide them through the residency application process?

There are two surveys of orthopedic surgery program directors available to applicants to guide them through the process of securing a residency position:

- In 1999 Wagoner and Suriano surveyed program directors about the residency selection process. Of the 149 surveys sent, responses were received from 46 directors.

Orthopedic surgery residency program rankings of academic criteria used in the residency selection process		
Criteria	Mean	Standard deviation
Grades in senior electives in specialty	4.24	0.87
Grades in required clerkships	4.02	0.77
USMLE Step 1 score	3.98	0.75
Number of honors grades	3.93	0.68

Orthopedic surgery residency program rankings of academic criteria used in the residency selection process

Class rank	3.89	0.64
Membership in AOA	3.89	0.71
USMLE Step 2 score	3.76	0.79
Medical school academic awards	3.54	0.69
Medical school reputation	3.54	0.72
Grades in other senior electives	3.50	0.89
Grades in pre-clinical courses	3.42	0.84
Published medical school research	3.41	0.86

Wagoner NE, Suriano JR. Program directors' responses to a survey on variables used to select residents in a time of change. *Acad Med* 1999; 74(1): 51-58.

- In 2002 Dr. Bernstein of New York University surveyed program directors about the importance of 26 residency selection criteria. Of the 156 surveys sent, responses were received from 109 directors.

Results of program director rankings of 26 residency selection factors (descending order of importance)
Rotation at director's institution
USMLE part I score
Rank in medical school
Formality/politeness at interview
Personal appearance of candidate
Performance on ethical questions at interview
Letter of recommendation by orthopedic surgeon
Candidate is a member of AOA
Medical school reputation
Dean's letter
Personal statement
Failed first attempt at orthopedic match
Telephone call placed on candidate's behalf
Candidate has published research
Candidate participated in a dedicated research experience
Letter of recommendation from non-orthopedic surgeon
Candidate is a M.D./Ph.D.
Reputation of undergraduate college
Undergraduate Grade Point Average
Appearance of CV
Letter of recommendation from senior resident
Candidate has a relative affiliated with director's program
Candidate has an undergraduate engineering major
Thank you letter from candidate
Performance on manual skills testing during interviews
Evaluation by psychologist/psychiatrist during interview

Bernstein AD, Jazrawi LM, Elbeshbeshy B, Della Valle CJ, Zuckerman JD. Orthopaedic resident-selection criteria. *J Bone Joint Surg Am* 2002; 84-A (11): 2090-2096.

Which criteria are ranked highest by program directors?

In Bernstein's survey, the three criteria ranked highest by program directors were performance during a rotation at the program director's institution, USMLE Step 1 score, and medical school class rank. Wagoner found that grades in senior orthopedic surgery electives were most important, followed by grades in required clerkships (core clerkships in third year of medical school) and USMLE Step 1 score.

How important are audition electives?

Performing an elective at the program director's institution was ranked as the most important residency selection factor. Bernstein further stated that "60% of programs reported that 50% or more of their matching residents over the previous three years had performed medical student orthopedic surgery rotations at the program prior to matching for residency." Drs. Peabody and Manning of the University of Chicago strongly recommend audition electives. "It's almost mandatory to do an away elective and shine."

How important are letters of recommendation?

Very important. In Bernstein's survey, letters of recommendation from an orthopedic surgeon were ranked seventh in importance among a group of 26 factors. Letters from non-orthopedic surgeons were less important, rated as 17th in importance. The most important aspect of a letter, according to 54% of the directors, was that it was written by someone they know. The University of Washington states, "input from senior orthopedists are particularly helpful" but only if the applicant is well known to the individual.

How important is the personal statement?

Bernstein found that the personal statement was ranked eleventh in importance among a group of 26 factors. Of note, it was ranked higher than having published research or participating in a dedicated research experience. It was also ranked higher than a letter of recommendation from a non-orthopedic surgeon. When asked, 43% of directors felt that the most important aspect of the statement was "to learn about the candidate's personal interests and background" while 32% felt that it was "to gain insight into an applicant's ability to write and communicate effectively." Dr. Coupe, former program director at the University of Texas-Houston, states that the "personal statement is read by each of our orthopedic faculty members, and is considered by our faculty to be a very important part of the application process. If is often used as a point of departure for interviewing the student."

How important is AOA?

Membership in AOA was eighth in importance. The NRMP reports that 30.5% of U.S. seniors who matched to orthopedic surgery in

2007 were members of AOA. Although AOA membership is valued, it is certainly not a requirement. According to Bernstein, only 1% of program directors agreed with the statement that "only applicants that are AOA are offered an interview," and 30% of program directors evaluate candidates regardless of their AOA status.

How important is the USMLE?

USMLE Step 1 scores are clearly important, ranking in the top three in both surveys. The average USMLE Step 1 score among U.S. seniors who matched in 2007 was 234. Of note, there are applicants with USMLE Step 1 scores below 200 who matched into orthopedic surgery in 2007, indicating that not all programs have a minimum score requirement of >200. However, the odds of matching with a lower USMLE Step 1 score significantly decrease. Only 12 of 42 applicants with a score <200 matched in 2007. There are also a number of applicants with scores > 230 who did not match (35 of 388).

How important is research experience?

Among 12 academic criteria, Wagoner found that published medical school research was last in importance. Its low ranking, however, may in part be due to the fact that so many applicants participate in research, and therefore it becomes a given. Among 2007 applicants, over 90% had participated in a research project, with over 60% claiming at least one abstract, publication, or presentation. Dr. Phipps, program director at the University of California-Irvine, states that doing research in the field will "definitely" improve the chances of obtaining a residency.

How important is the interview?

The interview is clearly of great importance. Three of the top six residency selection criteria were related to the interview, including formality/politeness at interview, personal appearance of candidate, and performance on ethical questions at interview. Once invited for an interview, 22% of programs place candidates on equal footing with ranking decisions based solely on interview performance. Interestingly, 18% of programs present applicants with clinical scenarios during the interview.

References

American Association of Orthopedic Surgeons. Available at www.aaos.org
American Board of Orthopedic Surgery. Available at www.abos.org.
American Orthopedic Association. Available at www.aoassn.org.
Bajaj G, Carmichael KD. What attributes are necessary to be selected for an orthopedic surgery residency position: perceptions of faculty and residents. *South Med J* 2004; 97 (12): 1179-1185.
Bernstein AD, Jazrawi LM, Elbeshbeshy B, Della Valle CJ, Zuckerman JD. Orthopaedic resident-selection criteria. *J Bone Joint Surg Am* 2002; 84-A (11): 2090-2096.

Brotherton SE, Etzel SI. Graduate medical education, 2006-2007. *JAMA* 2007;
  298 (9): 1081-1096.
Coupe K. Career counseling: orthopedic surgery. Available at http://
  www.uth.tmc.edu/med/administration/student/ms4/2003CCC.htm
Peabody T, Manning D. Pritzker residency process guide: orthopedic surgery.
  Available at http://pritzker.uchicago.edu/current/students/
  ResidencyProcessGuide.pdf
Phipps GJ. Residency selection handbook: orthopedic surgery. From
  www.ucihs.uci.edu.
Wagoner NE, Suriano JR. Program directors' responses to a survey on variables
  used to select residents in a time of change. *Acad Med* 1999; 74(1): 51-58.

Otolaryngology

How competitive is the specialty?

Otolaryngology is a highly competitive specialty. In 2007, out of 305 U.S. seniors applying to otolaryngology, 56 failed to match. In other words, 18.4% of U.S. seniors applying to otolaryngology failed to match.

What is the percentage of available positions filled by U.S. seniors? What about other applicants?

As of 2007 there were 1,292 residents training in a total of 104 otolaryngology residency programs (Brotherton). Of these, 96.0% were U.S. MDs, 2.8% were IMGs, 0.9% were osteopathic graduates, and 0.4% were Canadian graduates.

Otolaryngology: positions filled by U.S. seniors 2006-2008		
Year	Positions offered total	Percentage of positions filled by U.S. seniors
2008	273	92.7%
2007	270	93.0%
2006	264	92.0%
From www.nrmp.org		

How important are audition electives?

While there are no data available to guide these decisions, some programs suggest that an elective performed at the institution would be advantageous. For example, the website for the Boston University program states that "although it is not an absolute requirement that the clerkship be taken in our institution, it is advantageous to the candidate and to the program if it is taken in one of our hospitals." Dr. Suskind of the University of Chicago echoes these comments. "As an evaluator of the application process, it is hard to distinguish among the many strong medical student candidates. For this reason...we strongly encourage sub-internship...An away sub-internship at the program of your choice is recommended."

How important are letters of recommendation?

Letters of recommendation are very important. Follow the program's instructions carefully. Even if a chairman's letter is not required, ask your advisor about whether you should solicit one. Generally, at least two letters from otolaryngology faculty members are recommended.

How important is AOA?

AOA is important. The NRMP reports that 39.0% of U.S. seniors who matched to otolaryngology in 2007 were members of AOA. Some competitive programs will interview only applicants who are members of AOA, but most programs will consider the entire application.

How important is the USMLE?

Very important. The mean USMLE Step 1 score among 2007 matched applicants was 238.

How important is research experience?

While having research experience is not an absolute requirement for matching into otolaryngology, most applicants have participated in a research project and/or published. According to the NRMP, over 95% of U.S. seniors who applied in 2007 had some research experience, and 78% claimed at least one abstract, publication, or presentation. Highly academic or research-oriented programs may not extend interview invitations to applicants with no research experience.

How important is the interview?

As with other highly competitive specialties, the interview takes on considerable importance. Dr. Suskind states that "interviews are a major determinant in the decision process."

References

American Academy of Otolaryngology - Head and Neck Surgery. Available at www.entnet.org.
American Board of Otolaryngology. Available at www.abhpm.org.
Armstrong WB. Residency selection handbook: otolaryngology. From www.ucihs.uci.edu.
Brotherton SE, Etzel SI. Graduate medical education, 2006-2007. *JAMA* 2007; 298 (9): 1081-1096.
Pereira K. Career counseling: otolaryngology. Available at http://www.uth.tmc.edu/med/administration/student/ms4/2003CCC.htm
Suskind D. Pritzker residency process guide: otolaryngology. Available at http://pritzker.uchicago.edu/current/students/ResidencyProcessGuide.pdf

Pathology

How competitive is the specialty?

Pathology is among the less competitive specialties. However, securing a position in one of the top programs in the field is difficult.

What is the percentage of available positions filled by U.S. seniors? What about other applicants?

As of 2007 there were 2,310 total residents training in a total of 150 pathology residency programs (Brotherton). Of these, 64.5% were U.S. MDs, 29.9% were IMGs, 5.3% were osteopathic graduates, and 0.3% were Canadian graduates.

Pathology: positions filled by U.S. seniors 2004-2008

Year	Positions offered total	Percentage of positions filled by U.S. seniors
2008	508	58.7%
2007	513	57.7%
2006	525	60.0%
2005	526	62.0%
2004	477	61.2%
From www.nrmp.org		

Is there any literature available to applicants to guide them through the residency application process?

In 1999 Wagoner and Suriano surveyed program directors about the residency selection process. Of the 153 surveys sent, responses were received from 60 directors.

Pathology residency program directors' rankings of academic criteria used in the residency selection process

Criteria	Mean	Standard deviation
Published medical school research	3.77	0.98
Class rank	3.75	0.90
Grades in senior electives in specialty	3.73	0.99
Medical school academic awards	3.73	0.90
Membership in AOA	3.67	1.08
Number of honors grades	3.62	0.87
Medical school reputation	3.60	0.96
Grades in required clerkships	3.59	0.83
USMLE Step 2 score	3.41	1.02
USMLE Step 1 score	3.40	1.03
Grades in other senior electives	3.29	0.74
Grades in pre-clinical courses	2.98	1.21

Wagoner NE, Suriano JR. Program directors' responses to a survey on variables used to select residents in a time of change. *Acad Med* 1999; 74(1): 51-58.

How important are letters of recommendation?

Letters of recommendation are important, and applicants are urged to follow program directions carefully. While one letter from a pathologist may suffice for many programs, other programs, especially the more competitive programs, may prefer additional letters.

How important are audition electives?

Audition electives are not required but should be considered if you are seeking a position in one of the competitive programs.

How important is AOA?

The NRMP reports that 11.9% of U.S. seniors who matched to pathology in 2007 were members of AOA.

How important is the USMLE?

According to Wagoner, the USMLE Step 1 was third from last in importance. The mean USMLE Step 1 score among U.S. seniors who matched in 2007 was 223.

How important is research experience?

Among 12 academic criteria, Wagoner found that published medical school research was first in importance. Its presence may significantly strengthen your application. However, research experience is not necessary for matching. Among 2007 applicants, 58 of 64 claiming no research experience matched, and 131 of 143 applicants with no publications matched.

References

American Board of Pathology. Available at www.abpath.org.
American Society for Clinical Pathology. Available at www.ascp.org.
Association of Pathology Chairs. Available at www.apcprods.org.
Brotherton SE, Etzel SI. Graduate medical education, 2006-2007. *JAMA* 2007; 298 (9): 1081-1096.
College of American Pathologists. Available at www.cap.org.
Uthman MO. Career counseling: pathology. Available at http://www.uth.tmc.edu/ med/administration/student/ms4/2003CCC.htm

Pediatrics

How competitive is the specialty?

Pediatrics is one of the less competitive specialties.

What is the percentage of available positions filled by U.S. seniors? What about other applicants?

As of 2007 there were 7,964 total residents training in a total of 201 pediatrics residency programs (Brotherton). Of these, 68.8% were U.S. MDs, 23.9% were IMGs, 6.9% were osteopathic graduates, and 0.4% were Canadian graduates.

Pediatrics: positions filled by U.S. seniors 2004-2008

Year	Positions offered total	Percentage of positions filled by U.S. seniors
2008	2,382	67.6%
2007	2,328	72.8%
2006	2,288	72.9%
2005	2,269	74.0%
2004	2,261	71.3%

From www.nrmp.org

Is there any literature available to applicants to guide them through the residency application process?

In 1999 Wagoner and Suriano surveyed program directors about the residency selection process. Of the 196 surveys sent, responses were received from 70 directors.

Pediatrics residency program directors' rankings of academic criteria used in the residency selection process

Criteria	Mean	Standard deviation
Grades in required clerkships	4.32	0.62
Grades in senior electives in specialty	3.86	0.83
Number of honors grades	3.77	0.81
Class rank	3.60	0.90
Medical school academic awards	3.47	0.75
Grades in other senior electives	3.47	0.80
Membership in AOA	3.44	1.08
USMLE Step 2 score	3.42	0.95
USMLE Step 1 score	3.25	0.88
Medical school reputation	3.18	0.94
Grades in pre-clinical courses	2.85	0.79
Published medical school research	2.72	0.88

Wagoner NE, Suriano JR. Program directors' responses to a survey on variables used to select residents in a time of change. *Acad Med* 1999; 74(1): 51-58.

How important are audition electives?

Audition electives are not required, but should be considered if you are seeking a position in one of the competitive programs.

How important is AOA?

AOA members accounted for 11.6% of U.S. seniors who matched in 2007.

How important is the USMLE?

According to Wagoner, the USMLE Step 1 score was among the bottom four in importance. The mean USMLE Step 1 score for U.S. seniors who matched in 2007 was 217. Dr. West, program director at University of California-Davis, advises students "not to worry too much about boards, but to work very hard during their clerkships." He does note, however, that students "who barely pass" the USMLE may have difficulty with the pediatric board exam, and that failing the pediatric boards reflects poorly on a residency program.

How important is research experience?

Among 12 academic criteria, Wagoner found that published medical school research was last in importance.

How important is the interview?

A study performed at the Children's Hospital of Pennsylvania residency program offered some insight into the importance of the interview (Swanson). The authors wrote that "interview scores were the most important variable for candidate ranking on the NRMP list." The Department of Pediatrics at the University of Chicago encourages applicants to "prepare by familiarizing yourself with the program so that you can ask thoughtful questions."

References

American Academy of Pediatrics. Available at www.aap.org.
American Board of Pediatrics. Available at www.abp.org
Association of Pediatric Program Directors. Available at www.appd.org.
Brotherton SE, Etzel SI. Graduate medical education, 2006-2007. *JAMA* 2007; 298 (9): 1081-1096.
Kahana M, Fromme B, Schwab. Pritzker residency process guide: pediatrics. Available at http://pritzker.uchicago.edu/current/students/ ResidencyProcessGuide.pdf
Swanson WS, Harris MC, Master C, Gallagher PR, Maruo AE, Ludwig S. The impact of the interview in pediatric residency selection. *Amb Pediatr* 2005; 5 (4): 216-220.
West D. A guide to the perplexed: residency guide. From www.ucdmc.ucdavis.edu.

Physical Medicine and Rehabilitation

How competitive is the specialty?

Although physical medicine and rehabilitation (PM&R) is among the less competitive specialties, acceptance into top programs remains highly competitive.

What is the percentage of available positions filled by U.S. seniors? What about other applicants?

As of 2007 there were 1,167 total residents training in a total of 79 physical medicine and rehabilitation residency programs (Brotherton). Of these, 59.6% were U.S. MDs, 16.7% were IMGs, 23.5% were osteopathic graduates, and 0.2% were Canadian graduates.

PM&R: positions filled by U.S. seniors 2004-2008 (for PGY-1 positions)		
Year	Positions offered total	Percentage of positions filled by U.S. seniors
2008	83	62.7%
2007	78	57.7%
2006	82	57.3%
2005	78	48.7%
2004	75	68.0%
From www.nrmp.org		

PM&R: positions filled by U.S. seniors 2004-2008 (for PGY-2 positions)		
Year	Positions offered total	Percentage of positions filled by U.S. seniors
2008	287	46.7%
2007	274	50.0%
2006	270	45.2%
2005	278	53.6%
2004	268	49.6%
From www.nrmp.org		

Is there any literature available to applicants to guide them through the residency application process?

There are two surveys of PM&R program directors available to applicants to guide them through the process of securing a residency position:

- In 1994 Dr. DeLisa, chair of the department of physical medicine and rehabilitation at the UMDNJ - New Jersey Medical School sent questionnaires to all PM&R program directors in an effort to learn about the factors that programs use to select residents. Of the 75 surveys sent, 68 responses were received (88%). The importance of academic criteria used in the selection process is described in the following table

Importance of academic criteria in the PM&R residency selection process		
Criteria	Mean	Standard deviation
Grade(s) in PM&R clerkship in your facility	4.1	0.8
Grade(s) in PM&R clerkship in another facility	3.6	0.9
Grades in other mandatory clinical clerkships	3.4	0.6
Rank order in class	3.2	0.8
Grades in mandatory basic science clerkships	3.1	0.8
USMLE Step 2	2.9	0.8
USMLE Step 1	2.9	0.9
Research ability	2.8	0.8
Membership in Alpha Omega Alpha	2.6	3.4
PhD	2.0	1.0
Master's degree	1.9	0.7

DeLisa JA, Jain SS, Campagnolo DI. Factors used by physical medicine and rehabilitation program directors to select their residents. *Am J Phys Med Rehabil* 1994; 73(3): 152-156.

- In 1999, Wagoner and Suriano surveyed program directors about the residency selection process. Although 101 surveys were sent, only 10 directors responded. Grades in senior electives in the specialty and grades in required clerkships were found to be the two most important academic criteria used by programs to select residents.

How important are letters of recommendation?

DeLisa found that letters of recommendation were the second most important candidate criteria that directors use as they complete their rank list. Only the interview was rated higher in importance. Most highly valued was a letter from a faculty member in the program director's department, followed by a letter written by a chairman of a PM&R department.

How important is AOA?

Among academic criteria, DeLisa found that AOA membership was third to last in importance. However, the score had a large standard deviation, suggesting considerable variability in the importance that directors attach to it. Of U.S. seniors who matched in 2007, 5.5% were AOA members.

How important is the USMLE?

While USMLE scores are important, in DeLisa's survey, 78.1% of directors indicated that they would rank an applicant who failed Step 1 but passed on a subsequent attempt. The mean USMLE Step 1 score for U.S. seniors who matched in 2007 was 209.

How important is research experience?

Among 12 academic criteria, Wagoner found that published medical school research was fourth in importance. Please note, however, that only 10 of 101 programs responded to this survey.

How important is the interview?

The interview is clearly of great importance, ranking as the most important candidate criteria that directors use to rank their applicants. DeLisa also asked program directors about the importance of various applicant characteristics assessed during the interview.

Importance of applicant characteristics assessed during PM&R residency interview

Characteristic	Mean	Standard deviation
Compatibility with the program	4.4	0.8
Ability to articulate thoughts	4.2	0.6
Ability to work with the team	4.2	0.8
Ability to listen	4.1	0.7
Commitment to hard work	4.1	0.7
Ability to grow in knowledge	4.1	0.8
Maturity	3.9	0.7
Ability to solve problems	3.9	0.9
Fund of medical knowledge	3.8	0.7
Sensitivity to others' psychosocial needs	3.7	0.9
Relevant questions asked	3.7	0.7
Personal appearance and professionalism	3.6	0.7
Level of confidence	3.6	0.8
Realistic self-appraisal	3.6	0.9
Knowledge of the specialty	3.5	0.8

DeLisa JA, Jain SS, Campagnolo DI. Factors used by physical medicine and rehabilitation program directors to select their residents. *Am J Phys Med Rehabil* 1994; 73(3): 152-156.

References

American Academy of Physical Medicine and Rehabilitation. Available at www.aapmr.org.
American Board of Physical Medicine and Rehabilitation. Available at www.abpmr.org.
Association of Academic Physiatrists. Available at www.physiatry.org.
Amos DE, Massagli TL. Medical school achievements as predictors of performance in a physical medicine and rehabilitation residency. *Acad Med* 1996; 71: 678-680.

Brotherton SE, Etzel SI. Graduate medical education, 2006-2007. *JAMA* 2007; 298 (9): 1081-1096.

DeLisa JA, Leonard JA Jr, Smith BS, Kirshblum S. Common questions asked by medical students about physiatry. Brief report. *Am J Phys Med Rehabil* 1995; 74(2): 145-154.

DeLisa JA, Jain SS, Campagnolo DI. Factors used by physical medicine and rehabilitation program directors to select their residents. *Am J Phys Med Rehabil* 1994; 73(3): 152-156.

DeLisa, Leonard JA Jr, Meier RH III, et al. Educational survey: common questions asked by medical students about physiatry. *Am J Phys Med Rehabil* 1990; 69: 259-265.

Ogle AA, Garrison SJ, Kaelin DL, Atchison JW, Park YI, Currie DM. Roadmap to 'physical medicine and rehabilitation: answers to medical students' questions about the field. *Am J Phys Med Rehabil* 2001; 80(3): 218-224.

Wagoner NE, Suriano JR. Program directors' responses to a survey on variables used to select residents in a time of change. *Acad Med* 1999; 74(1): 51-58.

Plastic Surgery

How competitive is the specialty?

Plastic surgery is a highly competitive specialty. In 2007, out of 136 U.S. seniors applying to plastic surgery, 51 failed to match. In other words, 37.5% of U.S. seniors applying to plastic surgery failed to match.

What is the percentage of available positions filled by U.S. seniors? What about other applicants?

As of 2007 there were 609 total residents training in a total of 89 plastic surgery residency programs (Brotherton). Of these, 92.1% were U.S. MDs, 6.6% were IMGs, 0.3% were osteopathic graduates, and 1.0% were Canadian graduates.

Plastic surgery: positions filled by U.S. seniors 2004-2008 (for PGY-1 positions)		
Year	Positions offered total	Percentage of positions filled by U.S. seniors
2008	92	93.5%
2007	93	94.6%
2006	88	95.5%
2005	81	90.1%
2004	78	93.6%
From www.nrmp. org		

Is there any literature available to applicants to guide them through the residency application process?

In 2003 Dr. LaGrasso of the University of South Carolina surveyed 15 program directors to learn about the criteria that programs use to select residents. Program directors were asked to rank the importance of nineteen criteria used in the evaluation of applicants.

Objective resident selection criteria			
Rank	Objective resident selection criteria	Mean*	Standard deviation
1	AOA Honor Society membership	4.33	0.49
2	Publications	4.20	0.77
3	Letters from a plastic surgeon	4.20	0.94
4	USMLE scores	4.07	0.88
5	Letters from a friend or colleague	4.07	1.16
6	Letters of recommendation (overall)	4.07	1.22
7	Medical school class rank	4.00	0.85
8	Rotation at your institution	3.93	0.80
9	Medical school grade point average	3.87	0.74
10	Research performed	3.80	0.86
11	Medical school	3.73	0.59
12	Other honors	3.67	0.98
13	Extracurricular activities	3.53	0.83
14	Prior work experience	2.73	1.16
15	Personal statement	2.67	1.05
16	Dean's letter	2.60	1.35
17	Medical school rotations	2.47	0.83
18	Undergraduate institution	2.27	0.80
19	Absence of application photograph	2.07	1.44

*Survey participants were asked to rank each item on a scale of 1 (least important) to 5 (most important).
From LaGrasso JR, Kennedy DA, Hoehn JG, Ashruf S, Pryzbyla AM. Selection criteria for the integrated model of plastic surgery residency. *Plast Reconstr Surg* 2008; 121 (3): 121e-125e.

How important are letters of recommendation?

LaGrasso found that letters of recommendation from a plastic surgeon were ranked third in importance in the evaluation of applicants. Letters from a colleague or friend and letters of recommendation overall were ranked fifth and sixth overall among a group of 19 criteria.

How important is AOA?

Among objective resident selection criteria, LaGrasso found that AOA membership was most important; 36.5% of U.S. seniors who matched in 2007 were AOA members.

How important is the USMLE?

As shown in the previous table, USMLE scores are an important part of the application, ranking fourth in importance. The mean USMLE Step 1 score for U.S. seniors who matched in 2007 was 241.

How important is research experience?

Among 19 criteria, LaGrasso found that publications were second in importance. Having research experience was rated tenth in importance. Only 10 of the 136 U.S. seniors who applied in the 2007 match reported no research experience.

How important is the interview?

In LaGrasso's survey, program directors were asked to rank 20 items that were used in the evaluation of applicants during the interview process. The results are shown in the following table.

Subjective resident selection criteria			
Rank	Criteria	Mean*	Standard deviation
1	Leadership qualities	4.60	0.51
2	Apparent maturity	4.47	0.52
3	Answers to questions	4.07	0.88
4	Candidate's interest in teaching/academics	4.07	0.88
5	Attitude toward questions	3.93	1.39
6	Questions that candidate poses	3.80	1.01
7	Overall appearance	3.73	0.59
8	Statement of candidate's goals	3.73	0.96
9	General knowledge	3.47	0.64
10	Attire	3.00	0.76
11	Family obligations	2.87	1.30
12	Interest in specialty area	2.87	1.51
13	Age	2.47	1.19
14	Participation in ASPS activities	2.13	0.99
15	Family in plastic surgery field	1.73	1.10
16	Apparent ethnicity	1.53	1.13
17	Accent	1.47	0.74
18	Gender	1.40	0.83
19	Sexual preference	1.27	0.46
20	Religious preference	1.07	0.26

*Survey participants were asked to rank each item on a scale of 1 (least important) to 5 (most important).
From LaGrasso JR, Kennedy DA, Hoehn JG, Ashruf S, Pryzbyla AM. Selection criteria for the integrated model of plastic surgery residency. *Plast Reconstr Surg* 2008; 121 (3): 121e-125e.

The results of this survey indicate that most program directors place considerable emphasis on leadership qualities. Applicants having leadership experience in either academic or extracurricular activities need to incorporate this experience in their interview responses. Candidates are also encouraged to ask insightful questions, since questions posed by applicants were ranked sixth in importance.

References

American Board of Plastic Surgery. Available at www.abplsurg.org.
American Society of Plastic Surgeons. Available at www.plasticsurgery.org.
Brotherton SE, Etzel SI. Graduate medical education, 2006-2007. *JAMA* 2007; 298 (9): 1081-1096.
LaGrasso JR, Kennedy DA, Hoehn JG, Ashruf S, Pryzbyla AM. Selection criteria for the integrated model of plastic surgery residency. *Plast Reconstr Surg* 2008; 121 (3): 121e-125e.

Psychiatry

How competitive is the specialty?

Psychiatry is among the less competitive specialties. However, the top programs in the field are quite competitive.

What is the percentage of available positions filled by U.S. seniors? What about other applicants?

As of August 2007 there were 4,613 total residents training in a total of 181 psychiatry residency programs (Brotherton). Of these, 61.7% were U.S. MDs, 30.6% were IMGs, 7.3% were osteopathic graduates, and 0.4% were Canadian graduates.

Psychiatry: positions filled by U.S. seniors 2004-2008		
Year	Positions offered total	Percentage of positions filled by U.S. seniors
2008	1,069	55.7%
2007	1,057	59.9%
2006	1,037	62.0%
2005	1,026	63.6%
2004	1,020	62.8%
From www.nrmp.org		

Is there any literature available to applicants to guide them through the residency application process?

In 1999 Wagoner and Suriano surveyed program directors about the residency selection process. Of the 222 surveys sent, responses were received from 62 directors.

Psychiatry residency program directors' rankings of academic criteria used in the residency selection process

Criteria	Mean	Standard deviation
Grades in required clerkships	3.96	0.76
Number of honors grades	3.68	0.92
Grades in senior electives in specialty	3.67	0.93
Published medical school research	3.50	0.92
Medical school academic awards	3.47	0.94
Medical school reputation	3.42	1.12
Class rank	3.37	0.83
USMLE Step 2 score	3.23	0.95
Membership in AOA	3.07	1.15
Grades in other senior electives	3.03	0.82
USMLE Step 1 score	2.95	0.87
Grades in pre-clinical courses	2.76	0.86

Wagoner NE, Suriano JR. Program directors' responses to a survey on variables used to select residents in a time of change. *Acad Med* 1999; 74(1): 51-58.

How important are audition electives?

Audition electives are not important in residency selection. In the article, "Applying to Psychiatry Residency Programs," Bak and colleagues state that "a psychiatry externship at a program outside the student's medical school affords a student more accurate information about a program, and vice versa. Doing so is not, however, necessary in order to match at such programs ..."

How important are letters of recommendation?

Choose letter writers who know you well and can offer specific details about you. Avoid letters from senior professors, including psychiatrists, unless they can make meaningful and specific remarks.

How important is the personal statement?

Many applicants begin their statements by answering the question, "Why psychiatry?" Often, these statements start with the story of a patient that served as an impetus to pursue a career in psychiatry. Bak recommends that applicants not spend more than "a brief paragraph about such a vignette. Readers want the statement to give a sense of the applicant as a total person. Thus, applicants should feel empowered to expand on 'how,' in addition to 'why,' they ended up applying to psychiatry." In addition to answering "Why psychiatry?" Dr. Spitz, program director at the University of Chicago, encourages applicants to personalize the statement. "Why do you want to interview at a specific residency program?"

How important is AOA?

A total of 3.7% of U.S. seniors who matched in 2007 were AOA members.

How important is the USMLE?

According to Wagoner, the USMLE Step 1 was next to last in importance. The average USMLE Step 1 score for 2007 U.S. seniors who matched was 210. Dr. Servis, program director at University of California-Davis, states that USMLE Step 1 and 2 scores are less important. "We don't usually talk about scores in selection committee unless the students either have an unusually high score or failed their first time. If they failed first try, they may not be invited to interview." Dr. Lehrmann of the Zablocki VA Medical Center writes that "if a candidate failed two or more times, the application goes on a 'no interview' pile; however, if something else stands out positively on the application, it may end up on a 'maybe' pile. Applications showing scores of 200 or higher go on a 'yes' pile. Applications with passing scores less than 200 go on the 'maybe' pile" (Lehrmann).

How important is research experience?

Among 12 academic criteria, Wagoner found that published medical school research was fourth in importance. Bak writes that "most residents, even at top academic programs, primarily tend to become clinicians; thus, research experience is not essential for applicants to successfully match."

How important is the interview?

Dr. Reilly of the University of Texas-Houston states that interviews are "critical. The good interview can save someone with the less than perfect application. A bad interview cannot always be salvaged by a paper record. "

References

American Board of Psychiatry and Neurology. Available at www.abpn.com.
American Psychiatric Association. Available at www.psych.org.
American Association of Directors of Psychiatric Residency Training. Available at www.aadprt.org.
Bak MK, Louie AK, Tong LD, Coverdale J, Roberts LW. Applying to Psychiatry Residency. Acad Psychiatry 2006; 30(3): 239-247.
Brotherton SE, Etzel SI. Graduate medical education, 2006-2007. *JAMA* 2007; 298 (9): 1081-1096.
Lehrmann JA, Walaszek A. Assessing the quality of residency applicants in psychiatry. Acad Psychiatry 2008; 32(3): 180-182.
Reilly E. Career counseling: psychiatry. Available at http://www.uth.tmc.edu/med/administration/student/ms4/2003CCC.htm
Servis M. A guide to the perplexed: residency guide. From www.ucdmc.ucdavis.edu.
Spitz D, Penna N. Pritzker residency process guide: psychiatry. Available at http://pritzker.uchicago.edu/current/students/ResidencyProcessGuide.pdf

Radiation Oncology

How competitive is the specialty?

Radiation oncology is a highly competitive specialty. In 2007 out of 152 U.S. seniors applying to radiation oncology, 28 failed to match. In other words, 18.4% of U.S. seniors applying to radiation oncology failed to match.

What is the percentage of available positions filled by U.S. seniors?

As of 2007 there were 556 total residents training in a total of 79 radiation oncology residency programs (Brotherton). Of these, 96.0% were U.S. MDs, 2.9% were IMGs, 0.7% were osteopathic graduates, and 0.4% were Canadian graduates.

Radiation oncology: positions filled by U.S. seniors 2004-2008 (PGY-2)		
Year	Positions offered	Percentage of positions filled by U.S. seniors
2008	129	86.8%
2007	127	85.8%
2006	111	90.1%
2005	128	85.2%
2004	117	86.3%
From www.nrmp.org		

Of note, the data presented above do not include the few programs that incorporate PGY-1 years into their total residency.

Is there any literature available to applicants to guide them through the residency application process?

In 1999 Wagoner and Suriano surveyed program directors about the residency selection process. Of the 73 surveys sent, responses were received from 15 directors.

Radiation oncology residency program directors' rankings of academic criteria used in the residency selection process		
Criteria	Mean	Standard deviation
Grades in senior electives in specialty	4.33	0.72
Number of honors grades	4.00	0.93
Published medical school research	4.00	1.20
Grades in required clerkships	3.93	0.80

Radiation oncology residency program directors' rankings of academic criteria used in the residency selection process		
Class rank	3.67	0.98
Grades in other senior electives	3.67	0.72
Membership in AOA	3.60	1.24
USMLE Step 2 score	3.47	0.92
Medical school academic awards	3.47	0.99
Medical school reputation	3.27	1.10
USMLE Step 1 score	3.27	0.96
Grades in pre-clinical courses	3.07	0.88
Wagoner NE, Suriano JR. Program directors' responses to a survey on variables used to select residents in a time of change. *Acad Med* 1999; 74(1): 51-58.		

Which criteria are ranked highest by program directors?

Grades in senior electives in the specialty, number of honors grades, published medical school research, and grades in required clerkships are the four most important criteria for determining ranking.

How important are audition electives?

Dr. Kuo, program director at the University of California-Irvine, states that "audition electives … are considered very helpful by most students and residency program directors so that one can become acquainted with the other." Dr. Ryu, program director at the University of California-Davis, strongly recommends an audition elective, stating that "an elective rotation at the program of choice and a superb performance during that rotation is of foremost importance."

How important are letters of recommendation?

Dr. Kuo states that "program directors have come to expect at least one audition elective in clinical radiation oncology with two to three letters from radiation oncology faculty."

How important is the personal statement?

Dr. Connell of the University of Chicago states that the personal statement is "of moderate importance at some programs, while of major importance at others."

How important is AOA?

The NRMP reports that 24.2% of U.S. seniors who matched to radiation oncology in 2007 were members of AOA.

How important is the USMLE?

Very important. The mean USMLE Step 1 score for 2007 applicants who matched was 235.

How important is research experience?

Among 12 academic criteria, Wagoner found that published medical school research was tied for second in importance. Among 2007 U.S. senior applicants who matched, only 9 of the 152 applicants reported not having a single abstract, publication, or presentation. Dr. Ryu feels that research experience is highly desirable, increasing the strength of a candidate's application.

How important is the interview?

As is the case with other competitive specialties, the interview is given a great deal of importance.

References

American Society for Therapeutic Radiation Oncology. Available at
   www.astro.org.
Brotherton SE, Etzel SI. Graduate medical education, 2006-2007. *JAMA* 2007;
   298 (9): 1081-1096.
Connell P. Pritzker residency process guide: radiation oncology. Available at http:/
   /pritzker.uchicago.edu/current/students/ResidencyProcessGuide.pdf
Kuo, J. Residency selection handbook: radiation oncology. From
   www.ucihs.uci.edu.
Ryu J. A guide to the perplexed: residency guide. From ww.ucdmc.ucdavis.edu
Wagoner NE, Suriano JR. Program directors' responses to a survey on variables
   used to select residents in a time of change. *Acad Med* 1999; 74(1): 51-58.

Radiology, Diagnostic

How competitive is the specialty?

Diagnostic radiology is a highly competitive specialty. In 2007, out of 915 U.S. seniors applying to diagnostic radiology, 84 failed to match. In other words, 9.2% of U.S. seniors applying to diagnostic radiology failed to match.

What is the percentage of available positions filled by U.S. seniors? What about other applicants?

As of 2007 there were 4,368 total residents training in a total of 188 radiology residency programs (Brotherton); 89.6% were U.S. MDs, 6.5% were IMGs, 3.6% were osteopathic graduates, and 0.3% were Canadian graduates.

Diagnostic Radiology: positions filled by U.S. seniors 2004-2008 (PGY-1 level)		
Year	Positions offered total	Percentage of positions filled by U.S. seniors
2008	157	86.0%
2007	141	88.7%
2006	129	81.4%
2005	134	79.9%
2004	126	96.0%
From www.nrmp.org		

Diagnostic Radiology: positions filled by U.S. seniors 2004-2008 (PGY-2 level)		
Year	Positions offered	Percentage of positions filled by U.S. seniors
2008	928	81.7%
2007	902	79.7%
2006	882	80.3%
2005	884	77.0%
2004	855	80.8%
From www.nrmp.org		

Is there any literature available to applicants to guide them through the residency application process?

Three surveys of radiology program directors are available to guide applicants through the process of securing a residency position:

- In 1999, Wagoner and Suriano surveyed program directors about the residency selection process. Of the 270 surveys sent, responses were received from 66 directors.

Radiology residency program directors' rankings of academic criteria used in the residency selection process		
Criteria	Mean	Standard deviation
Class rank	4.21	0.90
Number of honors grades	4.09	0.69
Grades in required clerkships	4.08	0.77
Membership in AOA	4.00	0.97
USMLE Step 1 score	3.96	0.77

Radiology residency program directors' rankings of academic criteria used in the residency selection process		
Medical school academic awards	3.75	0.94
Medical school reputation	3.73	0.81
USMLE Step 2 score	3.67	0.96
Published medical school research	3.54	0.84
Grades in senior electives in specialty	3.45	0.89
Grades in other senior electives	3.24	0.89
Grades in pre-clinical courses	3.24	0.96

Wagoner NE, Suriano JR. Program directors' responses to a survey on variables used to select residents in a time of change. *Acad Med* 1999; 74(1): 51-58.

- In 2006, Dr. Otero of the Harvard Medical School surveyed 145 radiology residency program directors about the criteria that programs use to select their residents, and 77 directors responded to the survey.

Importance of ten criteria in selecting applicants for radiology residency interview	
Criteria	**Score***
USMLE scores	8.65
Dean's letter	7.52
Class rank	7.50
Recommendation	7.36
Honor society	7.24
Leadership	6.76
Research experience	6.35
Specific rotation	5.45
Employment experience	5.07
Volunteer experience	5.02

* based on a score of 0 (lowest) to 10 (highest)
Otero HJ, Erturk SM, Ondategui-Parra S, Ros PR. Key criteria for selection of radiology residents: results of a national survey by. *Acad Radiol* 2006; 13: 1155-1164.

- In 2005, the Association of Program Directors in Radiology (APDR) surveyed program directors, and 89 programs responded to the survey. USMLE Step 1 score and class rank were the two most important criteria used by program directors to decide whom to interview.

How important are letters of recommendation?

Otero found that letters of recommendation were the fourth most important criterion used to select residents for interview. In the APDR survey, 91% of programs considered letters to be extremely or somewhat important for selecting an applicant to interview. Dr. Amorosa, program director at the UMDNJ/Robert Wood Johnson Medical School, cautions applicants about obtaining letters from well known faculty. "Someone who is well known but who doesn't know the student very well may be less enthusiastic about her."

How important is the personal statement?

In the APDR survey, 79% of programs considered the statement to be extremely or somewhat important for selecting an applicant to interview.

In an analysis of personal statements submitted to one radiology residency program, Dr. Smith of the Wayne State University School of Medicine sought to determine the components of a statement considered most important to members of the selection committee (Smith). Most important was that an applicant clearly expressed his reasons for pursuing a career in radiology. Also considered important were the applicant's perception of radiology, defined as the applicant explicitly stating "what he/she feels are the important characteristics of either radiologists or the practice of radiology ... and mention of an applicant's personality traits or skills that would affect their training in a positive manner."

Dr. Rosenblum, program director at the University of Chicago, states that "if you are applying out of state, make sure it is clear why you would be interested in coming to that city or state. With the number of applicants, if a program does not think you are likely to want to come there, they probably will not grant you an interview." Consider using the personal statement to express your specific interest.

How important is AOA?

AOA members accounted for 25.8% of U.S. seniors who matched in 2007. According to Otero, being a member of AOA was fifth in importance when considering a radiology candidate for interview. Ranked higher were USMLE scores, Dean's letter, class rank, and recommendation letters. In the APDR survey, 17% of programs stated that AOA status was not important at all in deciding whom to interview.

How important is the USMLE?

USMLE scores are clearly important, ranking as the number one criterion programs use in selecting candidates for an interview (Otero). The mean USMLE Step 1 score for U.S. seniors who matched in 2007 was 235. Of note, there are some applicants, although not many, with USMLE Step 1 scores below 200 who matched into radiology in 2007. Of 45 applicants with Step 1 scores below 200, 21 matched. This indicates that not all programs have a minimum score requirement. Dr. Oldham, program director at the University of Texas-Houston, encourages applicants with low Step 1 scores to take the USMLE Step 2 CK exam. There are also some applicants with scores > 230 who did not match. In fact, the APDR survey revealed that 17% of programs stated that the USMLE Step 1 was not important at all for ranking applicants following an interview.

How important is research experience?

Among 12 academic criteria, Wagoner found that published medical school research was ninth in importance, above only preclinical course grades, grades in senior electives in specialty, and grades in other senior electives. In Otero's survey, research experience was sixth in importance among a group of ten factors used to select residents for interview. In the APDR survey, only 13% of programs considered research experience to be extremely important for selecting an applicant to interview. 66% felt that it was somewhat important. Dr. Amorosa states that "starting a research elective near the end of the third year in medical school can be challenging. If there is adequate infrastructure and close mentoring, it is possible to accomplish a project that may even be submitted to a national meeting and eventually be published."

How important is the interview?

The interview is clearly of great importance. Otero found that in 54.2% of programs, applicants are interviewed by all members of the interviewing bodies. Panel interviews were uncommon, with only five programs reporting their use. Three or more interviews took place in 87.1% of programs. Dr. Rosenblum emphasizes the importance of not asking "questions just to ask. ('What are the program's strengths?' or 'Is the faculty stable?' are turnoffs to most interviewers.)"

References

American Board of Radiology. Available at www.theabr.org.
American College of Radiology. Available at www.acr.org.
Association of Program Directors in Radiology. Available at www.apdr.org.
Amorosa JK. How do I mentor medical students interested in radiology. *Acad Radiol* 2003; 10: 527-535.
Brotherton SE, Etzel SI. Graduate medical education, 2006-2007. *JAMA* 2007; 298 (9): 1081-1096.
Oldham S. Career counseling: radiology. Available at http://www.uth.tmc.edu/ med/administration/student/ms4/2003CCC.htm
Otero HJ, Erturk SM, Ondategui-Parra S, Ros PR. Key criteria for selection of radiology residents: results of a national survey. *Acad Radiol* 2006; 13: 1155-1164.
Radiological Society of North America. Available at www.rsna.org.
Rosenblum J. Pritzker residency process guide: radiology. Available at http:// pritzker.uchicago.edu/current/students/ResidencyProcessGuide.pdf

Smith EA, Weyhing B, Mody Y, Smith WL. A critical analysis of personal statements submitted by radiology residency applicants. *Acad Radiol* 2005; 12: 1024-1028.

Wagoner NE, Suriano JR. Program directors' responses to a survey on variables used to select residents in a time of change. *Acad Med* 1999; 74(1): 51-58.

Surgery, General

How competitive is the specialty?

General surgery is a moderately competitive specialty.

What is the percentage of available positions filled by U.S. seniors? What about other applicants?

As of 2007, there were 7651 total residents training in a total of 251 general surgery residency programs (Brotherton). 78.0% were U.S. MDs, 19.1% were IMGs, 2.6% were osteopathic graduates, and 0.3% were Canadian graduates.

<table>
<tr><th colspan="3">General surgery: positions filled by U.S. seniors
2004-2008 (categorical)</th></tr>
<tr><th>Year</th><th>Positions offered total</th><th>Percentage of positions filled by U.S. seniors</th></tr>
<tr><td>2008</td><td>1,069</td><td>83.1%</td></tr>
<tr><td>2007</td><td>1,057</td><td>78.1%</td></tr>
<tr><td>2006</td><td>1,047</td><td>83.3%</td></tr>
<tr><td>2005</td><td>1,051</td><td>80.4%</td></tr>
<tr><td>2004</td><td>1,044</td><td>84.8%</td></tr>
<tr><td colspan="3">From www.nrmp.org</td></tr>
</table>

Is there any literature available to applicants to guide them through the residency application process?

In 1999 Wagoner and Suriano surveyed program directors about the residency selection process. Of the 456 surveys sent, responses were received from 100 directors.

<table>
<tr><th colspan="3">General surgery residency program directors' rankings of academic criteria used in the residency selection process</th></tr>
<tr><th>Criteria</th><th>Mean</th><th>Standard deviation</th></tr>
<tr><td>Grades in required clerkships</td><td>4.22</td><td>0.62</td></tr>
<tr><td>Class rank</td><td>4.06</td><td>0.81</td></tr>
<tr><td>Membership in AOA</td><td>4.06</td><td>0.89</td></tr>
<tr><td>Number of honors grades</td><td>4.04</td><td>0.71</td></tr>
<tr><td>USMLE Step 1 score</td><td>3.90</td><td>0.84</td></tr>
<tr><td>Medical school academic awards</td><td>3.80</td><td>0.69</td></tr>
</table>

General surgery residency program directors' rankings of academic criteria used in the residency selection process		
USMLE Step 2 score	3.77	0.96
Grades in senior electives in specialty	3.57	1.05
Published medical school research	3.53	0.89
Medical school reputation	3.45	0.81
Grades in pre-clinical courses	3.15	0.85
Grades in other senior electives	2.94	0.98
Wagoner NE, Suriano JR. Program directors' responses to a survey on variables used to select residents in a time of change. *Acad Med* 1999; 74(1): 51-58.		

Which criteria are ranked highest by program directors?

Grades in required clerkships, class rank, membership in AOA, and number of honors grades were the top four academic criteria used by programs to select residents.

How important are audition electives?

Several studies have shown that audition electives in general surgery are not necessary for matching.

How important are letters of recommendation?

Letters of recommendation are important, with the most desirable letters coming from academic surgeons who know the applicant well.

How important is AOA?

Being a member of AOA was tied for second in importance. However, most U.S. seniors who match are not members of AOA. The NRMP reports that 12.1% of U.S. seniors who matched to general surgery in 2007 were members of AOA.

How important is the USMLE?

The mean USMLE Step 1 score for 2007 applicants who matched was 222. Dr. Potts, program director at the University of Texas-Houston, states that "many university programs screen out those who made less than the 50th percentile on the USMLE Step 1." Dr. Scherer, program director at the University of California-Davis, states that their program puts "significant value on Step 1 scores."

How important is research experience?

Among 12 academic criteria, Wagoner found that published medical school research was fourth from last in importance. A more recent survey of 134 general surgery residency program directors revealed that approximately 90% considered research experience almost always or all the time in their evaluation of applications (Melendez).

Nearly 30%, though, reported giving research experience little or no credit unless the work had been published. Respondents were also asked to rate the importance of research experience on a scale of 1 (low importance) to 5 (high importance). While eleven gave it a 5 score, 93 directors rated it a 3, showing that most directors attach moderate importance to this selection variable. Of note, in this survey an applicant's demonstrated interest in surgery was an important selection factor, with 78 directors giving this factor a 5 score. The authors wrote that a "student's participation in research demonstrates considerable interest in the surgical field, which is a selection factor at the top of most program directors' lists."

Among the 812 U.S. senior applicants who matched in 2007, 129 had no prior research experience during medical school, and 337 reported no abstracts, publications, or presentations.

How important is the interview?

Dr. Britt, chairman and program director at the Eastern Virginia Medical School, warns applicants to not underestimate the interview. He writes that "after selection for interview, this is your only time to make an impression." In Melendez's survey, among selection criteria, the interview received the highest ranking from 93 of the 134 program directors.

In a recent study, faculty at the Medical University of South Carolina found that faculty evaluations of personal characteristics through the interview were predictive of subsequent resident performance (Brothers). This study also provided some insight into the selection process at one program. Each applicant has three one-on-one interviews with faculty members, as well as shorter interviews with the chairman, program director, and chief of general surgery. Interviewers are then asked to complete a "personal characteristics" form describing and rating the applicant's "attitude, motivation, integrity, interpersonal relationships, and response to specific life challenges…During a designated meeting, all surgical faculty members are given equal input, with individual members providing insight into the applicants whom they interviewed."

References

American Board of Surgery. Available at www.absurgery.org.
American College of Surgeons. Available at www.facs.org.
Association of Program Directors in Surgery. Available at www.apds.org.
Association of Women Surgeons. Available at www.womensurgeons.org.
Britt, LD. How to interview for a residency position. From http://wwwfacs.org/medicalstudents/britt.pdf
Brothers TE, Wetherholt S. Importance of the faculty interview during the resident application process. J Surg Educ 2007; 64(6): 375-388.
Brotherton SE, Etzel SI. Graduate medical education, 2006-2007. JAMA 2007; 298 (9): 1081-1096.
Melendez MM, Xu X, Sexton TR, Shapiro MJ, Mohan EP. The importance of basic science and clinical research as a selection criterion for general surgery residency programs. J Surg 2008; 65: 151-154.

Potts JR. Career counseling: general surgery. Available at http://
www.uth.tmc.edu/med/administration/student/ms4/2003CCC.htm
Scherer L. A guide to the perplexed: residency guide. From
www.ucdmc.ucdavis.edu.

Urology

How competitive is the specialty?

Urology is a highly competitive specialty. In 2008, out of 404 applicants to urology, 158 failed to match. In other words, 39.1% of all
applicants to urology (including U.S. seniors and other applicants)
failed to match.

What is the percentage of available positions filled by U.S. seniors? What about other applicants?

As of 2007, there were 992 total residents training in a total of 118
urology residency programs (Brotherton), with 95.0% who were U.S.
MDs, 3.6% were IMGs, 1.3% were osteopathic graduates, and 0.1%
were Canadian graduates.

Urology: positions filled by U.S. seniors 2004-2008 (categorical)		
Year	Positions filled total	Percentage of positions filled by U.S. seniors
2008	246	70%
2007	239	79%
2006	235	77%
2005	232	78%
2004	218	80%
From www.auanet.org/residents/resmatch.cfm		

How important are audition electives?

Dr. Terris, program director at the Medical College of Georgia, states,
"participating in a urology rotation at an institution other than the student's home institution may be beneficial if it is a program at which the
student is particularly interested in completing residency training. A visiting student rotation can give students the chance to impress the urology faculty at another institution if their clinical skills outweigh their
academic record or who attend a medical school of lesser reputation."

How important are letters of recommendation?

Dr. Schmidt, chairman of the urology department at University of California San Diego, considers letters of recommendation to be one of
the most important components of the application. "They are especially significant when coming from practicing urologists and particularly important if those urologists are in academic health centers and

well known to my faculty or me." Dr. Brendler, chairman at the University of Chicago, states that it is not necessary to obtain all letters from urology faculty. However, he does recommend a chair's letter. Dr. Bahnson, chairman at the Ohio State University, considers "letters from individuals we know and trust" to be the most important factor in the ranking of applicants. Dr. Zaslau, program director at West Virginia University, feels that letters of recommendation are most important, followed by class rank, clinical rotation performance, and USMLE scores.

How important is the personal statement?

Dr. Brendler encourages applicants to "emphasize some unique aspect of your life which will catch the interest of the reader. Remember that the reviewer will probably be reading at least 200 of these statements." Dr. Ritchey of the University of Texas-Houston Medical School writes that "the personal statement should be short and concise. Some programs like applicants to indicate a preference for an academic career."

How important is the USMLE?

Dr. Ritenour, program director at Emory, states "honestly, at most programs, I believe board scores, as they are the only objective standard, carry the most initial weight."

How important is research experience?

Dr. Terris states that "participation in a research project will improve the chances of matching with a program high on their list. The more in depth the research, the more the application is enhanced. Research does not necessarily have to be in the field of urology to boost one's application." Dr. Fallon, program director at the University of Iowa, encourages applicants to participate in research. Starting early in medical school is preferable, with the goal being to "get at least one publication from this involvement." Dr. Low, program director at the University of California-Davis, writes that "research is highly desirable; most invited for interview are involved in past research."

How important is the interview?

Very important. Dr. Shalhav, program director at the University of Chicago, urges applicants to "listen carefully to the information provided and presented by the program prior your actual interview and formulate your questions based on the information presented."

References

American Board of Urology. Available at www.abu.org.
American Urological Association. Available at www.auanet.org.
Brotherton SE, Etzel SI. Graduate medical education, 2006-2007. *JAMA 2007*; 298 (9): 1081-1096.
Low R. A guide to the perplexed: residency guide. From www.ucdmc.ucdavis.edu.

Ritchey M. Career counseling: urology. Available at http://www.uth.tmc.edu/med/
    administration/student/ms4/2003CCC.htm
Shalhav AL. Pritzker residency process guide: urology. Available at http://
    pritzker.uchicago.edu/current/students/ResidencyProcessGuide.pdf
Society of Women in Urology. Available at www.swiu.org/resources/
    students.aspx.
http://www.urologymatch.com/Program_Survey.htm (Includes statements from
    residency program directors)

Chapter 3

The Basics

The residency application process starts with some basic yet essential information. You may have chosen a specialty, but have you realistically evaluated your chances of matching into that field? How do you decide which programs you should apply to? How do you locate and actually work with a specialty specific advisor? How do you actually start the application process? In this chapter, we consider basic information needed to start the application process.

Choice of specialty

Your residency application starts with your selection of a specialty. Once you identify your specialty choice, you must determine the following:

- The competitiveness of your chosen specialty
- Your competitiveness for that specialty
- The matching program that administers the match process in your chosen field
- The right advisor to help you reach your career goals

Assessing the competitiveness of your chosen specialty

To develop the optimal match strategy, you must take into account the competitiveness of your chosen specialty. Listed in the following table are the numbers of U.S. seniors who failed to match in each specialty. We've also included the percentage of positions in the specialty filled by U.S. seniors, as opposed to international medical graduates or graduates of U.S. medical schools.

The other columns present the mean USMLE Step 1 scores among matched and unmatched U.S. senior applicants, followed by the percentage of applicants in the Alpha Omega Alpha Honor Medical Society (AOA) for each specialty.

Specialty	U.S. seniors who failed to match*		Fill rate, U.S. seniors#	Mean USMLE Step 1 score, U.S. seniors*		% in AOA*
				matched	un-matched	
Anesthesiology	66	(6.2%)	78.7%	220	200	7.5%
Dermatology	158	(38.8%)	86.7%	238	226	47.0%
Emergency medicine	89	(7.5%)	77.4%	220	208	12.4%
Family medicine	13	(1.2%)	43.9%	211	198	5.7%
Internal medicine/ pediatrics	25	(8.4%)	68.5%	221	211	16.8%
Internal medicine	61	(2.1%)	54.8%	222	199	12.6%
Neurology	12	(3.9%)	59.3%	219	202	14.5%
Obstetrics/ gynecology	102	(10.9%)	72.1%	214	200	11.8%
Orthopedic surgery	142	(19.7%)	93.1%	234	216	30.5%
Otolaryngology	56	(18.4%)	92.7%	238	224	39.0%
Pathology	19	(6.1%)	58.7%	223	207	11.9%
Pediatrics	46	(2.6%)	67.6%	217	200	11.6%
PM&R	23	(11.2%)	62.7%	209	193	5.5%
Plastic surgery	51	(37.5%)	93.5%	241	222	36.5%
Psychiatry	22	(3.4%)	55.7%	210	194	3.7%
Radiation oncology	28	(18.4%)	86.7%	235	219	24.2%
Radiology (diagnostic)	84	(9.2%)	86.0%	235	212	25.8%
Surgery (general)	93	(10.3%)	83.1%	222	204	12.1%

*From Charting outcomes in the match: characteristics of applicants who matched to their preferred specialty in the 2007 NRMP Main Residency Match (2nd edition). Available at www.nrmp.org #From www.nrmp.org (2008 data)
The fields of neurological surgery, ophthamology, and urology are not included because this data is not available through the San Francisco and Urology match programs.

Using the previous information, specialties can be loosely divided into three groups:

- Highly competitive
- Moderately competitive
- Less competitive

Competitiveness of specialties		
Highly competitive	**Moderately competitive**	**Less competitive**
Dermatology Neurological surgery Ophthalmology Orthopedic surgery Otolaryngology Plastic surgery Radiation oncology Radiology (diagnostic) Urology	Anesthesiology Emergency medicine Obstetrics/gynecology Pediatrics Surgery (general)	Family Medicine Internal Medicine Neurology Pathology Physical medicine & Rehabilitation Psychiatry

Among the highly competitive specialties, dermatology, orthopedic surgery, otolaryngology, plastic surgery, and radiation oncology had the highest failure to match rates, ranging from 18.4% (otolaryngology) to 38.8% (dermatology).

Note …

For highly competitive specialties, you must have a back-up plan. What do you plan to do if you don't match? Interviewers often ask about back-up plans to learn about the depth of your commitment to the specialty. A well thought out back-up plan that allows reapplication implies a deeper commitment to the specialty. Some students apply to two different specialties, using one as a back-up to the other. However, in a survey of general surgery residency program directors, 75% felt that knowledge of an applicant interviewing in multiple specialties would have a negative effect on the applicant's rank order (Anderson).

Assessing your competitiveness for your chosen specialty

Of critical importance in the residency application process is a realistic assessment of your academic credentials and qualifications. In other words, what are your chances for a successful match? In 1999, Wagoner and Suriano surveyed program directors in 14 specialties (Wagoner). Program directors were asked to rank the importance of the following twelve academic criteria in the residency selection process:

- Grades in required clerkships
- Grades in senior electives in specialty
- Grades in other senior electives
- Grades in pre-clinical courses
- Number of honors grades
- Class rank
- USMLE Step 1 score

- USMLE Step 2 score
- Membership in Alpha Omega Alpha
- Medical school academic awards
- Medical school reputation
- Published medical school research

Although nearly ten years have passed since the results of this survey were published, the information remains valuable as a tool to assess applicant competitiveness. The importance of these criteria varies from specialty to specialty. The results of this survey are summarized in chapter 2, Specialty Specific Information.

Also important is a discussion of your academic credentials and qualifications with those who are knowledgeable about the residency selection process. It is both necessary and important to seek the opinions of your dean, department chairman or program director in your chosen specialty, your advisor, and other key faculty. With their assistance, you can develop a more informed and objective view of your competitiveness for the specialty. Through this process, some applicants will recognize the necessity of a back-up plan.

Just as some specialties are more competitive than others, some programs within a specialty are far more selective than others. Again, discussions with those in the know can help you learn about program selectivity. In developing a list of programs to apply to, we encourage you to apply to those programs which you consider your "dream" programs. Every year, applicants match to programs for which they thought they had little or no chance. However, your list needs to include a sufficient number of programs which are sure bets.

Tip # 1

Ask key faculty members at your school for their thoughts on the number of programs to which you should apply. Based on your credentials, have you considered enough programs for which you are competitive?

Tip # 2

Strategize about concrete steps that you can take to strengthen your application. Should you take the USMLE Step 2 CK exam before applying? Can you participate in research? Should you do an elective with a distinguished professor to secure another strong letter of recommendation? Would an audition elective help?

As you review your competitiveness for the specialty and for particular programs, you must strategize on how to strengthen your candidacy. If you are reading this book early in your medical education, you have the advantage of time. However, even if you're in the midst of the

application process, there are multiple ways to enhance y   **86**
tials.

Tip # 3

Make sure you apply to enough programs. If you receive a plethora of interviews, you can always cancel some.

Matching programs

While most specialties participate in the National Resident Matching Program (NRMP), the ophthalmology and urology matches are handled by the San Francisco Matching program and the American Urological Association, respectively.

National Resident Matching Program (NRMP)

In 1952 the National Resident Matching Program, commonly referred to as NRMP, was established through the efforts of its sponsoring groups, which included the American Medical Association (AMA), the Association of American Medical Colleges (AAMC), and the American Board of Medical Specialties (ABMS). Before its inception, the residency application process was similar to the present college or medical school application process. Medical students were pressured by residency programs to accept residency training contracts early in their medical training, sometimes as early as the second year of medical school. Many students were forced to make specialty decisions before they were ready.

With the establishment of the NRMP the process became much more ordered, and today there is general agreement that the process is much easier. What did the NRMP do to improve this process? The NRMP requires both applicants and programs to create a rank list. Applicants submit a list of programs they would be willing to attend, in order of preference. Programs also submit their own lists, ranking the candidates they have interviewed in the order in which they would extend offers to fill their residency program. Sometime in February, the Match takes place, during which a computer matches each applicant to the highest ranking program (on the applicant's rank list) which has offered him or her a position in their residency program. The results are announced throughout the country in mid-March on "Match Day."

Programs and applicants are expected to honor the results of the Match. To participate in the Match, applicants must agree with the policies and rules of the Match Participation Agreement. When a match occurs between a program and an applicant, both parties have a binding commitment to one another. If either party does not honor the commitment, it is considered a breach of the Agreement and results in a NRMP investigation.

Every year, over 25,000 applicants participate in the Match. Over 15,000 are U.S. medical school seniors. The remaining applicants are considered "independent" applicants and include graduates of U.S. medical schools, students at osteopathic schools, Canadian students, and international medical graduates.

To participate in the Match, applicants must first register for the NRMP (http://www.nrmp.org/res_match/index.html). Applicants can register at the site by completing a form, agreeing to the terms and conditions of the Match, and paying the registration fee.

Other matches

Ophthalmology and urology specialties do not participate in the NRMP. The ophthalmology match is administered by the San Francisco matching program (www.sfmatch.org) while the urology match is handled by the American Urological Association (www.aua.net).

Both matches take place earlier than the NRMP match and are often referred to as "early matches." Results of the ophthalmology and urology matches are announced in January.

Note ...

Applicants participating in other matches (i.e., San Francisco Matching or urology matching program) will often register in the NRMP for several reasons. First, many of these residency programs require applicants to arrange for their first year of training (preliminary year) separately. Second, since both specialties are highly competitive, applicants will often apply to a second choice specialty as a back-up plan in the event that they fail to match.

Electronic residency application service (ERAS)

In 1995 the Electronic Residency Application Service (ERAS) was founded by the Association of American Medical Colleges (AAMC). Through ERAS, applicants can complete a single application which is transmitted electronically to designated programs. Presently, all specialties participate in the ERAS program, with the exception of ophthalmology, which participates in the San Francisco match program.

ERAS allows for transmission of all application components, including the common application, personal statement, Dean's letter, letters of recommendation, and transcripts.

Note ...

All specialties with the exception of ophthalmology use ERAS. Note that, while the urology match is administered by the American Urological Association, urology programs also use ERAS. Ophthalmology, however, participates in the Central Application Service (CAS). A few programs within ERAS participating specialties do not use ERAS. If so, you will need to obtain the application directly from the program.

Note that registering for the NRMP or other match services does not automatically register you for ERAS. Learn more about ERAS at http://www.aamc.org/students/eras/start.htm.

Note ...

It is to your advantage to apply as early as possible. At many programs, interview invitations are extended on a first come, first-served basis. Well-qualified applicants are sometimes rejected because applications were received after all available interview slots were taken.

Selecting an advisor

Insider advice is invaluable. Students recognize that the help of an advisor in guiding them through the complex residency application process can be an important factor in boosting the strength of their application. In a survey of third- and fourth-year medical students at UCSF, 96% of all participants rated mentors as important or very important (Aagaard). Unfortunately, recognizing the value of a mentoring relationship is a far cry from developing such a relationship. Although 96% of the participants rated mentors as important, only 36% actually reported having a mentor.

The value of advising is recognized in all fields. The literature in the fields of business, education, and medicine all support its value. Although they are at an advanced level in their career, even medical school faculty describe the need for advisors. Comments made by medical school faculty emphasize the value of an advising relationship (Jackson):

- "I had a difficult time learning the rules of the game."
- "Without a mentor...I had no idea really what to expect from academic medicine. I have been feeling my way through the tunnels because I don't know where the roadblocks are. I just kind of deal with them when I get there."

These comments mirror those we hear from applicants. It is difficult to learn the rules of the game when they're not written down. "I didn't know you could customize your personal statements for different programs." "I didn't know I should have sent an e-mail thank you immediately after the interview, especially since I was planning to send a note later."

Particularly difficult is when you learn the rules of the game too late to make a difference. "I didn't know that 95% of matched applicants to otolaryngology in the NRMP data from 2007 had reported one or more abstracts, publications, or presentations. I'm in my fourth year now, and it's probably too late."

As you'll see throughout this book, we often recommend seeking the opinions and advice of your advisors. Their insider advice and specific knowledge about the specialty is clearly very valuable. However, how do you, as an applicant, actually locate such an advisor?

Some medical schools recognize the importance of advising students and have responded with the development of mentoring and advising programs. These programs differ widely in structure and scope. At some schools, highly organized programs have been developed. At other schools, the mentoring process is more informal, consisting of students being given a list of faculty members willing to serve as advisors, and then encouraged to cultivate relationships. As one student in a survey of UCSF students stated, "I create the relationship, and then I follow it. I sort of take the risk" (Hauer).

While some students are able to create such relationships, it can be difficult, and some students blame themselves for not being assertive enough to find a mentor. "I just didn't know how to go about setting myself up for a good thing to happen" (Hauer). Other students maintain that the problem lies with the system, citing the short duration of courses and clerkships as impediments to developing relationships with faculty.

How have other students met potential mentors? In one study, 28% of students met their mentors during inpatient clerkships, 19% through research activities, and 9% during outpatient clerkships (Aagaard). If you are lucky, you will be assigned to an inpatient or outpatient clerkship in which you learn and excel, and through that process develop a relationship with your attending. If so, you may seek a letter of recommendation from your attending, or ask for advice with your career choices and application.

Many students won't find a mentor through randomly assigned clerkships and courses. One option is to choose a particular elective or clerkship for the chance to work with a specific attending. A discussion with other students, upperclassmen, or residents in your chosen field should help identify those faculty members who are known to be excellent advisors. If you're not able to work with these individuals directly in a clinical setting, you may be able to contact them for opportunities to work on research projects or publications. In some cases, potential advisors may be willing to meet with you outside of clinical activities.

It can be difficult to ask a faculty member for their help. Understandably, students often hesitate to burden faculty members who are already clearly very busy. However, while faculty members have many demands placed on their time, there are faculty at every medical school who find mentoring and advising students enjoyable and rewarding. While these individuals are sometimes recognized publicly for their work, it is more typical that they go about their work diligently but quietly. You should make every effort to identify these types of motivated, dedicated individuals.

In many departments, students applying to a particular field will be advised that they should start the process by setting up a meeting

- 4% were asked how they planned to rank the advisor's program.

Students reported varying degrees of discomfort with these queries. One respondent stated that "it felt very uncomfortable to talk to him about my own strengths and weaknesses and about which programs I preferred knowing that he would later be evaluating me in comparison with many other applicants and deciding whether or not to advocate for me to be accepted." Faced with such dilemmas, some students felt pressured to make misleading statements. Miller went on to raise some important questions. "What is safe for applicants to tell their advisors? Can applicants be sure that their advisors will put their interests first in these situations?" You need to consider how you would respond to these types of queries, since you may be placed in a similar situation.

Studies of medical students, advising, and the match are sparse, but our experience has demonstrated that having an effective advisor is invaluable. Advisors can help students with career decisions, evaluate potential residency programs, review *curriculum vitae* and personal statements, write letters of recommendation, and conduct mock interviews. Since faculty members often sit on residency selection committees, many can offer insight into the selection process that is not available elsewhere. By analyzing and comparing your credentials with those of students who have matched in previous years, advisors can identify ways in which you can strengthen your application and work with you to develop an overall strategy for success. Applicants should work hard to identify the right advisors, since these relationships can be invaluable in ensuring a successful match.

Adapted with permission from the column, "The Successful Match," available at www.studentdoctor.net.

Medical School Resources

If you are currently in medical school, you can and should take full advantage of the resources available at your institution. The scope and quality of these resources vary greatly, and you'll need to research to discover what resources are available. Many schools will offer meetings on the residency application process, with a particular emphasis on deadlines. These meetings typically review the institutional resources available to help students match successfully.

However, the support offered by medical schools varies greatly. In speaking with students and residents, we've heard of schools that cover the whole spectrum of relevant issues. In one school, no group meetings were offered, and no individual meetings with the Dean were arranged. Instead students were reminded of application deadlines by e-mail. "The information was handed down from the residents and upperclassmen, and you pretty much were expected to arrange for your own advisors."

with the clerkship director, program director or chairman of the department. The intent of this meeting is to state that you're planning to apply to the field. From there, the meeting can go in several directions. You can ask for recommendations on potential advisors. You can ask for recommendations on the application process, given the strength of your credentials. You can seek opportunities to work on a case report, to work on a research project, or to arrange a research elective.

Some schools lack residency programs in certain specialties. That poses obvious difficulties for students applying to that specialty. One option would be to seek advisors elsewhere, such as during an audition elective. In addition, local or national organizations may provide assistance. The Society of Academic Emergency Medicine (SAEM) has a virtual advisor program open to medical students at all institutions. Through this program, students can query experienced individuals about a variety of issues, including the EM residency application process.

Finding the right advisor can be difficult. Even with a formal system for assigning advisors, the advisor won't necessarily be the right fit for the student. If you encounter this problem, seek guidance from other faculty members. Even classmates, upperclassmen, and residents can serve as additional advisors, although they should not be your sole source of information. Few advisors have the answers to every question, and it is often to your advantage to have several opinions on certain issues. As one student told us, "My faculty advisor was very helpful when it came to writing my letter of recommendation, and giving me advice on where to apply. However, two of the upperclassmen who had matched into my field were very helpful when it came to my application itself. They told me which faculty members were the ones to work with, who might have papers that I could work on, and how I should be customizing my personal statement. I wish that I'd had the guts to approach the other faculty that I had worked with for their thoughts on the subject. I also really wish I had asked one of them to help me with a mock interview."

As you consider possible advisors, you should be aware of problems that can occur in the advisor-advisee relationship. Chief among these is the potential conflict of interest that can occur with a faculty member who advises a student and also serves on the residency selection committee at a program affiliated with the student's medical school. In a survey of 740 graduating medical students from 10 U.S. medical schools, Miller found that nearly half met with their advisors during or following the interview season (Miller). The results indicated that:

- 31.8% were encouraged to rank the advisor's program highly.
- 10.3% were asked which programs they planned to rank highly.

At another institution, every student meets with the Dean during the third year. The strengths and weaknesses of the candidacy are reviewed, particularly as it relates to the student's chances of matching into his or her chosen field. An annual workshop is offered, which pairs a group of students with a recently matched applicant in their chosen field who offers informal advice. At another school, a series of lectures reviews deadlines and the application process itself.

Some schools provide more extensive resources. Case Western University has a specific Office of Residency and Career Planning. The University of Chicago Pritzker School of Medicine offers an online residency planning guide, which provides specific recommendations from each of the departments. Some schools offer formal mentorship programs. Others offer workshops or assistance with writing a CV or personal statement. Some offer interview skills workshops or mock interviews.

It reflects well on a medical school when their students match well. Therefore, the administration is interested in providing the necessary resources to help their students achieve that goal. Interest expressed by the students can spur the development of further resources. You can also be involved in the creation of additional resources. You can approach the Dean's office. Would they be able to suggest a faculty member to give a lecture on interviewing skills? Would they be able to suggest several advisors to run a mock interview workshop? What about arranging for an annual workshop that takes place after Match Day and provides a forum for matched applicants to advise students applying to the same field? Can the student government approach the Office of Student Affairs about the feasibility of offering these types of programs?

Such programs can also be offered within individual departments. We've interviewed the founders of internal medicine or dermatology interest groups at individual schools. Such interest groups are ideal platforms from which to approach the department. Would the chairman or program director be able to suggest residents who could participate in an informal workshop with the students to offer their insights into the process? Is there a faculty member who would be interested in participating?

Timeline

To match successfully with the specialty and program of your choice, it is crucial that you remain well organized throughout the entire process. Of key importance is making sure critical deadlines are not missed. The following timeline outlines the process.

Application timeline	
Months	**Task**
February – April	Plan fourth year schedule Determine if you want to do any away electives; if so, obtain information from schools' websites
April – May	Attend any school meetings with dean regarding residency selection process Attend specialty-specific workshops (if offered by your school) and/or meet with specialty-specific advisor to develop application strategy Begin writing CV and personal statement Request letters of recommendation Request and complete applications for away electives Download ERAS applicant manual from www.aamc.org/students/eras Register for urology match (www.auanet.org/residents)
June – August	Research programs Develop a preliminary list of residency programs Identify each program's application deadline (aim to submit application as early as possible to maximize chances) Meet with advisors to discuss programs you wish to apply to Continue writing CV and personal statement Review CV and personal statement with advisor Review transcript for accuracy Request letters of recommendation Arrange for application photo MyERAS website opens on July 1 (earliest date on which you can begin preparing your ERAS application) Register with NRMP Register for San Francisco match (ophthalmology) in June
August – September	Request letters of recommendation, if not yet done Applicants may begin transmitting applications on September 1 Residency programs can begin downloading applications on September 1
October	Review MSPE Check that letters of recommendation have been submitted by writers and received by programs Participate in mock interviews with faculty advisors Schedule interviews (accept interview invitations quickly) Specialties participating in early matches may begin interviewing
November 1	National release date for Medical Student Performance Evaluation (MSPE), also known as Dean's letter
November – January	Interview (send thank-you notes following) Submit rank order list for San Francisco (ophthalmology) and urology matches (deadline usually in January) Early Match results announced in January

Application timeline	
January – February	Complete last interviews Review rank order list with advisor Submit rank order list to NRMP
March	Match day usually in mid-March Applicants notified of their status (matched vs. unmatched) three days before Match Day Scramble takes place two days before Match Day for unmatched applicants

Researching programs

Once you determine your specialty choice, you can consider individual residency programs. Applicants utilize a variety of resources to research individual programs:

- **American Medical Association—Fellowship and Residency Electronic Interactive Database Access (AMA-FREIDA)**

  AMA-FREIDA has been a principal source of residency program information for many years. Applicants can access this directory at www.ama-assn.org at no charge (select med school and residency tab). Information contained in the directory comes directly from residency programs. Every year, programs are surveyed by the AMA and AAMC and the data is loaded onto FREIDA.

  Through FREIDA, applicants can identify the program director and obtain contact information for both the director and coordinator. Generally, applicants are asked to contact the program coordinator for additional information. A link to the program's website is generally included. Applicants may also learn about a program's size, primary teaching sites, interview period, earliest and latest dates for submitting applications, work and call schedules, educational conferences and lectures, employment policies/benefits, compensation and leave, and medical benefits.

Did you know ...

The program director is a M.D. or D.O. physician who is accountable for all aspects of the residency program. As you might expect, overseeing a residency program is labor intensive and requires a team approach. No team member is more valuable than the program coordinator, a member of the residency program staff who works closely with the program director. In fact, the Accreditation Council for Graduate Medical Education has required that each residency program have a program coordinator. The program coordinator is typically a non-physician, administrative staff member. He or she is heavily involved in all aspects of resident recruitment. Coordinators handle requests for information from applicants, download applications from ERAS, and schedule candidates for interviews. On the interview day, coordinators greet applicants, provide them with informational materials, get candidates to their interviews, and arrange for lunch and transportation. Following interviews, coordinators are available to answer candidate questions, provide additional information, and arrange for follow-up visits. In February, coordinators submit the program's rank order list to the NRMP.

- **Graduate Medical Education Directory**

    Known as the "Green Book" because of the color of its cover, this resource is published annually by the American Medical Association. It is a comprehensive listing of accredited programs in each specialty.

- **Specialty organizations**

    Specialty organizations often have a section on their websites for medical students. In some cases, links to residency programs are included.

- **Printed brochures**

    Before the internet age, programs routinely printed brochures with program information. With the advent of the web, fewer programs are producing brochures. This information has now been moved to program and departmental websites. Some programs have made brochures available online.

- **Residency program websites**

    AMA-FREIDA often contains links to program websites. However, these links are not always functional. In a 2004 study of general surgery residency program websites, only 71% of programs listed in FREIDA had viable links (Reilly). When links are nonfunctional, program websites can still be found through search engines. Applicants have found these websites to be useful. In a survey of applicants who were invited for interviews at the Oregon Health and Science University internal medicine residency program, 79.6% of respondents found these sites helpful in deciding where to apply, while 68.5% found the sites useful in deciding where to interview (Embi). As you peruse websites, learn about how the program processes applications. Programs typically make clear what they consider to be a complete application and the steps involved in securing an interview.

- **Accreditation Council for Graduate Medical Education (ACGME)**

    At the ACGME website, www.acgme.org, applicants can determine the accreditation status of residency programs, including the date of the most recent site visit.

- **Advisors/colleagues**

    Faculty and resident advisors as well as colleagues can be a valuable source of information about residency programs. Advisors can provide insider information not readily available elsewhere.

Did you know ...

During the 1998 match season, applicants who were invited for an interview to the University of Pennsylvania internal medicine residency program were surveyed. While 92% claimed to have access to the internet, only 77% of respondents reported looking at the program's home page (Bellini).

Using these resources, develop a list of residency programs that are of interest. Base your list on the factors that are most important to you. Consider reputation, competitiveness of the program, geographic location, type of hospital (university affiliated, community), program emphasis (academic), setting (urban, rural, suburban), future plans (desire to pursue fellowship training), and your family's needs, in addition to a host of other factors.

Review your list of residency programs with your advisor. Ask if your list is realistic. While you shouldn't hesitate to apply to a program that would be considered a long shot, there should be a sufficient number of programs on your list which are within reach. Your advisor can estimate your chances of matching with programs on your list, taking into account the competitiveness of the specialty, the competitiveness of the programs on your list, and your academic qualifications and non-academic credentials.

Did you know ...

As you research programs, take note of whether the program is a categorical or advanced program. In categorical programs, residents complete their first year, or internship, as part of the training program. After completing your internship, you remain there to finish your training. Contrast this with advanced programs in which trainees are required to arrange for a preliminary or transitional year separately (see below). In other words, advanced programs do not include an internship year.

Did you know ...

Some specialties require applicants to do a preliminary year in internal medicine or surgery. Following this preliminary year, applicants then begin training in their chosen specialty. You must apply separately for preliminary year training.

Did you know ...

Applicants who are unsure of specialty choice may elect to do a transitional year. During the transitional year, the trainee rotates through various specialties, including internal medicine, surgery, pediatrics, and emergency medicine. Of note, some specialties allow their trainees to complete a transitional year in lieu of a preliminary year. For example, prior to starting dermatology residency, trainees can complete either a transitional or a preliminary year.

Tip # 4

To remain organized, we recommend that you start a filing system. Keep a file for each residency program with program information, application requirements, deadlines, and copies of all correspondence and communication.

The Basics: Common Sense Rules

> Why would an applicant approach an attending for a letter of recommendation, and then say "By the way, the deadline is next week." Why would a student ask to work on a case report, take from the attending the case details, photos, and preliminary literature on the topic, and then never turn in an actual case report? Why would an applicant interview at a program and not send a thank-you letter?

One would think that the actions in the box would be obvious mistakes. *We* would think that these would be obvious mistakes. And yet...we can quote from actual experience and anecdotes from colleagues, each of these mistakes made by multiple applicants. A student asking for a LOR and then not providing the attending any time to work on it. Was the applicant thoughtless, or desperate? Never turning in a final product? Was the applicant paralyzed by perfectionism? In the case of thank you letters, only 39% of applicants in one study sent a thank you letter to every program with which they interviewed. Did they believe it wasn't worth the hassle because the program wasn't going to be high on their list anyway?

We can only guess and try to keep further applicants from making the same mistakes. Some of these mistakes may seem like violations of common sense, and we fully agree. We've included rules that start with "Don't lie," words one should never have to say to future physicians. However, we quote from multiple studies that indicate that dishonesty in the residency application process occurs, and more often than you would think. In a review of 134 applications to the emergency medicine residency program at Washington University, of the 14 applicants claiming AOA membership, five claims were found to be inaccurate (Roellig). In the same study, of the 15 applicants claiming advanced degrees, four claims were inaccurate.

We've included these obvious rules because we see them every year, and the literature supports the fact that they occur.

Pay attention to the rules that only an insider would know well. Pay equal attention to the rules that are so obvious that they may be overlooked.

Chapter 4

Selection Process

In order to plan the optimal strategy and position your application for maximum impact, you need to first understand the selection process. Strategizing for a successful match hinges on the answers to these three questions:

- Who chooses the residents?
- What do they care about?
- How can you convince them that you would be the right resident for their program?

Who chooses the residents?

This first question really should be broken down further.

- Who selects the applicants to interview?
- Who ranks the applicants?

The two processes are markedly different, and the criteria for interview selection and candidate ranking are markedly different as well.

Who selects the applicants to interview? The committee may be composed of one individual—the program director, the chairman, a designated faculty member, or another designee. In this case, one individual has the power to choose all of the applicants that will be asked to interview. Their criteria become all-important if you have any hope of making it past the screening process.

Alternately, the committee may be composed of several individuals. If so, the committee members decide how to review applications, and this process varies. In some cases, the committee members divide up the applications randomly. In this case, again, only one individual will see your application, and their criteria become all important. In other cases, the committee reviews applications jointly, and discusses the applicants as a group.

What criteria do these decision makers utilize?

In the process of reviewing hundreds of applications, screening criteria are used frequently. It is a daunting task to review over 400 applications in order to choose 30 candidates to interview, as is the case at some programs. In a sea of qualified applicants, it's difficult to choose a small fraction to interview.

Personal knowledge of an applicant's skills and strengths can trump numbers alone. In highly competitive programs, applicants who are personally known to the program and its faculty have an advantage from that standpoint alone. The sole faculty member deciding whom to interview, out of hundreds of excellent applicants, will naturally give preference to a student she personally knows and respects. In fact, excellent performance on an audition elective at the program is frequently mentioned as an important resident selection criterion. Personal knowledge may also come in the form of a strong letter of recommendation from a program's own faculty member. A strong letter of recommendation from a faculty member outside the program, but well-known to the members of the selection committee, can also be very persuasive.

However, when personal knowledge of an applicant is not available, objective criteria, of necessity, take on more importance. Particularly when screening large numbers of applications, objective data is more easily mined. As a broad generalization, objective data is typically more important when making decisions on which applicants to interview. Subjective criteria take on more importance when making decisions on how to rank applicants.

By objective data, we mean factors that are easy to determine and quantify, such as grades in the specialty rotation, USMLE scores, clerkship grades, number of honors grades, and AOA status. Although grades in rotations themselves are based on a combination of objective and subjective factors, the grade itself is easily compared.

- In 2000, researchers surveyed program directors in internal medicine to determine which factors were most important in deciding whom to interview and how to rank applicants (Adams). Of 407 program directors, data was received from 81.5%. When deciding whom to interview, 94% of program directors found USMLE scores to be highly or moderately useful for making interview decisions. 85% of program directors found the medical school transcript to be highly or moderately useful for interview decisions.

  However, when it came to ranking decisions, the interview was found most useful. 96% of respondents found the interview to be highly or moderately useful.

- In 2006, a survey of 77 radiology residency program directors was performed to determine the criteria that programs use to select their residents (Otero). Directors ranked the importance of ten criteria in selecting applicants to interview. The highest ranked factor was USMLE score, followed in order by the Dean's letter, class rank, and letters of recommendation.

- In 2005, the Association of Program Directors in Radiology (APDR) surveyed program directors, and 89 program directors responded to the survey. The two most important criteria used by program directors when deciding whom to interview were the USMLE Step 1 score and class rank (www.apdr.org).

  The survey also revealed that 17% of programs stated that the USMLE Step 1 score was not important at all for ranking applicants following an interview.

- In 1995, researchers surveyed 205 obstetrics and gynecology program directors to determine which factors were most important when deciding whom to interview and when deciding how to rank applicants. The medical school transcript, Dean's letter, and USMLE scores ranked highest when making decisions about whom to interview. Each of these provides objective data that can be easily compared. In distinction, the interview, a highly subjective factor, was considered most important for ranking decisions (Taylor).

- In 2002, Dr. Bernstein and colleagues surveyed 109 program directors of orthopedic surgery residency programs (Bernstein). The study found that once invited for an interview, 22% of programs place candidates on equal footing, with ranking decisions based solely on interview performance.

USMLE Scores

Students ask us all the time about the importance of the USMLE score, and whether they have what it takes to get into a certain field. USMLE scores do play an important role in some programs when deciding whom to interview. Particularly for competitive programs, when the typical applicant is scoring in the 230s and above, the applicant with a 210 stands out. Dr. Ellis, the program director of the dermatology program at the University of Michigan, wrote that "last year, more than 100 of our applicants had achieved the top percentile on the United States Medical Licensing Examination" (Kia).

- The Office of Residency and Career Planning of the Case School of Medicine states: "Board results are most important for the very competitive specialties…A number of the programs set a threshold Step I score level that must be achieved in order to receive an invitation for an interview, such as the national mean of about 220 or even one standard deviation above the mean. The same is true for some of the most outstanding and sought-after residency programs in less competitive specialties…For specialties which have become more 'popular' recently, board scores pose a problem only when they are significantly below the mean." (http://casemed.case.edu/CareerPlan/USMLE%20&%20The%20Matches.htm)

- Dr. Oldham, the program director at the University of Texas Medical School at Houston Department of Diagnostic and Interventional Imaging, gives this information on the process: "The ERAS applications are first viewed by the Program Coordinator who filters out those I should read from the many I don't need to read. Ms. Roberts looks at several things in each ERAS application—the dreaded USMLE Step 1 score and grades from the medical school transcript. We set the minimum USMLE Step 1 score each year as the main filter for which applications move on to my computer and which do not. This year, the minimum was 225" (http://www.uth.tmc.edu/med/administration/student/ms4/2003CCC.htm).

- The website for the radiology program at the University of California at San Francisco (UCSF) states: "We review each application as a whole, and we do not have a threshold value for USMLE scores. However, in recent years, most of our interviewees have had three-digit scores of 240 or higher on Step 1. The small number of our interviewees with Step 1 scores between 200 and 239 have had offsetting factors such as a combination of top clinical grades at a competitive medical school and extraordinary research experience and academic promise" (http://www.radiology.ucsf.edu/residents/apps).

Clerkship grades

Clerkship grades are also a major factor in the residency selection process. In 1999 Wagoner and Suriano published the results of a survey of approximately 800 program directors (Wagoner). These program directors represented 14 specialties and were surveyed about the importance of various academic criteria in the selection of residents. Grades in required clerkships were found to be the most important academic criteria used to select residents.

Many medical students underestimate the importance of clerkship grades. In fact, 44% of students surveyed at the University of Colorado, University of Utah, and Vanderbilt University felt that these grades were moderately, mildly, or not important at all (Brandenburg).

Particularly important is the number of honors clerkship grades earned. In Wagoner's survey, the total number of honors clerkship grades was one of the three most important factors in considering a candidate. Most students don't realize this; only 14.7% of students rated the number of honors grades as extremely important.

Clerkship grades are another major determinant of class rank. The most competitive specialties rate class rank among the three most important selection criteria. Here again, a significant difference was noted between program directors and students regarding its importance. Surprisingly, 49.3% of students felt that class rank was mildly important or not important at all.

AOA status

For highly competitive specialties, applicants have sometimes been told that programs will use AOA membership as a filter when reviewing applications. "Don't even bother applying unless you're AOA." While this practice may hold true at some individual programs, it is not in widespread use. AOA membership is certainly valued, and in highly competitive specialties a significant percentage of applicants who match are members of AOA. The NRMP reports that 30.5% of U.S. seniors who matched to orthopedic surgery in 2007 were members of AOA. However, it is not a requirement. A survey of orthopedic surgery residency program directors in 2002 found that only 1% of program directors agreed with the statement that "only applicants that are AOA are offered an interview." Thirty percent of program directors evaluate candidates regardless of their AOA status (Bernstein).

Other criteria

Criteria such as USMLE thresholds, AOA status, or class rank would typically be used by the most competitive specialties and programs to winnow down their applicant pool. Even in these types of programs, though, some decision makers will choose to look more thoroughly at an application, even during the initial screening process. They may give weight to a variety of different factors, such as the personal statement or letters of recommendation indicating leadership qualities or community involvement. As we stated earlier, personal knowledge of an applicant's skills and strengths can also be a powerful factor for those who decide whom to interview.

We emphasize that these types of objective criteria may not be in standard use by less competitive specialties or programs. The personal statement takes on more importance for family practice residency program directors, for example. At the website for the University of Washington Family Medicine residency program: The "personal statement is the primary component that will be used to select applicants who are invited for an interview. Please write a careful and thoughtful document." A 1993 study of family practice residency program directors showed that the personal statement ranked second only to the Dean's letter for making decisions about whom to interview (Taylor). With regard to the ranking of applicants, it was third in importance, following only the interview and the Dean's letter.

How can you determine if you have the minimum requirements to be selected to interview?

Chapter 2, on specialty-specific information, provides some concrete numbers to review, including average USMLE scores and the percentage of applicants below a threshold who still matched into the specialty. The NRMP data from 2007 indicated that for applicants to anesthesiology, the mean USMLE Step 1 score was 220. Of the applicants with Step 1 scores below 200, 142 of 184 matched. Of U.S. seniors who matched, 7.5% were members of AOA. Of 214 applicants reporting no prior research experience, 200 matched. Such concrete numbers can provide perspective on the strength of your own application (www.nrmp.org).

A review of program websites may also provide very useful and specific information. Even within a competitive specialty, some programs are far more competitive than others, and criteria such as USMLE thresholds or AOA status may vary greatly. These criteria may not matter at all for less competitive specialties.

Probably the most important advice on this subject will come from your residency advisor. Advisors who participate in the residency selection process have a well-informed sense of the qualifications of other applicants, and how you compare with your competition. Therefore, an advisor who is a program chairman, a residency program director, or a faculty member of the residency selection committee can provide valuable insight into your chances. Other advice may come from the Dean's office, residents in the specialty, or recently matched students or upperclassmen who have researched the issue.

However, selecting applicants to interview is a very different process from ranking those who interview. In speaking with students and reviewing the discussion forums, we don't think enough students grasp this critical point. Great USMLE scores may get you in the door, but when it comes to ranking, they often don't play as much of a role. From the UCSF Department of Radiology: "Once an applicant is selected for an interview, USMLE scores have little bearing on the final rank" (http://radiology.ucsf.edu/residents/apps).

Who is actually ranking the applicants?

In 2006, researchers surveyed 145 radiology residency program directors about the process for ranking candidates (Otero). A total of 77 directors responded to the survey. In 88.1% of the programs, all members of the interviewing body vote in the ranking of candidates. Of interest, in 76.5% of programs, residents and fellows serve as interviewers. While the interviewing body is responsible for making the final ranking in 62.9% of the programs, the program director has the final word in 33.8%.

Some programs have published information about their own selection process.

- At the general surgery residency program at the Medical University of South Carolina, Brothers wrote that "...all surgical faculty are given equal input, with individual members providing insight into applicants whom they interviewed" (Brothers).

- Dr. Cruz, the chairman of the department of dermatology at the University of Texas Southwestern Medical Center (UTSW), stated "Because we are committed to a democratic process, each faculty member who participates in interviews (residents as well as the chief resident) has an equal opportunity to influence the match ranking...During a dedicated meeting, each applicant is discussed and her or his ranking is refined by consensus" (Cruz).

- The website for the department of radiology at UCSF states that "the selection committee meets in late January...we formulate our rank order list based on consensus."

- The department of anesthesiology at the University of Pittsburgh states that their selection committee meets as a group, discusses each applicant, and then ranks the applicant. The scores are then averaged to yield a final score which is used to form the program's rank list (Metro).

- Creation of the rank list for the University of Washington otolaryngology residency program "involves all members of the residency selection committee. Each member will develop his or her own rank list... A meeting of the residency selection committee will be held in February to develop a consensus rank order and which candidates will not be ranked. The program director and Chair may review and revise the final list if needed" (http://depts.washington.edu/otoweb/training/residency/policies/index.shtml).

What do these decision makers care about?

The short answer to this question is that it varies from program to program, and from individual to individual. In some programs, the decision makers have made an effort to provide objective grading of subjective criteria. In these programs, deciding criteria are identified, and a standard scoring system is used to grade the applicant on each criteria.

In other programs, the process of ranking applicants can be very subjective. In the study by Otero cited above, 15 directors stated that the "fit" of the candidates and a "gut feeling" were the most important criteria for admission decisions. Dr. Moore, chair and program director at the University of California-Davis department of anesthesiology, feels that an applicant's performance during the interview "is the deal breaker/maker."

Remember that every candidate invited to interview has already met the standards for acceptance. At this stage subjective measures of personal characteristics become more important. Studies have shown that behavioral and noncognitive skills have significant value in predicting resident performance, while measures such as USMLE scores may be poorly predictive of clinical performance (Brothers, Boyse, Bell). Therefore, at this stage of residency selection, indicators of noncognitive skills become very important. The Office of Residency and Career Planning at the Case School of Medicine states: "Remember it is performance on the clinical services reflected by your grades and, above all, by the evaluation comments that program directors consider most important in ranking their applicants. These parameters are considered to be the best predictors of how well an applicant will do as a resident.... the highest board scores will not guarantee a position in a program if the comments from your attendings are negative..." (http://casemed.case.edu/CareerPlan/USMLE%20&%20The%20Matches.htm).

The earlier studies we cited emphasized the importance of the interview in ranking decisions. A number of additional published studies have surveyed decision makers about the importance of criteria in the residency selection process. Although these additional surveys don't make the distinction between selecting applicants to interview and ranking applicants, they do provide additional insight into the criteria that decision makers value.

- Which criteria are most important to program directors when considering a candidate? A survey of 800 program directors in 14 specialties, as cited earlier, attempted to answer this question (Wagoner). The responses were separated into specialties that were very competitive, moderately competitive, or mildly competitive, based on fill rates of the residency programs. In this study, respondents were not asked to separate out criteria for interviewing versus ranking. The most competitive specialties ranked grades in required clerkships, total number of honors grades, and class rank as the three most important factors in considering a candidate. These criteria were not to the exclusion of other criteria; these specialties, predictably, also placed great importance on membership in AOA and scores on USMLE Step 1.

- As described earlier, a survey of 109 program directors of orthopedic surgery residency programs was published in 2002. Directors were asked about the importance of 26 residency selection criteria. Ranked highest was a rotation at the director's institution. Next was USMLE Step 1 score, followed by rank in medical school and formality/politeness at interview (Bernstein).

- As we alluded to earlier, interview performance is the one criterion that becomes magnified in importance at this stage of the process (ranking). The interview is of such importance that one study found that one third of internal medicine residency applicants were actually ranked less favorably following an interview (Gong). In a 2002 survey of orthopedic surgery residency program directors, researchers found that once invited for an interview, 22% of programs place candidates on equal footing, with ranking decisions based solely on interview performance (Bernstein). A survey of 361 U.S. family practice residency program directors found that the interview was the most important element of the resident selection process (Galazka). One study performed at the Children's Hospital of Pennsylvania pediatrics residency program, a highly competitive program, offered insight into the importance of the interview at their program (Swanson). The authors wrote that "interview scores were the most important variable for candidate ranking on the NRMP list."

What are the qualities that programs seek in a resident and are therefore searching for in the application components and interview?

Further chapters delineate these qualities more thoroughly, but in short, the qualities that make for an outstanding clinician are the same as those that make for an outstanding resident. Programs look for evidence that a student not only possesses high levels of intelligence, but has a very strong work ethic, is compassionate, is enthusiastic about their chosen field, and is able to handle an intense workload. Beyond that, the criteria for each program and for each individual decision maker at that program will vary.

Furthermore, the evidence required to demonstrate those criteria will vary for each decision maker. For example, what evidence best demonstrates a strong work ethic? Is it clinical grades, or letters of recommendation? What evidence best demonstrates high levels of intelligence? Is it USMLE scores, or overall grades in clerkships?

Your research should begin with a review of the individual program websites. These may provide insight into the program's goals and criteria for residency selection.

- The website for the radiology program at UCSF states that "One of our primary goals is to train academic radiologists, especially clinician-scientists...Most of our interviewees have had research experience...We should emphasize that because ours is a clinically rigorous program, we prefer applicants who have shined on the wards as well as in the laboratory" (http://radiology.ucsf.edu/residents/apps).

- Dr. Flemming, program director of the Penn State Hershey radiology program, states, "As for the qualities we seek, most of you will have demonstrated more than adequately, your academic abilities with success in exams, good board scores...Beyond academics, there are two important qualities we expect. These are creative thinking and character. Radiology is divorcing itself from the descriptive nature of the art. It is becoming one in which it is important to analyze, develop an opinion, and express this thought process to our other clinical colleagues. It is imperative that you possess the ability to communicate and to understand your role as a communicator...Character is equally important in our resident selection process. We expect trainees to understand their professional responsibility as a physician radiologist, their pivotal role in patient care, and their commitment to fulfill these expectations. It is clear then that we not only look at the merit of your application, but the interview process is all-important" (http://www.pennstatehershey.org/web/radiology/education/residency).

• The website for the psychiatry department at the Stony Brook University Hospital states that applicants should have "high intelligence, excellence in both written and verbal self-expression, superior ability to understand both verbal and non-verbal communications from others, exceptional curiosity about the human mind and human behavior, and psychological mindedness." (http://www.hsc.stonybrook.edu/som/psychiatry/selection_procecess.cfm) The website provides further information on the members of the selection committee, interview questions, and a copy of the residency applicant rating form used by evaluators.

• The department of anesthesiology at the University of Pittsburgh outlines the criteria that interviewers use to rank the applicants, which include such diverse criteria as "grades and honors," "knowledge of Pitt program," "quality of answers," "quality of questions," "enthusiasm, energy, liveliness" and "articulateness, communication skills" (Metro).

After sitting through years of resident selection committee meetings, we can state that the impact of selection factors varies markedly from faculty member to faculty member. Beliefs about which types of evidence prove certain traits also vary markedly. Meetings of the residency selection committee can be heated, and arguments about the importance of the different selection factors are common. What best predicts how well a candidate will perform as a resident? Our arguments during the ranking process can be as heated as any discussion forum on the topic.

The following paraphrased comments provide an insider's look at a residency selection committee meeting:

"Her USMLE score is the lowest score of all the students we've interviewed this year." "Who cares? Her USMLE score is high enough that we don't have to worry about her passing the boards. I don't care about the numbers, as long as the enthusiasm and work ethic is there."
"That letter of recommendation was lukewarm, and I consider that a red flag." "But are you taking that comment out of context? The evaluations from his senior electives were outstanding."
"That interview was great, but the letter of rec from Dr. Grant wasn't exactly gushing. Sylvia, don't you know him? Can you e-mail him to find out more?"
"You all know that work ethic is my number one priority, and the fact that this student couldn't even write a case report after two derm electives is a bad sign." "I know that everyone else we've interviewed today has been published, but maybe you need to cut him some slack. Maybe at their institution, there just aren't many opportunities to work on case reports." "That doesn't mean that much to me, because there are opportunities everywhere if you try hard enough."
"Based on that interview, I just don't think he'd fit in well here." "I know what you mean, but I think you're jumping to conclusions. Take a look at the letter from Dr __. He worked with him for one month, and that's a much more meaningful impression than one interview." "After that interview, I don't think any letter is going to convince me."
"Did you see what the attending on his Internal Medicine rotation wrote about him? That's very concerning." "Maybe there were personality issues? I certainly didn't see that repeated anywhere else, so I think we need to take that into account."
"That personal statement, to me, seems to emphasize lifestyle factors." "I certainly didn't see it in that light."

In the following chapters, we delve more deeply into these questions. What do the individuals making the decisions care about? What are the qualities that they seek in a resident? More importantly, how can you demonstrate that you embody those qualities? *How can you convince them that you would be the right resident for their program?* The remainder of this book is devoted to maximizing the impact of your application. Each component of your application can be created, modified, or influenced in order to significantly strengthen your overall candidacy. We devote the following pages to showing you, in detail, exactly how to do so.

Chapter 5

The Right Fit

In this chapter we focus on the final question of the application process:

How can you convince the decision makers that you would be the right resident for their program?

In order to convince those making the decisions, you need to strategize, and you need to start early. Strategic planning begins and ends with outstanding patient care. If you want to match at the residency program of your choice, then the first step is to learn how to be an outstanding clinician. Your ultimate message for any residency program is that you will be an outstanding physician, and that you would make an outstanding house officer. Our advice is to start by being the absolutely best clinician. You came to medical school to be a doctor. Learn how to be the best.

Excellence in patient care translates to better clinical evaluations and stronger letters of recommendation. These translate to a stronger transcript, a more positive Dean's letter, a higher class rank, and AOA candidacy. Evidence of outstanding patient care in an audition elective may even translate to a match at that program.

How do you excel at patient care? The process starts with the recognition that the skills needed to excel in clinical rotations are very different from those required for the basic science years. Our companion book, *250 Biggest Mistakes 3rd Year Medical Students Make and How to Avoid Them,* lays out in full detail how to perform at an outstanding level in the clinics and on the wards. Chapter 10 of this book, "The Audition Elective," provides further information on how to excel during your clinical experiences.

We outline the strategizing that continues throughout the application process. Your ultimate goal is to convince those making the decisions that you would be the right resident for their program. In order to do so, you need to confirm that you would be the right fit for their program.

"Fit" is one of those concepts that students don't realize is such an important criterion. In a survey of radiology residency program directors, 15 directors stated that the "fit" of the candidates in the program along with a "gut feeling" were the most important criteria for deciding admission (Otero). In another survey, program directors wrote that they sought to find applicants who were "people like us" (Villanueva).

Other residency programs use the term "compatibility with the program." In a survey of physical medicine and rehabilitation program directors, DeLisa found that compatibility with the program was one of the three most important candidate traits, along with the ability to articulate thoughts and work with others (DeLisa). In yet another study, program directors in 14 different specialties were asked to rank the importance of six personal and professional characteristics (Wagoner). Compatibility with the program was highest. This was followed by commitment to hard work, fund of knowledge, empathy and compassion, and communication skills.

What are program directors looking for when they search for applicants with the right fit for their program? "Fit" can refer to qualities of the applicant that the faculty feel are essential to success in their program. In one study done by faculty in the department of radiology at the Baylor College of Medicine, the five qualities "deemed most appropriate for training radiologists" at Baylor were interpersonal skills, recognition of limits, curiosity, conscientiousness, and confidence level (Lamke).

"Fit" can also refer to qualities of the applicant that would help the program reach its goals. Some programs are committed to training future clinician-educators. Students with a stated interest and experience in areas of teaching and education, such as through their work or volunteer experience, would more convincingly demonstrate their fit with the program.

When strategizing for your application, you should plan to utilize techniques that will confirm your fit with a program. This begins with thorough research to determine the traits valued by the specialty. This is followed by thorough research of individual programs to determine valued traits and departmental goals. Although you've already performed a thorough self-evaluation in the process of preparing your application, you need to repeat this step. What strengths do you exhibit that are highly valued by your specialty and targeted programs? At this point, you can formulate a compelling message as to why you would be the right resident for the program. Of course, your message doesn't mean anything without evidence to back it up. You must locate and present the evidence that confirms your fit with a program in the most compelling fashion possible.

Rule # 1   Research the specialty: What traits are valued by the specialty?

What traits are necessary to excel in your chosen field? What traits are valued by the members of the specialty? The following chart shows some of the essential attributes that the future resident in anesthesiology, emergency medicine, and radiology must possess.

Essential skills and personal qualities for the future resident in selected specialties	
Anesthesiology	Good manual dexterity Skillful at procedures Meticulous Ability to remain calm during stressful situations Ability to make quick decisions Warm and caring
Emergency medicine	Good manual dexterity Ability to work with and manage a team Compassionate Ability to establish rapport quickly with variety of people Ability to multitask Strength to make tough decisions Ability to make quick decisions Prioritizes well Ability to remain calm during stressful situations Recognizes one's own limits and is not afraid of seeking help
Radiology	Ability to interact effectively with a wide variety of clinicians and patients Good written and spoken communication skills Intellectual curiosity Willingness to seek help when necessary Meticulous Thorough Good problem-solving and decision-making skills

By speaking with specialists in the field and researching specialty-specific websites, you can generate a similar list for your chosen specialty. Analyze your list. Which qualities do you share, and how have you demonstrated those qualities?

Rule # 2   Research the individual programs.

By virtue of training many residents over the years, directors of residency programs have identified qualities they believe are essential to a resident's performance at their institution. Your application should emphasize the fact that you embody the traits that the residency program seeks in a resident.

Following is a partial list of personal qualities that are valued by residency programs (also included in Chapter 12: Before the Interview). In each section of this book, we've reviewed these traits, and how to successfully emphasize them. These traits form the foundation of how well you would fit with a residency program.

Personal qualities valued by residency programs

Ability to work with a team	Willingness to admit error	Responsibility
Ability to solve problems	Perseverance	Poise
Ability to manage stress	Initiative	Positive attitude
Enthusiasm	Intelligence	Reliability
Energy	Maturity	Honesty
Flexibility	Motivation	Dedication
Effective time management	Communication skills	Compassion
Efficient problem-solving	Conscientiousness	Curiosity
Confidence without	Listening skills	Determination
arrogance	Professional competence	Work ethic
Recognition of limits		Sense of humor
		High values

All programs value these personal qualities, and your application in its entirety should project them. Some programs will further delineate qualities they find most valuable in a resident. For example, the department of orthopedic surgery at Duke University states that "residents are selected for interview on the basis of preparedness, ability, aptitude, academic credentials, communication skills, and personal qualities such as motivation and integrity...Important intangibles which are fundamental to the selection process include leadership, work ethic, communication skills, and enthusiasm."
(http://ortho.surgery.duke.edu/modules/div_ortho_rsdncy/index.php?id=5)

For many programs, valued qualities won't be that clearly defined. You will need to determine any distinguishing characteristics that are not clearly stated. For example, a program centered in a multi-ethnic community serves a diverse population. Obviously, this program would value individuals with experience or an interest in serving a diverse population. Excellent communication skills and the ability to handle added obstacles in this type of population are critical. Characteristics of a program's patient population may be described on the program's websites or in informational brochures. You may be able to determine the traits most valued by the program based on its features and the areas where the program's resources are concentrated.

Unique features of selected residency programs

Cooper University Hospital Internal Medicine Residency
Among the unique features of this program is its "Resident as Teacher Curriculum." This curriculum "covers a range of topics, including team leadership, bedside teaching, leading effective rounds, and giving and receiving feedback...Resident-led work rounds are frequently observed by medical educators, after which residents are provided with brief and focused feedback designed to foster leadership and management skills that would otherwise not be addressed in any formal curriculum" (http://www.cooperhealth.org/content/)

Mt. Sinai Hospital Pediatrics Residency
The program encourages third year residents to do an "elective month as a rotation in a Third World country. This can be an opportunity for residents to experience providing medical care in a community different from any they have previously experienced" (http://sinai.org/education/pediatric/unique_features.asp).

East Carolina General Surgery Residency
"One year of the residency is devoted to research. The research year sharpens technical skills, provides rigorous training in research methodology, ensures an academically competitive curriculum vitae, fosters national research networking opportunities, and provides time for reflection and creativity. In cooperation with the ECU School of Business we have implemented a program to allow the optional use of the surgery research year to obtain the MBA degree" (http://www.ecu.edu/surgery/residency.cfm).

Another component of fit is dependent on the goals of the department. For example, if the program is committed to producing future clinician-educators, would you be the ideal candidate to help them reach their goal? If the program is committed to an understanding of the mind-body dynamic in treating medical illness, would your strengths and achievements suggest that you could help the program attain this goal? Other goals may include the training of future leaders in the specialty, enhancement of physician-patient communication, enhancement of care for rural populations, or enhancing the practice of evidence-based medicine, among a host of other goals. These goals may be reflected in the program's mission statement, may be described in their informational materials, or may be voiced by their faculty.

Rule # 3   Evaluate your experiences in order to emphasize your unique, individual qualities.

In a sea of extremely well-qualified applicants, how do you distinguish yourself? You can't rely on your class rank and great USMLE scores, because for competitive programs, those alone won't set you apart and won't make application reviewers sit up and take notice. You need to emphasize your individual strengths. Ideally, you will emphasize to residency selection committee members that you embody all the traits that they are seeking in a resident.

One of the first steps in the application process is an analysis of your career to date. What have you accomplished? What have your attendings written about you in your formal evaluations? What comments have residents or attendings made about your performance on rotations? (For example, "highly inquisitive" "very compassionate" "excellent teacher to junior students" "dedicated" "meticulous.") What have you been recognized for by your attendings? By your peers? What have you studied? Where have you worked? What did you bring to your work? What did you accomplish at work? Where have you volunteered? What did you learn about yourself from your volunteer experience? What extracurricular activities have you been involved in? What leadership positions have you held? What activities do you participate in outside of medicine?

At the end of this analysis, you need to answer this question: What types of qualities do these activities highlight? Rules 1 and 2 delineate some of the qualities valued by specialties and programs. Use these lists as a springboard for performing your self-evaluation.

Corollary to this rule

The corollary to this rule is just as important. You can ask yourself, "What I am known for?" However, you also need to ask yourself, "What do I wish to be known for?"

What do you envision as the qualities of the ideal physician? What would you like others to say about you as an individual and as a physician? The processes of self-evaluation and striving for improvement should always remain a priority.

Rule # 4   Formulate your message. Make sure that each component of your application reinforces this message.

"We have so many good applicants this year. Tell me why we should accept you."

The entire residency application process boils down to this one question. And yet, when we've asked this question in interviews, we've received so many truly unconvincing answers:

- "I think you'll find that I'm a real team player."

- "I realize that everyone today has great scores, or they wouldn't have been invited to interview. I think you should accept me because I have a very strong work ethic, and I've always brought 100% to whatever I do."

- "I'm sure it must be very difficult for you to decide, because everyone going into derm is so strong. I'm a very hard worker, and I would do whatever is needed to be done."

- "I'm very enthusiastic, and I would get along very well with the other residents."

- "I'm a very fun person to be with, and I would bring that to the program."

- "Well, you're right, you have excellent applicants. I'm sure everyone has great credentials. You'll find that I'm a real people person, and I work well with my colleagues no matter where I am."

- "I'm a very hard worker, and you'll find that I would come to work every day on time, ready to get the work done."

- "I'm a real team player."

Are some of these sounding pretty good to you? Decent answers, the kind you yourself might give? Sorry, but no. These answers could be given by just about any applicant, and they tell us nothing about you as an individual. They provide no evidence. They don't tell us *why* you would be an ideal fit for our program. They don't tell us specifically what you as an individual could bring to our program.

In our dermatology residency program, we have well over 100 applicants for each residency position. We're not thinking about what we can do for each individual applicant. Our focus is on the program. How well will this applicant match the goals of our program? How well will they fit with our program? What can this applicant bring to the specialty? Certain baseline qualities are assumed. To have gotten this far in your career, you are assumed to be hard-working, enthusiastic about your work and calling, and able to get along well with others. To stand out from other applicants, you must have an individual, convincing message.

As you start the application process, one of your primary goals is to formulate your message. Give a concise answer as to why the program should accept you. *Every aspect of your application must reinforce this message.*

Many books and articles have been written about creating a compelling message, and there are many different ways of approaching the same basic objective. Marketers write entire books on the subject. What makes your product so special? Can you convince a customer to buy your product? For entrepreneurs they call it the "elevator pitch." You meet a venture capitalist in the elevator. Can you convince him to invest in your company? Workplace experts call the same process "self-branding." What are you known for? How can you bring value to a company?

When formulating your message for a residency selection committee, you need to convince them that you would be the right resident for their program. What type of physician will you be? Compassionate, hard-working, focused, driven? Will your goals mesh with those of the program? What unique strengths and qualities do you possess that can help the residency program achieve its goals?

Your message may not gel until you've done the initial work of the application process. Brainstorming for your CV and your personal statement are critical components, especially as this process will highlight your own strengths and accomplishments. The substance of the message will be based on the work you've already done. If you're in your fourth year, you may not recognize the evidence that exists in your past experiences and evaluations. If you're still in your third year, even better: you have time to provide tangible evidence to support your message about your fit for the program.

Case 1

Joyce is a student from a middle tier medical school with an average transcript and an average USMLE score. She's applying to several competitive internal medicine residency programs. When asked why the program should choose her, she could say that she's a very hard worker, and would get along well with the other residents, and that would be entirely true. Instead, her response:

"You'll find that I give 100% to my patients, and I try very hard to involve the patient and their family in their own care. Several of my attendings have half-jokingly commented on my 'second job' in the patient education resource center at our teaching hospital, but several of the letters I've gotten back from former patients have made it worth it. I know that Lutheran General emphasizes an understanding of the family and community dynamic in the care of each individual patient, and that's one of the reasons that I would love to be here."

Her message: She is passionate about the care of her patients and works very hard to see that they're taken care of. She is very interested in patient education as part of that process.

Each piece of her application reinforces this message:

- Several of her attendings have included supporting comments in the written section of her formal clerkship evaluations. "Joyce works very hard to see that her patients are well taken care of, in all respects. I saw one of my patients in the clinic, and he related to me how much Joyce had helped him with the materials that she provided from the American Cancer Society."

- Joyce asked for letters of recommendation from two of the attendings who had commented on this quality in her end of clerkship meeting.

- The Dean's letter, in the narrative section summarizing attending evaluations, included two such comments verbatim.

- In her CV, she highlighted her past experiences of volunteering for the American Cancer Society on an ongoing basis for two years and her involvement in multiple health fairs.

- She did an elective with a well-regarded preventive medicine attending and specifically asked for opportunities to participate in a case report or other publication. Dr. Sveta asked her to author a patient information brochure that was to be published in a nursing journal, and it was accepted for publication.

- Her personal statement discussed a memorable patient who was only partially compliant with diabetes care recommendations.

- She came prepared to reinforce this message during her interviews. What's your greatest strength? Tell us about a memorable patient. What are you looking for in a program? Where do you see yourself ten years from now? Each of her answers was supported by evidence.

Case 2

Ria was a very soft-spoken student with average grades and average scores. During the interview, when asked about her publications, she simply replied that one was a review article on reactions to chemotherapy, and one was a case report about an interesting patient she had seen in clinic.

When asked where she saw herself in ten years, she simply replied that she wanted to go back to her hometown rural community, which lacked dermatologists. She stated that she would have liked to be more involved in academics and teaching, but there were no academic programs in the area. The overall impression she created was that of a nice, average applicant.

I quizzed her more extensively in an informal meeting, and here her message came across much stronger. She was very nice and soft-spoken, but was also passionate about patient care and the field of dermatology. Her strong work ethic was already evidenced by her letters of recommendation and her publications, but she needed to send that message more clearly during the interview. She was ready to emphasize that her goal was to practice in a rural, underserved area, and to become a source of expertise for the primary care physicians in the area.

Tell me about one of your publications.

> One of the most interesting publications I worked on was the review article on cutaneous reactions to chemotherapy. Dr. Sentry needed to submit the final publication in four weeks, and I was concerned because it was the first dermatology article I had worked on. But once I got started, the information was fascinating, and even though it was a challenge, we submitted it on time. The finished publication had over 100 references, and I'm very proud that it was such a thorough review.

Tell me about interesting patient you had.

> Stella was a one-year-old girl with a large hemangioma on her face. She was seen by her pediatrician in a rural area that didn't have any dermatologists, and the pediatrician was used to dealing with dermatology cases on his own. The parents were told that hemangiomas eventually resolve on their own, and no treatment was needed. However, the hemangioma was obstructing her vision, a key criterion for aggressive therapy. Stella was now blind. I was so saddened to think that this was

an entirely preventable case of blindness, and it really emphasized to me how much access to a specialist would have
helped that baby and that pediatrician, and how there are still
underserved areas in this country.

Where do you see yourself in ten years?

I've always wanted to go back to my rural community to practice. I really see myself serving as a source of information to
the primary care physicians and nurse practitioners in the area.
I've spent a lot of time working and volunteering in tutoring and
educational programs, as you can see from my CV, and I'd like
to create some formal programs of education in the area.

Rule # 5   Your message doesn't mean much without the evidence to back it up.

If you're applying to a competitive specialty, you'll hear statements
like the following:

- "Don't even bother to apply unless you're AOA."
- "They screen out applications based on minimum USMLE scores."
- "You need to have an outstanding transcript, or they won't even look at your application."

There is some truth to these statements.

Programs that receive an overwhelming number of applications
are forced to seek out tangible evidence of a student's qualifications.
Membership in AOA, USMLE scores, the Dean's letter summary
statement; all of these provide easily quantified data.

However, students sometimes focus exclusively, and erroneously,
on such academic criteria. The assumption is that once you've
reached a certain academic level, getting into the residency program
of your choice is guaranteed. However, personal traits are given
greater weight than applicants often believe.

Programs want residents who can learn the material and pass the
boards. However, it takes a lot more than that to be an outstanding
resident. Programs seek residents who are hard-working, excited
about patient care, compassionate, involved in patient education,
interested in improving their communities, exhibit manual dexterity,
are able to handle the pressures of residency, will contribute to the
specialty in some meaningful fashion, and on and on. All of these criteria are important to programs, and none can be easily quantified.
How do you prove you're hard-working? How do you prove you're
passionate about the field of anesthesiology? How can a program
know how well you get along with others?

Your job is to provide the evidence that backs up each of these claims. A program isn't going to just take your word for it. Anybody can say that they're hard-working, and pretty much everyone does. You are going to have to provide tangible evidence. Many of the most important criteria are those for which tangible evidence is not easy to come by. That's why students who can convincingly capture the presence of these qualities and support them with evidence are so notable.

Your past experiences contain many such examples of evidence. It can be difficult to initially recognize them as such. Your work as an anatomy teaching assistant, for example, was far more than just employment experience. Analyze your work experience. What did your experience reveal about your strengths and about you as an individual? How can you successfully highlight this evidence? Do the same with all of your honors, work experience, volunteer experience, research experience, publications, presentations, and outside activities.

Following are examples of how applicants presented information in ERAS and the message that this information conveys. By changing the emphasis, adding crucial details, or expanding upon the information, the applicant can substantiate their message. The information can then serve as evidence to back up their message. In the following examples, the use of evidence sends a message with greater impact.

Information in ERAS: Work experience September 1999-December 1999 Served as an anatomy teaching assistant
Message: This student has teaching experience.
Evidence: September 1999-December 1999 Anatomy teaching assistant; position awarded to two students per year by invitation of anatomy faculty. Instructed first year medical students in anatomy lab, created 10 dissection lesson plans, and led an additional 10 discussion sessions.
Message: This student has successfully emphasized that he values teaching, and was recognized for his abilities to teach. The preparation of ten lesson plans is a significant commitment of time, energy, and effort, and his transcript confirms that he was able to maintain excellent grades during this time period.

Information in the personal statement: I'm a very hard worker, and one of my strengths is attention to detail. I bring these qualities to everything that I do, especially in issues of patient care.
Message: This student believes she is a hard worker.

Evidence: *With all my might, I tightened the knob one last time. Bending over the gas tank, I placed my nose just millimeters away from the connection site and took in a deep breath. No smell of gas could be detected. With drops of water on my palms, I rubbed a bar of soap for a couple of minutes. I coated the soap suds over the connection site and waited for signs of bubbling but saw none. Gingerly, I turned on the stove and lit a match. What a sigh of relief! No explosion.*

I am always systematic and detailed in my work. Whether the job is a routine replacement of the portable gas tank for the stove, gathering data for my research projects, or taking care of my patients at the hospital, my performance has always been thorough.

Message: This student is systematic and detailed, and has demonstrated these traits in multiple ways.

Information in the interview: What is your greatest strength? I'm a very hard worker, and I bring 100% to everything that I do.

Message: This student believes she is a hard worker.

Evidence: What is your greatest strength? I think my perseverance. When I first conceived of the idea of the pre-natal and post-natal classes in the city school district, the faculty were on board immediately, but we hit a lot of logistical issues with the school administration. I had to work through a number of issues, but I'm very proud of the fact that our first classes started this year.

Message: This student is innovative, persistent, and willing to work hard to reach a goal.

Information in ERAS: Work experience 2003-2004 Physician director, Karachi Ob/Gyn Associates, Karachi, Pakistan. Supervised a team of healthcare professionals.

Message: This physician has clinical experience as an Ob/Gyn.

Evidence: Work experience 2003 - 2004 Physician director, Karachi Ob/Gyn Associates, Karachi, Pakistan
Supervised a team of 20 healthcare professionals in a clinic responsible for the care of 3000 obstetrics and gynecology patients

Message: The concrete numbers and action verbs used in this CV provide evidence of the responsibility she was entrusted with as a physician director, and documents her significant clinical experience and the type of heavy workload to which she is accustomed.

Information in ERAS: Hobbies and interests: Varsity college volleyball player

Message: This student played college volleyball.

Evidence: In the personal statement, this student fleshed out the lessons she learned from her time in collegiate athletics. She wrote about her work ethic, ability to handle a challenging schedule, her lessons in prioritizing, and lessons on teamwork.

Message: The traits she developed and displayed through her time in varsity college volleyball are the same traits that a program seeks in its residents, and are the traits that have contributed to her reputation as an excellent clinician, as per her Dean's letter and clinical evaluations.

Information in ERAS: Participant in the Susan A. Albert junior-senior high mentor program 9/2007-5/2008.
Message: This applicant served as a mentor.
Evidence: Invited by the faculty panel to serve in the Susan A. Albert junior-senior high mentor program. Mentored two adolescent middle-schoolers with learning disabilities. Met weekly with mentee, discussed any personal or academic school issues, and tutored in the subjects of English and science.
Message: The applicant was invited to serve, and thus this is a recognition of his abilities. He gained tutoring experience. Serving as a mentor to a child for a one year time period, and meeting weekly, is a significant effort and demonstrates commitment.

Information in ERAS: The Erin Kelley award 2006
Message: This student won an award.
Evidence: The Erin Kelley award 2006—awarded to one student per year who embodies compassion in patient care; voted on by peers.
Message: This student is known for her compassion, to the point that she was the single individual recognized by her peers for her compassion in patient care.

The concept of presenting evidence in your application is easy to understand. It sounds great. And we make it sound so easy. However, we do recognize the difficulties involved. How can you identify and present evidence when you're not even sure what you're really known for? What if it seems as though you're not that outstanding?

Each section of this book walks you through this process. Your experiences in patient care provide the best opportunities to demonstrate those qualities that would make you an outstanding house officer. Each rotation provides multiple opportunities to demonstrate your work ethic, your compassion, your commitment to patient education, your ability to work well with a team, and many other traits. After you've demonstrated your skills in patient care, add in other experiences that can serve to illustrate your best traits. Make presentations during your rotation. Look for opportunities to be published in your field. Reflect on your past work experiences. Seek out opportunities for clinical or basic science research, depending on your interests. Continue your volunteer commitments. Don't neglect your outside pursuits.

We discuss how to strengthen your application in this type of concrete fashion in much greater detail throughout the book. Our companion book, *250 Biggest Mistakes 3rd Year Medical Students Make And How To Avoid Them,* reviews how to excel in clinical rotations. In this book, Chapter 10, "The Audition Elective," goes into further detail on how to excel during an audition elective. Opportunities to give talks may arise during clerkships or audition electives and should be fully utilized. Our companion book also provides explicit directions on how to give an outstanding talk. In this book, Chapter 11, "The Competitive Edge," starting on page 253, provides further guidance on how to locate opportunities to participate in publications and research, and how to make the most of those opportunities. If you're applying to a competitive residency program, these sections are a must. Strengthening your application is much easier if you have sufficient lead time. If you're reading this book in your third year, you can make significant strides in improving your candidacy. However, even as a fourth year student, you can actively create and present further evidence. These same opportunities exist for residents applying to a different field, or for practicing physicians seeking additional training.

Rule # 6   Present it all in a powerful package.

In each section of this book, we discuss how to create a perfect package. By perfect, we mean *perfect*. This is a painstaking process, and you need to follow the guidelines exactly. Your CV and personal statement must be in the proper format, the correct length, and completely free of any grammatical or spelling errors. When members of a residency selection committee are reviewing hundreds of applications, even a single such error can be grounds for exclusion. If this applicant made a mistake on such an important document, how are they going to handle the tenth admission of the night?

The perfect package also means that your application is noticed. You may have great grades and great scores, and your application may be free of errors, but that won't always be enough to make members of the residency selection committee notice your application. You need to include the type of information that convinces committee members that you would be the right resident for their program, and you need to highlight that information in such a way that they notice it.

We've discussed how to formulate your message and how to collect the evidence that backs it up. In Rule #5, we've given examples of how the same experience, presented in a different manner, can send a completely different message. The remainder of the book goes over, in comprehensive detail, how to prepare each component of your application so that your candidacy is presented in a powerful package.

Chapter 6

Curriculum Vitae (CV)

Curriculum vitae is a Latin expression, meaning the "course of one's life." Known as CV for short, this document provides an overview of a candidate's academic and professional background. While similar to a resume, a CV includes additional information such as research experience, publications, and presentations. It is typically used in medical, research, and other academic fields.

Reviewing a vast number of CVs from applicants is a difficult process. In many cases, your CV will be skimmed. You only have 1-2 pages to impress the residency selection committee, and therefore every line, word, and number becomes important. When your CV is skimmed, reviewers may not even note significant achievements, unless they're described and positioned well. In addition, particularly with competitive programs, mistakes of any sort may justify discarding an application. We review how to create a professional CV, and how to maximize the impact of every word, line, and number.

Rule # 7   Your CV must create maximum impact.

Creating a good CV requires time, effort, and a thorough examination of your training and achievements. The overall appearance of your CV needs to be impeccable. The proofreading must be perfect. Each individual line should be positioned for maximum impact. Every pertinent aspect of your achievements must be included.

Students don't always recognize the importance of creating an outstanding CV. Many residency programs now require applicants to submit applications through ERAS, the Electronic Residency Application Service of the Association of American Medical Colleges. Students aren't permitted to attach their CV to the ERAS application. However, you are allowed to enter information from your CV directly by computer into the ERAS CV format. Program directors can then print out this information in a CV format.

Even though you won't be able to attach your CV to your ERAS application, you still need to create a professional-looking paper version of your CV for the following reasons:

- Some residency programs don't participate in ERAS. These programs will request a paper CV.
- The CV will help you fill out your Medical Student Performance Evaluation (MSPE) Data Form. Medical schools use this form

to help them create your MSPE (Dean's letter), an important component of the residency application.

- The CV will help you complete different sections of the residency application.
- The CV can be of considerable help as you begin to draft your personal statement.
- When students apply for an elective rotation at another institution, they may be required to submit a CV first. Such "away" or "audition" electives are often helpful for students applying to competitive residencies. Obtaining such an elective can be a competitive process in and of itself.
- Reviewing your CV prior to the interview will remind you of your strengths and accomplishments, helping to boost confidence.
- Interviewers may request a copy of your CV at the start of an interview in order to help structure the interview. This provides an ideal opportunity to emphasize your strengths and highlight the skills you would bring as a resident.

Your CV will continue to be an important document even after you match into a residency program. It is not a static document, but rather one that needs to be updated regularly as you progress through your career.

Tip # 5

Program directors are able to view and print your application information in an ERAS CV format. You can, and should, do the same prior to submitting your application.

Tip # 6

For programs that don't participate in ERAS, you may have to submit a paper CV. While you may be an intelligent, enthusiastic, and charming applicant, you won't have the opportunity to showcase these qualities during an interview if a poorly written, or even average, CV eliminates you from further consideration. If done well, your CV has the potential to position you above other applicants, even those who may be more qualified.

Rule # 8   Utilize only the correct CV format and structure.

All CVs begin with your name and contact information. Since these items will be at the top of your CV, they can contribute to a positive first impression, and so should be visually appealing. Many applicants use the same font size for the name and contact information. However, your name should be a bit bigger and even bolder than the rest of the contact information. Don't add the words "curriculum vitae" to the top of the page, as many students tend to do. The reader recognizes a CV. Why waste valuable space stating the obvious?

Tip # 7

Double-check your contact information to ensure that a program director could reach you quickly and easily if necessary. Since most programs will communicate with you entirely by e-mail, double check your e-mail address.

Tip # 8

Is your e-mail address professional? The inappropriate and immature examples we have encountered include partygirl@hotmail.com and ralphlaurenmd@aol.com. You've worked hard to create a specific image throughout the entire application. Need we say more? If you don't have a professional e-mail address, now is the time to create one. Your e-mail address should simply be your first and last name (e.g., meljackson@hotmail.com, jayapatel@yahoo.com).

Tip # 9

While most communication between an applicant and program occurs via e-mail, sometimes applicants are contacted by phone. Make sure that your answering machine or voice mail message is professional. "Hey dude, you know what to do at the tone" might suffice for your buddy, but replace this with something more professional during the residency application process: "Hello, this is Rodrigo Martin. Thank you for calling, but I'm not available to take your call right now. Please leave your name, telephone number, and message, and I'll return your call as soon as possible."

Tip # 10

In the event that a program director calls you at home while you are away, educate those at home in how to answer the phone politely. Ask them to note the name of the person calling, the return phone number, the name of the residency program, and a good time to call back. Afterwards, have them contact you as soon as possible so you can return the phone call.

Following your name and contact information should be an "education" section. From here, you have considerable latitude in the order in which you present the remaining categories. It is preferable, however, to lead with your strengths. If you have earned honor after honor in medical school, have the "honors/awards" section follow "education" rather than placing it second to last. Weigh the impact of each section before deciding where to place it. Below are the standard sections of the CV.

Standard sections of the CV

Name
Contact information
Education
Postgraduate training
Employment experience
Honors/awards
Professional society memberships/affiliations
Teaching experience
Research experience
Publications
Presentations
Licensure and certification
Extracurricular activities
Volunteer activities
Personal interests

Tip # 11

The order in which you present the elements of your CV is important. Program directors are no different than you or I. They will read your CV from top to bottom and from left to right. Don't place your most important accomplishments at the end.

Incorrect ordering is among the most common CV mistakes. In all sections of the CV, information should be presented in reverse chronological order. Using this order, one would list items such as jobs and awards with the most recent item first.

Education

2005 to present	University of Texas Medical Branch, Galveston, TX M.D. anticipated in 6/2009
2001 – 2005	Baylor University, Waco, TX B.Sc., Chemistry

Rule # 9   Every section and line of your CV must impress.

If you have a section with just one item, plan on eliminating it, unless it's an impressive accomplishment. A category with a single item looks decidedly unimpressive. It also wastes valuable lines of CV space. A single item can always be woven into another category. For example, a single honor earned during medical school can be listed in the "education" section.

Rule # 10   Each line of your CV must serve as evidence of your skills and accomplishments.

Each line of your CV must pack the maximum impact. Study your CV line by line. In many cases, a description or explanation of an item will maximize its impact.

Honors and Awards

2004	George Lambert Scholarship

Do you know what this scholarship is? The residency selection committee has no idea, either. For all we know, it is a $250 scholarship given to 35 students per class who are from a particular geographic district in the state.

This version makes a far greater impression:

2004	George Lambert Scholarship
	Awarded to the student with the highest academic performance during the freshman year of medical school (1/200)

Tip # 12

As you read through your CV, question whether the reader would understand the significance of what you have written. If not, it may be assumed to have little to no value.

Tip # 13

Avoid unfamiliar acronyms or abbreviations. An abbreviation that is readily apparent to you may have no meaning to a program director. CMSC is short for the Chicago Medical Student Council, a student government organization. While a University of Illinois-Chicago medical student might recognize this, a program director at the Texas Tech University School of Medicine would have no idea what it stands for. If an organization is not readily recognizable, a brief explanation of the group and its purpose should be included in the CV.

Rule # 11   The structure of your CV should be used to highlight all accomplishments.

While students review CVs with an obsessive attention to detail, the typical member of the residency selection committee is forced to more quickly review a CV. Part of refining your CV, then, should be the two-minute glance over. Have you captured the reviewer's attention and conveyed your accomplishments?

Professional Membership

2005 (summer)	American Medical Association, Medical Student Section (President)

Reading this, you could easily miss the fact that the applicant was president of the organization. Faculty members don't have the time to ferret out all the small print on every CV. You must structure your CV to highlight all accomplishments.

Professional Membership

2005 (summer)	President, American Medical Association, Medical Student Section

Rule # 12   Use the personal interests section to catch a reviewer's attention, but with caution.

Programs are interested in an applicant's hobbies and interests. "What is this person like? Is he or she well rounded? Interesting? What would it be like to work with this person?" Provide this information in the personal interests section of your CV, which is usually the last section.

Don't take this section lightly. Faculty often start the interview with some discussion of your interests as a way to break the ice. You may also find that you share an interest with your interviewer. This can quickly build rapport.

Certain interests are viewed positively and may enhance your candidacy. The ability to speak Spanish fluently would be a noted positive at a residency program whose institution serves a large Hispanic population. Interests may also be viewed negatively. While there are certainly student and physician members of the organization People for the Ethical Treatment of Animals (PETA), some physicians don't agree with the organization's stance against medical testing in animals or the way in which the organization conducts itself.

Rule # 13   The language style you use makes a difference. Use only action verbs.

Use words that capture the reviewer's attention. The use of action verbs acts to strengthen your CV. Placed at the beginning of sentences, these verbs make more powerful statements.

In writing about your work, extracurricular, volunteer, and research experiences, use action verbs to emphasize your accomplishments. Many applicants simply describe their duties and responsibilities. It is far more powerful to stress what you accomplished.

Research Experience

2004-2005   Research Assistant, Department of Pharmacology,
                 National Institute of Mental Health, Bethesda, MD
                 ● Assisted professor in research related to receptors
                   in the hippocampus
                 ● Helped collect data

Note the impact of the changes in the revised version:

Research Experience

2004-2005   Research Assistant, Department of Pharmacology,
                 National Institute of Mental Health, Bethesda, MD
                 ● Isolated and characterized several receptors in the
                   hippocampus
                 ● Elucidated the functions of these receptors
                 ● Sequenced the amino acid composition of these
                   receptors

Utilize the following extensive list of action verbs in order to highlight your accomplishments:

Action Verbs	
A	Abridged, accelerated, accomplished, accounted for, achieved, adapted, adjusted, administered, advanced, advised, allocated, analyzed, answered, approved, arranged, assembled, assimilated, assisted, attained, augmented
B	balanced, broadened, built
C	calculated, calibrated, cared for, categorized, catalogued, chaired, charted, clarified, classified, coached, collaborated, collected, compared, compiled, completed, composed, conceived, condensed, conducted, consolidated, constructed, consulted, contributed, coordinated, counseled, created, critiqued
D	debated, defined, delegated, delineated, delivered, demonstrated, derived, designed, detected, determined, developed, devised, diagnosed, directed, discovered, displayed, distributed, documented, drafted
E	edited, earned, educated, elicited, enabled, encouraged, enhanced, ensured, established, estimated, evaluated, examined, exceeded, exhibited, expanded, expedited, explained, explored
F	facilitated, followed, formulated, found, founded, furthered
G	gathered, generated, guided
H	handled, headed, helped
I	identified, illustrated, implemented, improved, increased, initiated, innovated, inspected, installed, instituted, instructed, interacted, interpreted, interviewed, invented, investigated
J	judged, justified

L	launched, lectured, led, logged
M	made, maintained, managed, mastered, measured, met, modified, monitored, motivated
O	observed, obtained, offered, operated, organized, oversaw
P	participated, performed, pinpointed, pioneered, planned, prepared, presented, presided, prioritized, processed, produced, programmed, proposed, proved, provided
Q	quantified
R	raised, realized, received, recommended, recorded, redesigned, reported, researched, revamped, received, revised
S	scheduled, screened, searched, secured, selected, served, set up, simplified, solved, spearheaded, started, streamlined, strengthened, studied, submitted, succeeded, summarized, supervised, supplied, supported, surpassed, surveyed, synthesized
T	tabulated, tallied, taught, tested, traced, tracked, trained, translated, transmitted, tutored
U	uncovered, undertook, updated, upgraded, used
V	validated, verified, volunteered
W	widened, won, worked, wrote

As you review this list, note the following:

- Some action verbs are more powerful than others. Use the most powerful verb you can without exaggerating your accomplishments.

- Do not downplay, diminish, or deflate your contributions by using verbs such as "assisted" or "helped."

- Avoid the much too commonly used phrases "Responsible for ..." or "Duties included ..."

- Avoid repeating the same verb if possible.

- For those activities or experiences with which you are currently involved, use the present tense. Use the past tense for completed work or past experiences.

Tip # 14

You need not, and should not, write your CV in complete sentences. Instead, use short phrases that make your points as quickly as possible. The words "I" or "me" do not belong in a CV. Articles such as "the" "a" and "an" are typically omitted as well.

Rule # 14　Use numbers to provide concrete evidence.

Provide tangible evidence whenever possible to support your claims. This means including numbers and facts to emphasize your accomplishments. Numbers can often drive home key points in ways that words can't.

Work Experience

2003-2004　　　Physician director, Karachi Ob/Gyn Associates,
　　　　　　　　Karachi, Pakistan
　　　　　　　　● Supervised a team of healthcare professionals

In this more powerful version, note how the applicant was able to describe her experience quantitatively and specifically:

Work Experience

2003-2004　　　Physician director, Karachi Ob/Gyn Associates,
　　　　　　　　Karachi, Pakistan
　　　　　　　　● Supervised a team of 20 healthcare professionals
　　　　　　　　in a clinic responsible for the care of 3000 obstetrics
　　　　　　　　and gynecology patients

Rule # 15　Utilize multiple reviewers.

It doesn't matter how many times you review and revise your own CV. You should have several individuals review your CV prior to submission. We recommend having your CV reviewed by two faculty members, if at all possible. Ideally, one would include the residency program director of your chosen specialty at your medical school. The director is likely to be an authority in this area, having seen hundreds or even thousands of CVs over the years. Don't submit your CV for review to faculty, though, until you feel that it is perfect.

You should ask someone with excellent writing and editing skills to review your CV. This type of careful review may lead to the discovery of spelling or grammatical errors, mistakes that can be very damaging to your candidacy.

Finally, consider the benefits of having a family member or close friend critique your CV. Those who know you well on a personal level may point out accomplishments that you'd forgotten.

After collecting reviewer comments, consider them carefully. Compare reviewer comments with another. While you don't need to agree with all comments, if several of your reviewers make the same recommendations, take these comments seriously. If there is disagreement, solicit more opinions to help you make a more informed decision.

Tip # 15

Applicants from other countries should recognize that CV and resume styles differ from one country to another in terms of style and tone. What may be considered appropriate in your home country may be too casual or too stiff in the United States. Herein lies the importance of having the CV reviewed by someone with experience in the United States.

Tip # 16

While there is a benefit to having your CV reviewed by someone close to you, such as your mother, roommate, or significant other, understand that loved ones are usually not the best reviewers. Always have your CV reviewed by qualified individuals such as a faculty member, the residency program director at your institution, or advisor.

To maximize the value of others' opinions, use the following CV review form to check your own work prior to their review.

CV review form		
	Yes	No
Does the overall appearance make an excellent first impression?		
Is the length of the CV appropriate?		
Is the CV easily read?		
Is the CV well organized?		
Is the font type easy to read?		
Is the font type and size consistent?		
Is the font size appropriate?		
Is the spacing consistent throughout the CV?		
Is the name and contact information presented in an appealing manner with the name being most prominent?		
Is the contact information correct and complete?		
Are the section headings lined up and consistent (i.e., font size/ style, bold)?		
Is the formatting within each section consistent (spacing, font size, bullets, etc.)?		
Are the margins on each side equal?		
Are underlining, italics, and bolding used appropriately?		

Are there any grammatical errors?		
Are there any spelling errors?		
Is there any use of *I, my, me, a, an,* or *the*?		
Are the most important sections listed first?		
Is information presented in reverse chronological order?		
Are action verbs used consistently?		
Are the dates correct?		
Are there any time gaps in the work or school history?		
Is there anything in the CV that is irrelevant?		
Is the CV printed on professional, high-quality paper?		

Rule # 16 Avoid even a single spelling, typographical, or grammatical error.

Spelling, typographical, and grammatical errors are among the worst mistakes you can make on the CV. Even one misspelled word can make you look careless. Residency programs are searching for individuals who are motivated and compulsive. If your CV shows that you lack attention to detail, program directors fear that this will spill over into your work as a resident. Otherwise well-qualified applicants have been removed from consideration because of these errors.

Ensure your CV is free of errors:

- If you created your CV using word processing, use the spell checker. However, the spell checker won't help if you misuse a word (e.g., substituting "there" for "their"). International medical graduates should avoid British spellings.
- Take the time needed to proofread your CV. Read it aloud, and sound out each word, syllable by syllable. Errors not apparent during a silent read may be picked up by this method.
- Read the CV backwards one word at a time, a technique used by many professional proofreaders. This allows you to focus on each individual word.
- Set the CV aside for a day before looking at it again. This allows you to look at your work with fresh eyes.

Rule # 17 Use the correct length.

As a general rule, the CV should not exceed 1 or 2 pages. Program directors don't have the patience or time to review a long CV. Occasionally, the CV may be longer, particularly if an applicant has published a considerable number of articles. If you can't place all of your information on one or two pages, ask yourself if you've been too verbose. Don't use a smaller font size or shrink the margins in order to fit more text onto a page. We've seen students attempt this technique, and it doesn't work well. Instead, use fewer words and omit information that doesn't support your application. A CV reviewer can help you edit out repetitive or unnecessary information.

Tip # 17

Placing too much information in a CV is among the most common mistakes applicants make. For most applicants, the CV should not exceed 1-2 pages.

Tip # 18

If your CV extends to a second page by a line or two, adjust the margins to fit the CV onto one page. If your CV extends to a second page but takes up only half of the second page, spread the text over the two pages to eliminate excess white space.

Tip # 19

Mark each page of your CV clearly. Place "Page 1 of 2" at the bottom of the first page. Place your name followed by the page number at the top of the second page
(e.g., Reza Hourhani - page 2 of 2).

Rule # 18   First impressions matter, even for a piece of paper.

The overall appearance of your CV is important as well. Residency selection committee members must whittle down a large group of applications, and therefore every piece of the application becomes magnified in importance. Before reviewing your CV, the reader will form an initial impression of you based on its overall appearance. These recommendations should be used to create a CV with a professional appearance:

Margins

Allow for generous margins at the top, bottom, and sides of your CV. A margin of at least 1 inch is often recommended. Shrinking the margins to anything less than an inch will make the CV difficult to read.

Font

Use a font that is easy to read. Times New Roman or Arial are appropriate choices. After selecting a particular font, stick with it. The use of multiple fonts can appear unprofessional.

Font size is also an important consideration. Avoid a font size less than 10-point or one greater than 12-point. It is acceptable to use two font sizes, a larger one for headings and a smaller one for the content under each heading. The use of more than two font sizes is discouraged.

Spacing

Be consistent with spacing. Maintain enough white (open) space, especially between sections. If you use one line space between the end of one section and the beginning of another, maintain this with all sections. Rather than striking the space bar twice after each sentence, strike it only once to save space. If your CV exceeds one page in length, avoid splitting a section when going from page 1 to 2.

Design elements

It is acceptable to use the bold function to highlight your name and section headings (e.g., education). You can also consider bolding certain awards and leadership positions as a way to highlight these achievements. However, excessive use of the bolding technique can overwhelm the reader. If you bold an element such as "education," then you should bold similar elements as well (e.g., honors/awards). Keep headings consistent in style and size.

Limit the use of italics to the names of journals and foreign phrases such as *magna cum laude.* Underlining should also be used sparingly. The excessive use of underlining tends to focus the eyes on the underlined portion of the CV only. Occasional use of all caps may be acceptable, but some consider it to be rude, akin to shouting.

Paper quality

Print your CV on one side only of high quality 8.5" X 11" bond paper (e.g., 24 to 28 lb). Do not use unusual or multicolored paper that may appear unprofessional. Select a white, off-white, natural, or cream colored paper.

Print the CV using a laser printer. If you don't have a laser printer, make a copy of your CV on disk, take it to a local copy store, and have them print it. CVs should not be printed on both sides of the paper. If you will be mailing the CV to a program, send it in an envelope that matches the paper.

Characteristics of an outstanding CV	Characteristics of a poor CV
Visually appealing, professional look	Weathered look (e.g. bent corners, stains)
Brief and concise	Long sentences/paragraphs
Easy to read	Lack of organization
Uniform margins with none <1 inch	Too little white space ("crowded look")
No misspelled words or typos	Typos or misspelled words
Use of action verbs	Handwritten corrections
Moderate use of bolding/underlining/ italics	Poor paper or printing quality

Rule # 19   Some information has no place in a CV. Learn what to leave out.

We have seen many CVs that include unnecessary information. The following information has no place in the CV:

- Age
- Gender
- Height/weight
- Race/ethnicity
- Social security number
- Marital status
- Name of spouse/significant other
- Children
- Religion
- Description of health

Rule # 20   Start your CV now.

Your CV plays a key role in the residency application process. It also serves a key role in creating other components of the residency application. It is used to prepare the general application, MSPE, personal statement, and letters of recommendation. When should you start working on your CV? Some advisors will tell you to begin sometime between May and July of your third year of medical school. We don't recommend that you wait that long for two main reasons.

Starting early provides the time needed to create a powerful CV. Because the medical student CV tends to be a one or two-page document, many applicants mistakenly assume that they can create a CV in a matter of minutes or, at the very most, a few hours. However, if you wish to create a CV that makes a strong impact, both in content and appearance, you need sufficient time. Your reviewers also need sufficient time, especially busy individuals such as residency program directors.

Starting early also highlights areas in your CV that can be maximized. Students who have no items to place under the heading of presentations or publications can remedy this situation with enough lead time.

There are a few other reasons to have your CV prepared now, wherever you are in the application cycle. As we discuss later, when you approach a faculty member for a letter of recommendation, you will provide a packet of information to assist them. Your CV is a standard component of that packet. The CV you provide must be in its final, perfected form, even at this stage. You need to make an impact with these individuals, who are advocating for your candidacy and have the power to sway program directors.

If you're planning to do an audition elective, recognize that competitive programs may require an application, including a CV. You may also seek to approach faculty members for career opportunities, as we discuss in Chapter 11: The Competitive Edge. "Dr. Vo, I'll be applying for anesthesiology residency, and I have a one-month research elective in July. The residents suggested that I speak with you. Do you have a clinical research project that I could work on during this elective month?" Some faculty members will request a copy of your CV before entrusting you with such an opportunity. Even the simple e-mailed query about working on a review article may require further information on a faculty member's part.

Rule # 21   Don't exaggerate.

We don't include this rule lightly. However, candidates seeking residency positions in competitive specialties or programs have been known to exaggerate their research experience or even misrepresent themselves in an attempt to gain a competitive advantage. The literature is replete with studies that prove that lying on a CV is much more commonplace than students would suspect. It is also caught more often than students would imagine. In a study of applications to the radiation oncology residency program at the Roswell Park Cancer Institute, 49 applicants claimed authorship of a publication. Of those claiming authorship, 22% listed inaccurate citation information (Yang). In a review of applications to the orthopedic surgery residency program at Wright State University, 20.6% of the 131 articles listed as published were in fact misrepresented (Konstantakos).

"I would never lie. This is just a slight exaggeration." "I think this should be fine—my name *is* mentioned in the article. If anyone ever asks me about it, I'll just explain that I didn't understand I wasn't an author." "I did work on the project, and I deserved to be listed as an author, but they couldn't include everyone due to the rules of the journal."

Most students don't set out to lie on their CV. If they do exaggerate or lie, they don't expect to be caught. While there is no universal agreement regarding the actions that should be taken if an applicant is caught in an act of misrepresentation, the possible consequences are many. At the very least, you won't be matching into that particular program. Other potential consequences include notification of the NRMP as well as the applicant's medical school and letter writers.

In some cases, applicants have claimed authorship of a publication based on participation in the research project. You cannot call yourself an author unless your name appears with the rest of the author group. Similarly, having your name cited in the acknowledgements section of an article is not synonymous with authorship.

Did you know …

You might assume that only desperate applicants would exaggerate or lie. However, Yang found that among radiation oncology residency applicants, CV misrepresentation was more common among applicants with higher USMLE scores (> 235).

Other examples of misrepresentation discussed in the literature include the following:

- Claiming authorship of an article that does not exist in the medical literature
- Claiming authorship of an existent article when, in fact, the applicant was not listed as an author
- Moving one's name further up in the author list (i.e., listing your name as second author when, in fact, you were the sixth author)
- Listing a publication in a more prestigious journal rather than the actual journal
- Claiming membership in the AOA honor medical society when, in fact, the applicant was not a member
- Claiming receipt of an advanced degree when, in fact, the applicant did not earn the degree

The following table summarizes the literature regarding misrepresentation.

Misrepresentation among residency applicants

Study	What was found
134 applications to the emergency medicine residency program at Washington University (Roellig)	Of the 47 applicants claiming published citations, ten were found to be inaccurate. Of the 14 applicants claiming AOA membership, five claims were found to be inaccurate. Of the 15 applicants claiming advanced degrees, four claims were inaccurate.
493 applications to nine emergency medicine residency programs (Katz)	9.8% contained at least one error. Inaccuracies were found on 41% of all publications. 3.7% of advanced degree claims were inaccurate.
404 applications to the pediatric residency program at the University of Washington School of Medicine (Bilge)	147 applicants claimed authorship of a journal article, abstract, book chapter, or book but authorship could not be confirmed in 19.7% of this group.
350 emergency medicine residency applications (Gurudevan)	23 of 113 applicants claiming authorship were found to misrepresent citations. Interestingly, the number of inaccuracies increased as the number of publications cited increased.
213 applications to the orthopedic surgery residency program at the University of Tennessee (Dale)	76 publications were checked and verified. Of this group, 14 were found to be misrepresented. The misrepresentations included the citing of an article which did not exist in an actual journal and erroneous claims of authorship of an existing article.
379 applications to the radiology residency program at the University of Indiana (Baker)	Of the 73 applicants who listed articles on their applications, misrepresentation occurred with eight applicants (11%).
102 applications to the neurosurgical residency program at the Mayo Clinic (Cohen-Gadol)	73 applicants reported published citations. Possible misrepresentation was found in six applicants (6%).
497 residency applications to two John Hopkins-affiliated internal medicine residency programs (Hebert)	Of the 224 applicants who reported authorship, 4 applicants were found to misrepresent citations (1.8%).
138 applications to the dermatology residency program at Vanderbilt University (Boyd)	Of the 52 applicants claiming published articles, 3 applicants claimed authorship but were not listed as an author.
117 applications to the radiation oncology residency program at the Roswell Park Cancer Institute (Yang)	Of the 49 applicants claiming authorship, 11 listed inaccurate citation information (22%).
396 applications to the orthopedic surgery residency at Wright State University (Konstantakos)	27 of 131 articles listed as published were misrepresented (20.6%).
697 applications to the Harvard Longwood psychiatry residency program (Caplan)	Of the 196 applicants reporting publications, 18 (9.2%) were found to have misrepresented their publications.

To guard against difficulties, we recommend that you bring copies of published, accepted, or submitted publications with you to the interview. Obtain your mentor's permission before bringing copies of publications that have been submitted. If you have listed an article as "in press," obtain a copy of the journal's letter of acceptance from your research mentor and bring it with you to the interview.

Did you know ...

Residency programs do verify publications. In one instance, Dr. Schwartz, chief of dermatology at the New Jersey Medical School, came across an applicant who claimed coauthorship of a paper when in fact he had only received an acknowledgment (Schwartz). When Dr. Schwartz informed him that he had requested the paper through interlibrary loan for verification, the applicant withdrew his application.

Rule # 22   Take adequate time to reflect on your experiences and accomplishments.

Most students dread the process of writing their CV; many feel they have nothing to make them stand out from other applicants. However, every applicant has individual, unique qualifications. On the other hand, the process of identifying your unique characteristics, experiences, and accomplishments is not an easy one. It is critical that you take adequate time to reflect on your experiences and accomplishments. Start with brainstorming. Begin the process by writing down absolutely everything; this is not the time to edit your thoughts. Start by taking each section of the CV, and make a list of everything that you've done that relates to that category. The standard sections of the CV are outlined in Rule # 8.

In the pages that follow, we describe each section in detail and provide worksheets to complete. As you complete each section, write down everything that you can possibly think of. After several initial brainstorming sessions, you should seek out other sources to help you come up with more ideas. Look at other books, websites, other examples of CVs, and speak to friends, family members, and colleagues. All of these sources may provide you with ideas. Later, you can edit this information.

Note: You can use the worksheets to take notes or scribble ideas. You can also use a handheld recorder to brainstorm ideas, which has the added benefit of traveling with you and being accessible whenever inspiration hits. You can also enter all of this information directly into your word processor.

After completing the worksheets, you may find that you don't have anything to list in a particular category. Don't be alarmed-- you're in good company. If you don't have anything to list under a section, then omit the section. However, if you are reading this book well in advance of application season, you do have time to improve your situation. Discuss with your residents, your attendings, and your faculty advisor your wish to strengthen your CV. Seek out opportunities, responsibilities, or experiences that would enhance your application. The chapters on audition electives and the competitive edge outline further ways to enhance your CV.

Rule # 23   Don't obsess over your first draft.

Once you have reviewed and written down your experiences and accomplishments, you can use this information to create the first draft of your CV. The ultimate goal is to present the information from the worksheets in such a way that it captures the interest and attention of the reader. However, your first draft doesn't need to be perfect.

Instead of agonizing over small details related to phrasing or formatting, take the information you have generated, transfer it to your word processing software, and arrange it in an organized manner. Once you've completed your first draft, you can then start agonizing over revisions.

Education Worksheet

Detail your education in reverse chronological order (i.e., with your most recent or current place of learning first). Include the following:

- Name of institution
- Location of institution
- Area of study or concentration (major/minor)
- Dates of enrollment (month/year)
- Degree(s)

For applicants in medical school, list the anticipated degree and expected graduation date. Include information about any graduate and undergraduate education. High school education is generally omitted.

If you received an honor, you can list it here (e.g., Dean's list, *magna cum laude*). If you have multiple awards, you can list them together in an "honors/awards" section. If you have completed a thesis or dissertation for a particular degree, you may wish to include it in this section.

Education
Medical school
Institution
Location
Date
Degrees

Areas of concentration
Medical school
Institution
Location
Date
Degrees
Areas of concentration
Graduate school
Institution
Location
Date
Degrees
Areas of concentration
Graduate school
Institution
Location
Date
Degrees
Areas of concentration
Undergraduate school
Institution
Location
Date
Degrees
Areas of concentration
Undergraduate school
Institution
Location
Date
Degrees
Areas of concentration

Honors and Awards Worksheet

In this section, the focus should be on awards received during medical school. If you have a significant number of honors grades, you can list clerkship honors in your chosen specialty first, followed by honors in other clerkships, and then basic science honors.

Awards and scholarships earned during the undergraduate years can also be included here, particularly if they are of great significance. You need not limit this section to academic awards. It is appropriate to include organizational, community, institutional, and departmental awards. If the honor is one that you feel a program director might value, then you should include it.

For awards that are not self-explanatory, include a single-sentence description to ensure that the reader understands the award's significance. Also include the date that you received the award.

What about high school awards? As a general rule, these should be omitted. An exception to this rule would be an extraordinary honor or accomplishment such as valedictorian or National Merit Scholarship Finalist.

Honors and Awards
Honor/Award
Bestowing Organization
Date:
Honor/Award
Bestowing Organization
Date:
Honor/Award
Bestowing Organization
Date:
Honor/Award
Bestowing Organization
Date:

Employment Experience Worksheet

List jobs you held during medical school, along with the dates of employment. For most traditional medical students, this is generally not an extensive section. Some students will have no work experience whatsoever.

However, this can be an important section for medical graduates who are switching residencies, are returning to residency after practicing in another specialty, or for IMGs. In these cases, it is vital that this section is complete, and you must avoid any time gaps.

If you had extensive work experience prior to starting medical school, you should include those jobs as well. Military service can also be placed in this section. Include your branch of service, number of years served, highest rank achieved, and any awards earned.

Volunteer work is very important as well. Applicants often forget to include volunteer work, but this is important information that demonstrates your interest and commitment to the community.

For each work experience, list the employer, location (city/state), job title, duties/responsibilities, and dates of employment. Give a brief description of your responsibilities using action verbs. In particular, focus on skills you gained that would enhance your value to a residency program (transferable skills). For example, tutoring may have helped you develop skills in directing, guiding, or supervising.

Employment Experience
Position
Organization or business
Location
Duties/responsibilities
Position
Organization or business
Location
Duties/responsibilities
Position
Organization or business
Location
Duties/responsibilities
Position
Organization or business
Location
Duties/responsibilities
Position
Organization or business
Location
Duties/responsibilities
Position
Organization or business
Location
Duties/responsibilities

Professional Memberships/Affiliations Worksheet

List all professional organizations of which you are, or were, a member, along with the dates of your membership. It is especially important to include membership in an association that is relevant to your chosen specialty. If you are planning to pursue a career in obstetrics and gynecology and are a member of the American College of Obstetricians and Gynecologists (ACOG), you should include this in your CV. Some applicants elect not to list relevant memberships, citing their infrequent attendance at events or meetings. Even if you attended nothing more than an occasional meeting, don't let this stop you from listing membership in that organization on your CV. The fact that you are a member demonstrates a commitment to the specialty.

If you have not yet become a member of the professional organization of your chosen specialty, do so as soon as possible. Lack of membership may indicate a lack of enthusiasm for the field. Professional memberships offer students concrete advantages, including subscription to the organization's journal and the opportunity to attend meetings at a substantial discount. This will keep you abreast of the major issues in the field.

Leadership or committee positions within an organization are significant. If you no longer hold the position, attach the word "past" to the title of the position you held.

When listing the organization's name, do not use its abbreviation. If any organization to which you belong is considered controversial, such as PETA, leave out any mention of it.

Professional memberships/affiliations	
Professional organization	
Position	Dates
Professional organization	
Position	Dates
Professional organization	
Position	Dates
Professional organization	
Position	Dates
Professional organization	
Position	Dates
Professional organization	
Position	Dates

Research Experience Worksheet

You should list all research experience, even if it did not lead to a publication or presentation. Be specific in describing your duties and responsibilities. If your project was funded, list the amount and source of funding. You should always list your research mentor and principal investigator on the project.

Research Experience	
Project title	
Description/Responsibilities	
Institution	Dates
Mentor	Funding
Project title	
Description/Responsibilities	
Institution	Dates
Mentor	Funding
Project title	
Description/Responsibilities	
Institution	Dates
Mentor	Funding
Project title	
Description/Responsibilities	
Institution	Dates
Mentor	Funding

Publications Worksheet

List all abstracts and articles that you have published. The most recent publication is listed first, followed by all others in reverse chronological order. Applicants often forget to include articles published in newsletters, newspapers, magazines, or the Internet. Contributions to a book, not just authorship of a book, may be listed as well. List publications in the standard format used by medical journals. Most commonly, citations are listed using the American Psychological Association or American Medical Association format.

Publications
Publication
Authors
Title
Journal/book
Date, volume, page
Publication
Authors
Title

Journal/book
Date, volume, page
Publication
Authors
Title
Journal/book
Date, volume, page
Publication
Authors
Title
Journal/book
Date, volume, page
Publication
Authors
Title
Journal/book
Date, volume, page
Publication
Authors
Title
Journal/book
Date, volume, page

Presentations Worksheet

Although "presentations" can be combined with "publications" in one category, you may wish to create two separate categories. If you've only given one presentation, however, then use the joint category.

With presentations, it is particularly important to document the title, name of organization, location, and date. Include presentations given to academic societies and professional associations at the regional, national, and international level. Poster presentations should be listed here as well.

What about presentations you have given at your medical school? Presentations you were required to give should be omitted. However, occasionally a student may be asked to give a presentation because of exceptional performance. For example, if you were selected to be the sole presenter during psychiatry grand rounds, then you should include this experience on your CV.

Presentations	
Title	
Organization	
Location	Date
Title	
Organization	
Location	Date
Title	
Organization	
Location	Date
Title	
Organization	
Location	Date

Teaching Experience Worksheet

For each teaching experience, include your position, subject taught, audience, location, frequency of teaching, and date. Don't forget about tutoring experience.

Teaching experience	
Position	Subject
Audience	
Institution	
Location	Dates
Position	Subject
Audience	
Institution	
Location	Dates
Position	Subject
Audience	
Institution	
Location	Dates
Position	Subject
Audience	
Institution	
Location	Dates
Position	Subject
Audience	
Institution	
Location	Dates

Position	Subject	
Audience		
Institution		
Location		Dates
Position	Subject	
Audience		
Institution		
Location		Dates
Position	Subject	
Audience		
Institution		
Location		Dates

Licensure/Certification Worksheet

Include any licenses or health-related certificates that you hold (PA, RN, EMT, ACLS). For international medical graduates, it is important to list USMLE and ECFMG status. If you have done very well on your USMLE exam(s), list the score as well. If your performance was not stellar, you can simply state "passed." Include the date of licensure or certification. If licensure application is pending, use the phrase "application pending."

Licensure/Certification	
License/certificate	Date
License/certificate	Date
License/certificate	Date
License/certificate	Date

Extracurricular Activities Worksheet

Residency programs take interest in an applicant's extracurricular activities. They respect the fact that students active in organizations have demonstrated an ability to balance a difficult course load with outside activities.

List activities you were involved in during medical school. Avoid listing activities prior to medical school unless they are of significance. If the type of activity is not obvious, include a description.

Extracurricular activities	
Extracurricular activity	Dates
Description, including any positions held	

Extracurricular activity	Dates
Description, including any positions held	

Extracurricular activity	Dates
Description, including any positions held	

Extracurricular activity	Dates
Description, including any positions held	

Extracurricular activity	Dates
Description, including any positions held	

Personal Interests Worksheet

Few applicants give enough thought to this section. Often, two or three hobbies or interests are placed here without any consideration of how best to present the information. However, if done properly, this section can provide readers with insight into your personality and interests.

Interviews commonly begin with discussion of an applicant's personal interests as a way to break the ice. Applicants have been surprised to learn that they share the same interests as the program interviewer. [Wow. You like to brew beer too?]

While this section should not be any longer than a line or two, make every word count.

Personal interests

    Running

Listing simply "running" is an understatement in this case, as seen below:

Personal interests

    Long distance running—Chicago Marathon 2007

Sample CV #1

SONIA AMIN
465 Stuyvesant Circle
Youngstown, OH 44555
(643) 844–7300
soniaamin@gmail.com

EDUCATION

Northeastern Ohio Universities College of   2005 – Present
Medicine (NEOUCOM)
Rootstown, OH
    M.D., Anticipated in 5/09

University of Akron,   2001 – 2005
Akron, OH
    B.S., Biology

HONORS & AWARDS

Irwin Jacobsen Scholarship, NEOUCOM   2008
    Awarded to student finishing first overall
    during third year
Liza Emerson Award, NEOUCOM   2006
Summer Research Grant   2005

EXTRACURRICULAR ACTIVITIES

NEOUCOM Medical Student Admissions   2006 – Present
Committee, Student Chair
Dermatology Interest Group, Founder   2006 – Present
International Students Association, President   2005 – Present

RESEARCH EXPERIENCE

Research Assistant   8/07 – Present

Case Western University School of Medicine,
Dept. of Dermatology

> Grace Lin, M.D.: Helped gather data on
> incidence of heart disease in psoriasis
> patients

Research Assistant   6/06 – 8/06

National Institute of Health, Bethesda, MD

> Francisco Giovanni, M.D.: Assisted in
> the characterization of G2 receptor
> function

PROFESSIONAL MEMBERSHIPS

American Medical Women's Association   2005 – Present

American Medical Association   2005 – Present

Student National Medical Association   2005 – Present

PERSONAL INTERESTS

Avid tennis player
Violin player in the medical school orchestra
Traveling

Sample CV # 1, comments

Contact information: Notice how Sonia's contact information (name, address, phone number, e-mail address) is presented. In particular, her name is bolded in a larger font. The e-mail address is professional and the contact information is separated from the rest of the CV by a single, clean line.

Education: With few exceptions, CVs of residency applicants should begin with the education section. Note that Sonia has provided an abbreviation for her medical school. Throughout the rest of her CV, Sonia uses this abbreviation when referring to her school.

Honors and Awards: Following the education section, Sonia has included her honors and awards. Although she has done research and participated in several organizations, the nature of her awards is impressive. For this reason, this section should clearly follow education. Remember that readers will read your CV from top to bottom. Don't bury important information at the end of your CV.

While Sonia has properly described the Irwin Jacobsen Award, she should have done the same with the other two awards—the Lisa Emerson Award and Summer Research Grant. We have no way of knowing the significance of these awards. Was the grant given to her by the school as one of twenty grants offered to students in her class, or was it a more prestigious grant offered to five students across the country by the National Institutes of Health?

Extracurricular activities: Following the honors and awards section, Sonia continues with her extracurricular activities. She has placed this section next because it is stronger than those that follow. Of note, she has been a member of several organizations. If we hadn't been looking closely, however, we might have missed the fact that she was student chair of the admissions committee and founder of the dermatology interest group. She could have bolded the words "founder" and "president" to highlight her leadership positions. An alternative approach would have been to lead with the leadership position rather than the organization name, as Robert did in sample CV # 2.

As an officer of several organizations, Sonia may have accomplished quite a bit. However, she chose not to describe her accomplishments. Her CV would have been strengthened had she done so. For example, as founder of the dermatology interest group, she could have listed her accomplishment in organizing a group of students to assist in a free skin cancer screening offered by the dermatology department.

Research experience: In the research experience section, Sonia chooses weak verbs such as "helped" or "assisted" to describe her role. We don't have any idea of her contributions to the research project. Contrast this with Robert's CV (CV # 2).

Note: Sonia's CV is spread over two pages. At the top right corner of the second page, she should have included her name and the page number, as Ashutosh did in CV # 3.

Sample CV # 2

ROBERT HERNANDEZ

| 1243 Huntington Drive | | Home: (734) 222-4164 |
| Chicago, Illinois 60611 | hernandezr@hotmail.com | Cell: (632) 489-3500 |

EDUCATION

University of Oklahoma College of Medicine, Oklahoma City, OK   2004 - Present
    M.D., Anticipated 5/09
    Class rank: Top 10% (through junior year)
University of Central Oklahoma, Edmund, OK   2000 - 2004
    B.S., Biochemistry

RESEARCH EXPERIENCE

Clinical Research Assistant   2006 - 2007
    University of Oklahoma College of Medicine, Dept.
    of Medicine
    Supervised by James Rainer, M.D.

- Developed studies investigating safety and efficacy of new antibiotic in the treatment of *Pseudomonas aeruginosa*
- Strategized with leading infectious disease experts on development of study protocols
- Recruited patients directly and indirectly through collaboration with other centers participating in multi-center study
- Collected, analyzed, and interpreted safety and efficacy data in preparation for publication and presentation
- Prepared progress reports on all aspects of study projects and presented results at monthly research meetings

PUBLICATIONS

Hernandez RL, Miner ZH, Costanzo TL, Rainer JK. The antimicrobial action of compound X5432. *J Pharm Infec Dis* 2007; 43 (4): 54 - 59.

Costanzo TL, Roberts RR, Varicao CN, Hernandez RL, Rainer JK. Susceptibility of *P. aeruginosa* to compound X5432. *J Antimic Thera* 2007; 22 (3): 456 - 462.

PROFESSIONAL MEMBERSHIPS

Vice-President, AMSA	2007 - Present
Member, IMIG	2005 - Present
Member, AMSA	2004 - Present

EXTRACURRICULAR ACTIVITIES

Intramural volleyball, soccer, and basketball   2004 - Present

Sample CV # 2, comments

Education: With few exceptions, CVs of residency applicants should begin with the education section. Robert has chosen to include his class rank here rather than in a separate honors and awards section. This is the preferred approach for applicants who have a single honor. For applicants with multiple honors and awards, a separate section is advisable. It is not necessary to include your class rank or GPA. If it's exceptional, though, it's worth mentioning.

Also important to note is that Robert will be finishing medical school in five years. Readers will want to know why. Unfortunately, Robert doesn't make that clear. Later, in the research experience section, we see that he has done one year of research. However, we still don't know if he took one year off to do this research or if he took time off for another reason. If time was taken for a one-year research experience, it should be clearly noted in the education section.

Research experience: Robert follows the education section with research experience. Since Robert's research experience is a strong point of his application, it is appropriate to follow with this section. Note the active verbs he uses to describe his responsibilities as a clinical research assistant. Many applicants use words such as "helped" or "assisted." In many cases, this minimizes their contributions, diminishing the impact of the CV.

Professional membership: In the professional membership section, note how Robert has led with his title rather than the organization name. In leading with his title of Vice-President of AMSA, Robert succeeds in highlighting his leadership role.

In addition to membership in AMSA, Robert is an IMIG member. Readers may not be familiar with IMIG, which is an abbreviation for the Internal Medicine Interest Group. It would have been better to avoid the abbreviation in this case.

Sample CV # 3

Ashutosh Verma, MBBS   342 Webster Ave
                                                             Detroit, MI 48231
                                                             313-834-6266
                                                             averma@gmail.com

---

EDUCATION

2007 (Sep)   Externship (Dermatology)
                  St. Joseph Hospital, Waco, Texas
                  • Interviewed and examined patients independently
                  • Formulated differential diagnosis and treatment plan
                  • Presented patients to faculty preceptor
                  • Wrote SOAP notes and prescriptions
                  • Delivered presentation on cutaneous leishmaniasis
                  • Published case report, "Pseudoporphyria due to
                    Sulindac"

2005-2007   Master of Public Health (MPH)
                  University of Missouri, Columbia, Missouri

1999-2004   MBBS
                  Bombay Medical College, Mumbai, India

LICENSURE/CERTIFICATION

2007 (July)   ECFMG certification
2007 (April)   USMLE Step 2 CS - passed
2007 (March)   USMLE Step 2 CK - passed (score of 238)
2006 (January)   USMLE Step 1 - passed (score of 245)

PUBLICATIONS

                  Verma AS, Silva I. Pseudoporphyria due to sulindac. *J Adv Derm*
                  2007; 31 (8): 41 - 43.

WORK EXPERIENCE

2004-2005   House Intern
              Bombay General Hospital, Mumbai, India
              • Rotated through the departments of internal medicine,
                surgery, pediatrics, obstetrics and gynecology, and
                emergency medicine
              • Conducted teaching programs for students

PROFESSIONAL MEMBERSHIPS

2005 - Present   American Association of Physicians from India—
                   Young Physicians Section

2005 - Present   Michigan Association of Physicians from India— Young
                   Physicians Section

2005 - Present   American Association of Family Medicine—
                   International Medical Graduate Section

EXTRACURRICULAR ACTIVITIES

Finished runner-up in the medical school table tennis competition

Sample CV # 3, Comments

Education: Note that Ashutosh is an international medical graduate. Since residency programs highly value U.S. clinical experience, Ashutosh has included his externship in the education section of his CV.

Note also that Ashutosh has used the term "externship" as the title of his rotation experience rather than "observership." The former refers to an experience in which there is hands-on patient care, while the latter is strictly observational. Make sure you use the proper term. If you are unsure, ask the institution through which you rotated.

He uses bullets as a professional way to organize his responsibilities at St. Joseph Hospital.

While he has used active verbs such as "interviewed," "formulated," and "published" to describe his responsibilities, he could have taken it one step further by also including numbers. In other words, how many patients did he interview and examine per half day? How many SOAP notes did he write?

In the education section, he elected to lead with his rotation or degree rather than the institution name. An alternative approach would have been to lead with the institution name. If the institution is highly regarded, consider starting with the name rather than the degree or rotation. If you choose this option, you must begin each educational experience in the same manner.

Licensure/certification: Ashutosh chose to follow the education section with the licensure/certification section. ECFMG status is of major interest to programs. Therefore, if you are ECFMG certified, it should be clearly stated in your CV.

If your USMLE scores are exceptional, as is the case here, include the scores in your CV. Otherwise, simply indicate that you have passed.

Work experience: Under work experience, he describes his responsibilities as an intern. Again, the inclusion of numbers would have strengthened this section.

Note: This CV is spread over two pages. At the top right corner of the second page, he has included his name and the page number. Contrast this with Sonia's CV (CV # 1).

Chapter 7
Letters of Recommendation

Letters of recommendation are a critical component of the residency application. The purpose of these letters is to demonstrate to programs that you have both the professional and personal qualities to succeed as a resident and, later, as a practicing physician. Since these letters are written by those who know you and the quality of your work, they offer programs a personalized view. In contrast to your transcript and USMLE scores, they supply programs with qualitative, rather than quantitative information, about your cognitive and non-cognitive characteristics. A number of studies have shown that behavior, attitude, and other non-cognitive skills are important predictors of resident success. As such, programs place great importance on these letters in evaluating your application.

Since you will not be directly writing these letters, it may seem as if you have no control over their content. In reality, you wield more influence than you realize.

Rule # 24   Letters of recommendation are extremely important in some specialties.

In a study of medical students at the University of Colorado, University of Utah, and Vanderbilt University, participants were asked to rate the importance of sixteen residency selection criteria (Brandenburg). While 65% of survey participants rated the letters of recommendation as extremely important, 35% felt that letters were either moderately, mildly, or not important at all. This underlines the misconceptions that students hold about the selection process.

A number of studies have looked at the importance of recommendation letters in the residency selection process. These studies have demonstrated that letters are an important factor in selecting candidates for interview and in the development of the program's rank list. These studies are summarized in the following table.

Letters of Recommendation: How important are they?

Study	What was found
In personal research performed by Greenburg, surgical residency program directors were surveyed (Greenburg). Directors were asked to rank the various factors they consider important when ranking candidates.	Recommendation letters from surgical faculty were the second most important factor following only the interview. Letters from nonsurgical faculty were fifth most important.
Questionnaire sent to all PM&R program directors in the United States asking about the relative importance of various application factors. Directors were asked to rate factors on a scale of 1 to 5 with 1 being unimportant and 5 being critical (DeLisa).	Letters of recommendation were the second most important candidate criteria (3.7 + 0.9) that program directors use as they complete their Match list, second only to the interview.
Questionnaire sent to 16 directors of psychiatry residency programs in Canada asking them to assess the importance of 32 criteria for selecting residents (Ross)	Most highly valued were the personal interview and letters of recommendation. Among the 32 criteria, recommendation letters from clinical faculty in the program director's specialty was 4th most important while letters from general clinical faculty were rated 9th in importance.
Questionnaire sent to emergency medicine program directors asking them to rank 20 application items on a scale of 1 to 5, with 5 being most important (Crane)	Letters of recommendation were fourth most important (mean score of 4.11) following emergency medicine rotation grades, interview, and clinical grades.
Review of every letter of recommendation for the emergency medicine residency program at the Christ Hospital during the 1998-1999 application cycle (Harwood)	Offered insight into the match list ranking process at one residency program. Letters of recommendation accounted for 16% of an applicant's score.
Survey sent to all radiology residency program directors asking them about the criteria that departments use for selecting their residents (Otero)	Letters of recommendation were the fourth most important criterion in selecting candidates for interview, behind USMLE scores, Dean's letter, and class rank.

Rule # 25   Read the instructions, because programs differ on their requested letters.

You must painstakingly read the instructions to determine exactly how many reference letters are needed. Programs, even within the same specialty, have different requirements. Programs may also ask applicants for a specific number of letters from faculty in the same specialty. For example, the otolaryngology residency program at the Loma Linda University Medical Center requires that at least two of the letters come from an otolaryngology faculty member. Check each program's website to ensure compliance with their policy.

Tip # 20

The number of letters you need may vary from program to program. Although most programs require three letters of recommendation, review the specific requirements of each program. Some programs request that a letter come from a particular department, rotation, or individual (e.g., chairman).

In general, I advise applicants NOT to submit more letters than are requested. In fact, ERAS only allows applicants to submit a maximum of four letters to any one program. If you are considering submitting an additional letter, make sure the letter will enhance your candidacy. In some cases, a compelling argument can be made for sending an additional letter:

> After submitting her ERAS application, Linda did an away elective at institution X. The faculty member Linda worked with was impressed with her performance and wrote a glowing letter of recommendation. Since the residency program at institution X was one of her top choices, I advised her to send this additional letter to the program as it was sure to carry great weight.

Although you can send no more than four letters to an individual program, you can send different combinations of letters to different programs. In other words, you can solicit as many letters as you like and then choose which three or four to send to a particular program. This is particularly helpful if you are applying to two different specialties.

Tip # 21

Don't assume that sending additional letters of recommendation will strengthen your application. There's an old saying—"The thicker the application, the thicker the student." If you "stuff your file" with extra letters, it may raise red flags. Programs may assume that you are trying to compensate for weak letters by offering quantity rather than quality. Before you send an additional letter, make sure you have a very good reason. Discuss it first with your advisor.

Tip # 22

While programs will often specify how many letters they require from faculty members in their specialty, some programs don't have any specific requirements. However, you must still send at least one letter written by a faculty member in that specialty. Programs like to see that you have worked with a faculty member in the field and impressed him. This may seem obvious, but some applicants fail to grasp this point.

Rule # 26   Request letters of recommendation at the end of the rotation, not in the summer following third year.

Most students start requesting letters of recommendation during the summer following the third year of medical school. While following the crowd is just fine, it is often to your advantage to ask earlier. Asking for a letter soon after a clerkship ends offers one major advantage. If the writer drafts the letter after the rotation, your accomplishments are fresh in the writer's mind. This letter can then be filed until needed. Don't worry if you haven't chosen a specialty yet. When it comes time to apply, you can always ask the writer to update the letter, incorporating information about your specialty choice and career goals. This plan avoids the following scenario:

"I'm sorry, but I won't be able to write you a letter of recommendation because I just don't remember you that well. After all, it's been almost a year since you worked with me. I hope you understand that, over the course of a year, I have 30 to 40 students. It's hard for me to remember all of them with enough detail to do the letter justice."

Tip # 23

Requests for a letter of recommendation may be denied if considerable time has passed since your last contact with the professor. To avoid this, ask for the letter at the end of the clerkship. An alternative approach is to keep in touch with the professor. Sending periodic e-mails about your progress and meeting to discuss your plans and goals are two easy ways to make sure you won't be forgotten.

I would add one caution. If you haven't met with your attending to review your performance, and haven't seen your evaluation, then you can't know for sure how he feels about you. A colleague of mine, as a student, felt that she had done an excellent job on her sub-internship. She worked hard, read extensively, and requested a letter of recommendation at the end of the rotation. She had never had a mid-rotation feedback meeting, or an end of clerkship meeting, nor had she yet received her written evaluation. The letter ultimately included this sentence: "Mary was a very enthusiastic, hard-working student. She received a high pass for the rotation."

The best time to request a letter is at the end of the rotation, after the end of clerkship meeting. During this meeting, your attending will review your performance and your grade. Some attendings don't initiate such meetings, but they're very important. You can always request this meeting yourself. "Dr. Thompson, Friday is my last day. I was wondering if you might have some time to meet with me to review my performance on the rotation?" If you confirm during the meeting that your attending was impressed with your performance, you can end by asking for a letter of recommendation.

Rule # 27   Your letter writers can make your career, so choose the correct ones.

Your goal is to secure a glowing letter of recommendation. You'll never know exactly what a potential letter writer would say about you, so this poses a challenge. First, seek out attending physicians who gave you an honors evaluation. Because most students will be able to review their clerkship evaluations at the end of the rotation, this is straightforward. However, it's only the start. You must take into consideration a number of other issues. If you can answer the following questions with a "yes," then consider the individual to be a potential letter writer:

- Did I do well in the letter writer's rotation?
- Does the writer think highly of me?
- Did I work closely with the writer?
- Can the writer include specific experiences from our work together that reflect my strengths?
- Does the writer care about me and my future?
- Can he or she write a letter that will best reflect my background and strengths?
- Does the writer have good communication skills?
- Is the writer known to reliably meet deadlines?

We agree fully with the advice of Dr.Greenburg of Brown University. In his article on recommendation letters, he writes that "students need to select someone whom they feel knows them and their performance well and who is concerned and committed enough to the student's career to write a well thought out, detailed, and positive appraisal of them. We have seen that some letters, written on behalf of excellent applicants, did not do them justice because their authors were brief, vague, and/or noncommittal" (Greenburg).

Did you know ...

In a survey of writers who wrote letters for applicants applying to a baccalaureate-M.D. program, participants were asked about how they would handle a request for a letter from an applicant with whom they had little contact (Mavis). 16% stated that they would write a letter, but that it would be generic, containing little detail. It's likely that many medical school faculty would do the same, an important point to note as you decide whom to ask for a letter.

Rule # 28   Request letters from medical school faculty.

Avoid asking residents, interns, family, friends, or basic science professors. Solicit letters from faculty members of U.S. medical schools who are familiar with your clinical skills. You may also choose to request a letter of recommendation from a faculty member you assisted in performing research, if he knows you well, and especially if you plan on making research a big part of what you do in the future. Faculty members in the departments of emergency medicine at the University of California San Diego and University of California Irvine wrote that "research mentors can provide effective letters of recommendation, assuming they also know the clinical skills of the applicant" (Loftipour). Your other letters of recommendation, however, must come from clinical faculty.

Tip # 24

Before you request a letter from a resident or a private physician, consider the words of Dr. Mark Farnie, director of the internal medicine/pediatrics residency program at the University of Texas Medical School at Houston, who wrote that "letters of recommendation from private physicians or part-time faculty, and letters from residents are generally discounted."
—2003 University of Texas-Houston Medical School Career Counseling Catalog

Did you know ...

Directors of 102 internal medicine residency programs were surveyed to determine the most important predictors of performance for international medical graduates (Gayed). Directors were asked to rate the importance of 22 selection criteria. Rated lowest were letters of recommendation from a foreign country. "Only 7% of the program directors disagreed with the statement that such letters are useless." In another words, 93% of the program directors agreed that such letters were useless. The results of this study confirm that international medical graduates are better served by submitting letters of recommendation from U.S. faculty.

Rule # 29   Choose a writer who knows how to write a letter of recommendation.

Writing effective letters of recommendation is both an art and a science. Unfortunately, few faculty members have received training in this area. Your letter writer should be aware of the norms of letter writing by persons of professional standing. Also of importance is the person's writing ability. A professor may have very positive things to say about you, but if he can't express himself well, he won't be able to effectively convey his favorable views.

How can you possibly learn about a professor's writing ability? Examine your clerkship evaluation. Pay close attention to how well the attending has worded your evaluation. A favorable evaluation that has been eloquently worded suggests a comparable letter. If at all possible, ask upperclassmen about their experience.

Rule # 30   Choose a writer who actually cares about your career.

When choosing among possible writers, select faculty members who care about you and your future. Such faculty members will spend the time and energy necessary to write an effective, well thought out, and carefully written letter. They will be committed to you and your goals, and will want to provide you with whatever assistance is needed in order to help you succeed. Ideally, they will also be available to handle any phone inquiries from the residency program.

At every medical school, there are many professors who have a sincere interest in mentoring, advising, and helping their students reach their professional goals. As you progress through clerkships, have your radar up for these faculty members. Some will be easy to spot, such as the professor who is so impressed with your performance that he volunteers to write you a letter of recommendation. With others, question if the professor has shown interest in your work, goals, and plans.

Tip # 25

If you haven't had the opportunity to work with someone whom you feel cares about you and your goals, ask upperclassmen and fellow students about faculty members who take an active interest in the careers of their students. Once you've identified these individuals, arrange to work with them.

Rule # 31   The professional status of a letter writer is important, but it isn't everything.

How important is the letter writer's professional status? Clearly it's an important consideration. A glowing letter written by a distinguished full professor carries more weight than one written by an associate professor. Likewise, a letter written by an associate professor is preferred over one written by an assistant professor. Clinical instructors and chief residents would be options of last resort. Many feel that an applicant should never request a letter from a resident.

Did you know ...

In one study, academic rank of the writer was found to be an important factor influencing the reviewer's ranking of the letter (Greenburg). 48% of the reviewers rated it as important.

Did you know ...

In a survey of program directors in four specialties (internal medicine, pediatrics, family medicine, surgery), it was learned that a candidate's likelihood of being considered was enhanced if there was a connection or relationship between the writer and residency program director (Villanueva). "In cases where there was both a connection between the faculty members and in-depth knowledge of the student (i.e., personal knowledge), the likelihood was that the student's application would be noted." In another survey, 54% of orthopedic surgery program directors felt that the most important aspect of a letter was that it was written by someone they knew (Bernstein).

Why does professional status matter? Acclaimed professors are likely to have developed relationships with faculty at other institutions. In fact, they often interact at conferences, collaborate on projects, and publish papers based on shared work. When program directors and members of the resident selection committee receive a strong letter of recommendation from a colleague whom they know and trust, it can make a tremendous difference. Obviously, the letter carries more weight than a similar letter from a junior faculty member whom they don't know. The following table taken from a survey of PM&R program directors supports this belief (DeLisa). This study showed that the "most important letters of recommendation were from a PM&R faculty member in the respondent's department, followed by the Dean's letter, and the PM&R chairman's letter."

Results of mean ratings of the importance of letters of recommendation in selecting residents		
	Mean	Standard deviation
Clinical PM&R faculty member in respondent's department	4.0	0.8
Dean's letter	3.7	1.0
Chairperson of a PM&R department	3.7	1.0

PM&R faculty member in a PM&R department other than the respondent's	3.6	0.9
Clinical faculty member in another specialty	3.0	0.7
Basic scientist's letter	2.6	0.8

From DeLisa JA, Jain, SS, Campagnolo DI. Factors used by physical medicine and rehabilitation residency training directors to select their residents. *Am J Phys Med Rehabil* 1994; 73: 152-156 - page 154.

Many people in the academic community also feel that it is easier to impress junior rather than senior faculty members. Although this isn't necessarily true, those reviewing your application may be operating under that assumption. If that's the case, a letter from a junior faculty member won't be given the same weight as one from a full professor.

Having said this, you may be tempted to request letters from renowned figures. Unless that individual knows you well, resist the temptation. A stellar letter written by a junior faculty member with whom you've had significant interaction is much better than a lukewarm letter written by a senior faculty member of high stature. Applicants often lose sight of this fact, thinking that a letter written by Professor Bigwig, irrespective of its content, will do wonders for their application. In reality, a lukewarm letter will weaken your application.

Requesting a letter of recommendation from a professor who knows you well may prevent a letter of "minimal assurance." Messner and Shimahara defined this as a letter "missing one or more of the following attributes: 1) specific distinguishing information about an applicant 2) information about an applicant's academic record 3) an evaluation or comparison of the applicant's traits or accomplishments" (Messner). In their study of letters written on behalf of 204 applicants to the Stanford University otolaryngology residency program, 13.2% and 10.8% of female and male applicants, respectively, had a letter of "minimal assurance."

Tip # 26

While name recognition and status is important, it does you no good to submit a neutral or lukewarm letter from a well-known or distinguished faculty member. It is far better to submit a strong letter from a less known junior faculty member.

Did you know …

In an article written by faculty in the departments of emergency medicine at the University of San Diego and University of California Irvine, the authors wrote that "an exceptional letter from a respected faculty member may sway residency program directors to offer an applicant with non-competitive scores and evaluations an interview due to the importance programs place on clinical abilities. Therefore, it is valuable for a student to orchestrate time to work with a well-known EM faculty member, such as program director or assistant program director, clerkship director, research director, or Chief/Chair" (Loftipour).

Did you know …

In the document titled "How to request a letter of recommendation," found on the website of the David Geffen School of Medicine at UCLA, advisors at that school state that "the ideal letter of recommendation is from an individual who:

Is a nationally recognized figure in your specialty of choice and is well known to other program directors in your field;

Has personally worked with you clinically;

Thinks you are a star; and

Came from the institution to which you are applying."

Rule # 32   Discuss your list of possible letter writers with your residency advisor or dean of student affairs.

Because they have counseled many students over the years, residency advisors and deans are often knowledgeable about professors who write great letters of recommendation. They may also steer you away from professors who are not good letter writers, including those who have missed deadlines in the past. Always discuss your list of possible letter writers with your advisor.

Tip # 27

Show your advisor or dean your list of potential letter writers. Ask them which of the professors on your list have been known to write timely, thoughtful, and positive letters.

Rule # 33 When asking for a letter, provide your writer with an out.

There is a right and a wrong way to request a letter of recommendation. Many students have approached us for a letter with "Could you write a letter of recommendation for me?" *Anyone* can write you a letter, but the key question is whether they know you well enough to write a *strong* letter of recommendation. The correct way to phrase the question is this: "Dr. Desai, do you feel you know me and my work well enough to write me a strong letter of recommendation?"

By phrasing the request in this manner, your letter writer can politely opt out if he doesn't feel comfortable writing you a letter. Don't despair. A negative or even lukewarm letter written and sent can sink your application. Count yourself lucky to avoid that fate.

Even if a writer says that he will support your application with a letter, gauge their level of commitment. If they seem hesitant or ambivalent, then the recommendation letter may not be as positive as it could be. In this case, simply thank them for their time and let them know that you will ask another professor.

Tip # 28

Don't just ask for a letter of recommendation. Ask for a strong letter. Otherwise, you might have a faculty member simply agree to your request, not because he is a fervent supporter of your application, but because he feels it is another one of his many job responsibilities. This could lead to a poor letter.

Tip # 29

Writing an effective letter of recommendation takes time and effort. Not all letter writers are able to make that type of commitment. You, of course, would like to know that up front. How can you find out?

Politely and delicately tell the letter writer that you realize he is busy, you understand how much effort and time it takes to write a letter, and you will understand if he can't make that commitment to you right now. This provides an easy way to opt out.

Rule # 34 Ask for a letter of recommendation in the correct fashion.

Never ask an individual for a letter of recommendation by:
- Asking in the hallway
- Passing a note under the door
- Leaving a note in the mailbox
- Asking him or her on the phone
- Leaving a voice mail message

- Sending an e-mail
- Approaching at a busy time, such as in between patients
- Making your request at the last minute

Doing any of the above is unprofessional and may make a difference in the strength of your recommendation letter. The best way to ask for a letter is by making an appointment.

"Dr. Murthy, I would like to meet with you for fifteen minutes to get some advice on my career plans. Would you be able to meet with me, and if so, when would be a good time?"

Remember that you are asking for a favor, one that takes time and effort. Don't take the request lightly. Be sensitive, polite, cordial, and formal.

Asking for a letter of recommendation in person also allows you another advantage—you can gauge the professor's level of interest in writing the letter. If you have any doubts at all about the letter writer, you must meet face to face. If there is any hesitancy, indifference, reluctance, or aversion on the letter writer's part, it will be more apparent to you in person than by phone or e-mail. Should this occur, simply thank the letter writer for his time and move on to the next potential writer on your list.

Tip # 30

Always ask for a letter of recommendation in person. Why? Not only is it more polite but it offers several other advantages. A face to face meeting reminds the faculty member of who you are and how you excelled. And last, but certainly not least, it allows you to gauge the person's response to your request.

Rule # 35   Empty praise means nothing. Your job is to provide the evidence that backs up the adjectives.

Unfortunately, many letters, while complimentary, are simply full of adjectives. They lack examples, stories, and anecdotes that support the adjectives used. Letters that include evidence to support the writer's opinions are much more effective and powerful than letters that simply praise. Details often convince the reader that the praise is actually true.

Typical recommendation: Lisa's intellectual curiosity was refreshing. In fact, few of my medical students have been as inquisitive. During rounds, this quality enriched the entire team's educational experience.

Powerful recommendation: Lisa's intellectual curiosity was refreshing. In fact, few of my medical students have been as inquisitive. During rounds, this quality enriched the entire team's educational experience. For example, she performed a literature search on a relatively newly described microorganism, Leclercia adecarboxylata, after our team took care of a pyelonephritis patient whose urine grew out this organism. Her search revealed that there were 21 published articles on this organism. She not only brought us each one of these abstracts, but she even had one article, which was published in French, translated to English.

To maximize the chances that your letter writers will provide evidence to support their opinions, choose writers who know you well enough that they can include specific anecdotes. Examples of evidence:

- She performed a literature search on a newly described microorganism.

- She was a great source of comfort to a family with newly diagnosed breast cancer. She provided patient information booklets from the hospital library, and when the patient expressed interest in attending a support group, investigated the options. The family wrote a heartfelt note of thanks at the end of the patient's stay.

- He was very enthusiastic about the learning process, and early in the rotation expressed his interest in writing a case report. When I identified a potential case, he had a first draft ready within 72 hours, with a full discussion, references, and very few revisions needed.

- I had asked for a volunteer to make a short presentation on diagnostic techniques for pulmonary embolism. He was the first to volunteer, and a few days later gave an outstanding presentation on the topic. He even provided handouts and an excellent reference article.

- As a sub-intern, she had a heavy case load and many duties. However, she clearly made quite an effort to help guide and educate the third year students on the team.

Rule # 36   You cannot tell your letter writer what to say. However, there are professional ways in which you can emphasize your strengths and the evidence that backs those up.

Most applicants assume that their letter writers know what to say. That's a dangerous assumption to make. In an analysis of 116 recommendation letters received by the radiology residency program at the

University of Iowa Hospitals and Clinics (O'Halloran), reviewers noted the following points:

- 10% of letters were missing information about an applicant's cognitive knowledge
- 35% of letters had no information about an applicant's clinical judgment
- 3% of letters did not discuss an applicant's work habits
- 17% of letters did not comment on the applicant's motivation
- 32% of letters were lacking information about interpersonal communication skills

In another review of recommendation letters sent during the 1999 application season to the Department of Surgery at Southern Illinois University, writers infrequently commented on psychomotor skills such as "easily performed minor procedures at the bedside," "good eye-hand coordination in the OR," "could suture well," and so on (Fortune).

If you simply assume that a letter writer knows precisely what to say about you, you may be doing yourself a disservice. To increase the chances that your letter writer will submit a letter commenting on those qualities valued by programs in your chosen specialty, you must first determine these qualities. In the following table, we have included qualities valued by program directors in four specialties (Villanueva).

Skills and personal qualities frequently identified by residency program directors in defining an applicant's "fit"	
Family Medicine	Good communicator
	Interpersonal skills
	Team player
	Lifelong learning skills
	Empathic
	Interested in community practice
	Non-judgmental
	Active in the program
	Experience with underserved populations
Internal Medicine	Good communicator
	Interpersonal skills
	Team player
	Hands-on patient care
	Potential positive impact upon program
	Reliable and stable
	Warm and humane
	Demonstrated commitment to specific area (music, sports)
	Well-organized
	Ability to get along with others
	Resourceful

Pediatrics	Good communicator
	Interpersonal skills
	Team player
	Well-organized
	Well-rounded
	Mature
	Independent
	Sense of professionalism
	Flexible (ability to change)
	Enthusiastic
	Ability to cope with stress and change
	Positive attitude (views glass "half full")
Surgery	Good communicator
	Compulsive
	Neat
	High energy
	Honest and straightforward
	Confident
	Hardworking
	Demonstrated commitment to specific area (music, sports)

From Villanueva AM, Kaye D, Abdelhak SS, Morahan PS. Comparing selection criteria for residency directors and physicians' employers. *Acad Med* 1995; 70(4): 261-271.

If you are applying to a surgical residency, it would be great if your letter writer commented on your ability to perform procedures, suture in the OR, and maintain a high level of energy. However, directly asking the writer to comment on your abilities in these areas is presumptuous, and will be viewed negatively.

A more professional approach is to list patient encounters from your rotation. Include those encounters that highlight your strengths in these areas, and emphasize how these patient encounters impacted your training.

Sample patient list

Dear Dr. Tung,

During our month together, I cared for a number of patients. Below are a few of these patients, along with my role in their care and the impact these patients had on my training:

1) Mr. Jordan—72 year old male with dementia who was hospitalized with small bowel obstruction due to adhesions from previous surgery. Managing the bowel obstruction was challenging because Mr. Jordan sometimes became agitated, particularly at night. On three occasions, he pulled out his nasogastric tube. I had the opportunity to reinsert the tube each time and became quite comfortable inserting these tubes.

I also learned how to better evaluate delirium in a patient with dementia.

2) Ms. Hernandez—52 year old female with alcoholic cirrhosis who developed spontaneous bacterial peritonitis following incision and drainage of a skin abscess. To confirm the diagnosis, I was given the opportunity to perform the paracentesis under the supervision of Dr. Jones. Analysis of the ascitic fluid revealed findings consistent with monomicrobial bacterial ascites, prompting us to repeat the procedure 48 hours later. After performing the second tap, we were able to diagnose him with spontaneous bacterial peritonitis when his neutrophil count returned > 250.

3) Mr. Fozio—64 year old male with history of intravenous drug abuse who was admitted with appendicitis. Shortly after admission, his IV fell out. The nurses on the floor had difficulty inserting a new IV. Understandably, Mr. Fozio was quite upset with these failed attempts and was reluctant to have anyone try again. After much discussion, he agreed to let me try. Having had considerable experience placing IVs as part of a hospital IV team before starting medical school, I was able to successfully insert the IV and build great rapport with the patient. I was thereafter known on our team as the "IV man."

I learned so much during my rotation, from these patients, from others, and from your teaching. Thank you very much for your teaching and for your letter of recommendation, and please let me know if you need any further information.

Sincerely,

Jorge Rubio

An attending reading the above might be inclined to comment on your ability to perform procedures. If he had forgotten about your involvement in Mr. Jordan's care, your list will help to jog his memory. You should never assume that the writer remembers as much as you do.

This approach may facilitate the development of a letter highlighting certain skills or qualities. Include these examples in the letter of recommendation packet you give to your writers.

Tip # 31

In a survey of program directors in 14 specialties, directors were asked to rank the importance of six personal and professional characteristics (Wagoner). Compatibility with the program was highest. This was followed by commitment to hard work, fund of knowledge, empathy and compassion, and communication skills. Provide your letter writers with patient examples that highlight your strengths in these areas.

Rule # 37 Faint praise is just as bad as no praise.

If your letter writer shares the letter with you, examine it carefully. It's a given that the writer will praise you. However, you need to be vigilant for faint praise. This is defined as praise that appears positive at first glance, but may not be viewed as such by a residency program. In an article discussing letters of recommendation for pediatric residency applicants, Dr. Morgenstern of the Mayo Clinic wrote that "some words, seemingly positive, are often considered red flags. Calling a student's performance very good, or solid, may be viewed by program directors as a warning to avoid ranking the student very highly" (Morgenstern). Below are other examples:

Faint praise—What does it really mean?	
Statement	**Translation**
"Shilpa's write-ups were solid."	Shilpa's write-ups were solid but not exceptional in any way.
"Roberto's knowledge base was above average."	Roberto's knowledge base was above average but not very far above average.
"Glen's oral case presentations clearly improved throughout the course of the rotation."	Glen's oral case presentations were subpar to begin with and required considerable work.
"As far as I am aware …"	I don't want to wholeheartedly back this applicant because I don't know him that well.

Using the word "improved" can also be considered a red flag. While every student would be expected to show improvement during the course of a rotation, apparently the inclusion of the word "improved" suggests that the writer did not feel that the applicant was very strong in that area.

Notice how these comments on the surface seem to say good things about an applicant. However, the use of the above adjectives, rather than stronger ones, may lead the reader to wonder why the writer wasn't more enthusiastic about his choice of words.

As an applicant, you may wonder why your letter writer would "damn you with faint praise." While faint praise may be intentional, more often than not its use is entirely unintentional. Some writers are simply unaware that an unofficial hierarchy of superlatives exists. These well-intentioned writers may wish to give their highest recommendation to an applicant, but may unknowingly use an adjective considered by program directors to be a second or third-tier superlative.

Dr. Fortune of Southern Illinois University, in his article analyzing the content of recommendation letters, described this unofficial hierarchy of superlatives (Fortune). He commented on the fact that letter writers will often sum up an applicant using a particular adjective as in "Randy will make an exceptional house officer." He categorized these adjectives as shown:

Single adjective summary	
Outstanding	Outstanding, superior, exceptional, best, phenomenal
Excellent	Excellent, superb, great, terrific, wonderful
Good	Good, strong, solid, fine, valuable, splendid
OK	Asset, successful, delightful, distinguished, capable, effective, qualified, well rounded
From Fortune JB. The content and value of letters of recommendation in the resident candidate evaluative process. *Curr Surg* 2002; 59 (1): 79-83.	

Fortune also writes about how writers generally provide, usually in the last paragraph, an indication of their comfort level of recommendation for the candidate. Examples include "enthusiastically recommend," "give my outstanding recommendation," and "without reservation I recommend." These qualifiers are categorized below:

Level of recommendation	
Highest	Highest, most enthusiastically, wholeheartedly, strongest, outstanding, stellar, superior
Strongly	Strongly, highly, enthusiastically, heartily, very highly excellent
Without reservation	Without reservation, no hesitation, unqualified
Recommend	Recommend, no hesitation, unqualified, comfortable, support, endorse, pleased
From Fortune JB. The content and value of letters of recommendation in the resident candidate evaluative process. *Curr Surg* 2002; 59 (1): 79-83.	

The risk of faint praise emphasizes two points. To avoid being the recipient of faint praise, always ask the letter writer if he feels comfortable writing you a strong letter of recommendation. While an enthusiastic "yes" does not offer any guarantees, it significantly reduces the risk. Secondly, if you view a letter that includes faint praise, seek out additional letter writers.

Did you know ...

In a study evaluating the content of recommendation letters, the comment, "I hope we can attract ___ to our own residency," was viewed very favorably (Greenburg). On the other hand, the commonly used phrase, "If I can provide any additional information, please call ..." was generally viewed as a negative comment. It was believed that its inclusion meant that the letter writer had additional things to say but did not feel comfortable discussing them in the letter.

Did you know ...

In a review of letters written on behalf of applicants to the Stanford University otolaryngology residency program, the authors wrote about how disclosure of a personal relationship between the letter writer and applicant could affect the way in which the letter is viewed. "Disclosed personal relationships... can also raise doubt in a reader's mind, constituting a doubt raiser (e.g., 'I coached him in little league,' 'I have known his parents for many years'). While the letter writer is appropriately stating his/her credentials to evaluate the candidate, revelations such as these lead to questions in the reader's mind whether the recommendation is impartial or based on a personal relationship" (Messner).

Rule # 38   Short letters of recommendation may harm you.

In a review of 966 letters of recommendation sent during the 1999 application process to the Department of Surgery at Southern Illinois University, the average length of the recommendation letter was 13.7 sentences, with a range of 4 to 36 sentences (Fortune). Is there any correlation between the length of a letter and its value to program directors?

In a study designed to determine the aspects of letters that programs find useful for screening and selection, the letters which received the best scores were generally twice as long (363 versus 150 words) as those letters rated lowest (Greenburg). This makes sense, as letters that contain stories and anecdotes to support a writer's praise will be longer than letters that simply praise.

Tip # 32

If your letter writer shares the letter with you, pay attention to its length. If it's too short, you may not wish to submit it.

Rule # 39   The chair's letter may be critical to your application. Plan accordingly, especially if you've never even met the chair.

Some residency programs either mandate or recommend that one of your letters come from the department chairman. If you have worked closely with the chairman during a clinical or research rotation and performed at a high level, this won't be a problem. Approach the chairman the same way you would any other faculty member.

However, many students haven't had the opportunity to interact with, let alone work with, the chairman. Don't worry if you've never met the chairman. Departments understand that many students interested in their specialty won't have had this opportunity. They typically have a policy in place for the writing of the chair's letter. To determine the policy at your school, call the department office.

Depending on the program, the chairman or his designee will write the letter. In order to do so, the chairman will typically ask for a CV, review your clerkship evaluation forms, and meet with you to learn more about you and your goals. Treat any meeting with the chairman as you would a formal interview. Bring with you any supporting materials that might be useful in the development of your letter, such as copies of journal articles or summaries of presentations.

Did you know ...

In a survey sent to internal medicine program directors, directors were asked to rate the usefulness of various components of the residency application (Adams). 79% of survey participants rated the chairman's letter as highly or moderately useful for interview decisions, and 77% rated it as highly or moderately useful for ranking decisions.

Why would programs place such importance on the chairman's letter, given that most students don't even work with the chairman? In the article "Factors used by program directors to select residents," Wagoner and Suriano offered some possible reasons (Wagoner). They "speculated that the chairman is perceived as feeling less compelled to act as an advocate for the student and can, therefore, present a more factual portrayal of the student's performance in courses of that specialty. Further, because department chairmen are often in personal contact with each other by telephone and at professional meetings, the authors believe that it is important to the program directors to maintain their credibility with each other by giving credible evaluations."

Rule # 40   Waive your right to review the letter.

In 1974, with the passage of the Family Educational Rights and Privacy Act (FERPA), students were given some important rights regarding their educational records. These rights, which also apply to letters of recommendation, include the following:

- Students have the right to inspect their educational records.
- Students have the right to challenge any information in the educational records that they feel is inaccurate or incorrect.
- Students have the right to keep the educational records private or confidential.

With the granting of these rights, no institution can force you to waive these rights. It is fairly standard, however, for students to be given a form in which they are asked to indicate whether they waive or retain the right to review the recommendation letter. Before making the decision, review the following table, which discusses the advantages and disadvantages of waiving your right to see the letter.

Advantages of retaining your rights	Advantages of waiving your rights
By knowing the content of the letter, you will know exactly what the residency program knows about you.	You will have no need to explain why you retained your rights, if asked in an interview.
You will have less stress and anxiety because you know the contents of the letter.	The letter writer may not write you a letter if you have retained your right to view the letter.
You will be able to identify mistakes before the letter is sent. You can then give the writer an opportunity to correct these errors.	The selection committee may feel that the letter is more candid because you waived your rights.
You can use the comments in the letter to maintain your strengths and work on your weaknesses.	The selection committee may feel that you have nothing to hide and that you are not concerned about what the faculty member might say.
You can make sure that an unfavorable letter is not sent.	The letter writer may be less inhibited in praising you if you have waived your right.

Most advisors, including ourselves, recommend that applicants waive their right to review the letter. In a study cited previously, a review of letters written on behalf of 204 applicants to the Stanford University otolaryngology residency program in 2006 found that only one applicant "was recorded as 'not waiving' her right to see the letters" (Messner). Many residency programs consider confidential letters to have greater credibility. Because of this, they may be given greater weight in the application process. When rights are not waived, programs may assume that you only sent letters that painted you in a very positive light.

If you are reluctant to waive your rights, consider the reasons for your reluctance. If you have heeded the advice in this chapter, you can be very confident that the letter writers you have chosen will write you a strong letter of recommendation, in which case you should feel comfortable waiving your right to review the letter. If there is any concern that the writer may submit a letter that is not flattering or frankly negative, then you shouldn't be asking that individual for a letter of recommendation.

Tip # 33

Waiving your right to see the letter of recommendation does not prohibit you from reading your letter if the writer chooses to share it with you. However, if you've waived your right to see the letter, then don't ask to see the letter. That would be poor etiquette, and you risk annoying the letter writer. If the writer offers to show it to you, however, then by all means accept.

Tip # 34

If you have applied for a research grant, award, or scholarship during medical school, you may have been asked to submit letters of recommendation as part of the application process. Think back to that time. Were you asked to sign a waiver? If not, you should have full access to the letters of recommendation. You may even have been asked to submit the letters along with the rest of the application, in which case you may have the letters in your possession. Review the letters to gauge their strength. Since writers will often use a previous letter as a template for future letters, you will know which letter writers will be most supportive of your residency application.

Rule # 41   Do not hesitate to ask for a letter of recommendation.

Students are often hesitant to approach professors to ask for letters. Some students feel they are imposing. However, faculty members realize that this is just one of their many professional responsibilities. Professors expect to be asked to write letters for good students. Other students are hesitant because they fear refusal. If the letter writer refuses, what's the worst that could happen? You just move on to the next person on your list of potential letter writers.

> **Did you know ...**
>
> Letter writers can do more than write a letter. If a writer ever asks you "Is there any other way I can be of assistance?" always respond with a "yes." Can they conduct a mock interview with you? Do they know anyone on the faculty of your top-choice programs? Would they be willing to give them a call on your behalf?

Rule # 42   In this section, perhaps more than any other, you cannot procrastinate.

In this section, perhaps more than any other, you cannot procrastinate. You do not have the ability to make up for lost time, as your letters are not under your direct control. Students often procrastinate when deciding whom to ask and how to ask for a letter of recommendation. Procrastination makes things much more difficult. Professors who may have been willing to write a letter may not be able to do so when asked on short notice. Provide the writer with adequate time, preferably one to two months, to write the letter. Professors have other tasks and responsibilities, so contact them as early as possible.

> **Tip # 35**
>
> Don't procrastinate when it comes to asking for letters of recommendation. Faculty members expect to be asked to write these letters. However, giving short notice is not only poor form; it also increases your risk of a suboptimal letter.

Rule # 43   Don't even bother asking for a letter unless the writer has sufficient time to do an outstanding job.

As a general rule, you should give the letter writer at least one to two months to write and send the letter. If possible, give the letter writer more time. Nothing is more irritating than being asked to write a letter of recommendation under pressure. Remember that letter writers do have other responsibilities. You don't want them to do shoddy work, which you risk if you don't provide enough advance notice.

Rule # 44   Always provide all of the relevant information.

Even if a professor tells you that he will write a strong letter of recommendation, the letter may turn out to be mediocre. Many professors are just not proficient at writing effective letters. They may lack a firm understanding of what residency programs are seeking, or may not know how to advocate strongly for their students. For example, a well-intentioned letter writer may produce a letter full of generalities. Although the overall tone and content will be supportive, a letter that is short on specifics that back up the praise will do little to differentiate you from other candidates.

Tip # 36

Larkin wrote that "some writers invest significant time and effort into writing an accurate narrative with examples and evidence to support their conclusions. Others write quickly and superficially, in generic, nonverifiable terms that seem to lack substance" (Larkin).

Therefore, you need to make it as easy as possible for the writer to produce a strong letter of recommendation. You can do so by providing the writer with a packet, containing the following:

- Cover letter thanking them for writing your letter, along with a summary of the packet's contents (see following example)

- Your reasons for applying to the specialty

- Anecdotes, stories, and examples from your rotation together (see Rule # 36)

- Curriculum vitae (CV)

- Personal statement

- Transcript

- Clerkship evaluation form completed by the letter writer

- Write-up or other assignment given a high grade or evaluation by the same professor

- Ways to reach you in the event more information is required or a question arises

- Deadline

If you are applying through the Electronic Residency Application Service (ERAS), you will also need to provide each writer with the ERAS Cover Sheet. On this sheet are instructions for the letter writer. The letter will be attached to the cover sheet and sent to your designated medical school office where it can be scanned into your electronic file. If you are applying through the Common Application Service (San Francisco Match), you will have to obtain your letter directly from the writer in a sealed envelope to include as part of your application. If you will need the letter writer to mail the letter directly, then you should provide stamped envelopes with neatly typed addresses of the residency programs.

Sample cover letter

Dear Dr. Egbert,

Thank you for writing me a letter of recommendation for orthopedic surgery residency. I know how busy you are, and I sincerely appreciate your support of my application. I am including additional information to help you as you write the letter. Included are the following:

- This cover letter
- CV
- Personal statement
- Two write-ups that you reviewed during my clerkship
- Handout from the talk I gave on pulmonary embolism
- Several cases from our month together that impacted my training

I am hoping to have my entire application completed by September 15. If you have any questions or require any other materials from me, please let me know. I can be reached by phone (555-1212) or e-mail (lisa.ray@gmail.com).

Thank you,

Lisa Ray

This packet provides the writer with all the facts needed to write an effective letter. The information in the packet will help the writer include specifics and examples that convince the reader that the praise is true. We agree with the words of Dr. Loftipour, a faculty member in the department of emergency medicine at the University of California Irvine, who wrote that "the easier the letter-writing process is, the more positive the letter is likely to be" (Loftipour).

Tip # 37

If you are applying to two or more specialties, make sure that your letter writer is recommending you for the right specialty.

Rule # 45   You may be asked to write your own letter of recommendation. We recommend that you don't.

Don't be surprised if you encounter a professor who asks you to draft your own letter of recommendation. While some students are disappointed or even insulted by this type of response, others view it as an incredible opportunity. If you are presented with the opportunity to write your own letter, you may choose to accept the offer. Do so with great caution, and only after deliberation, for the following reasons:

- By asking you to write the letter, the professor has already made it clear to you that he is not that enthusiastic about you and your application. What will this individual say if a selection committee member calls to ask more questions?

- You probably haven't been asked to write a letter of recommendation before. Having the ability to write a strong letter of recommendation is not an innate ability—it is one that is learned through practice. Letters of recommendation written by seasoned professors have a certain tone and perspective. Your inexperience may result in the development of a weak letter.

- A letter that you write may end up being similar to your personal statement and may not add much to your application. In contrast, letter writers who use their own words will offer multiple perspectives on your performance, achievement, and strengths.

- Some application reviewers view this act as unethical.

Tip # 38

If your letter writer asks you to draft your own letter of recommendation, consider the negatives. Program directors, having seen thousands of letters, may be able to spot a letter written by an applicant. This may lead the director to call the letter writer. If it is learned that you wrote the letter and the professor merely signed it, you risk having your application taken out of consideration. In a survey of family practice directors inquiring about candidate deception, it was learned that 15% of deceptive acts were related to the letter of recommendation (Grover). While the article did not describe these acts of deception in any detail, writing your own letter may be viewed as such.

Rule # 46 Your work does not end once you request a letter.

Your work does not end with requesting the letter. You must make sure the letter is sent, and sent by the deadline. When making your initial request, be clear about the deadline for receipt of the recommendation letters. To make sure that the letters are sent before the deadline, consider doing the following:

- Stopping by the professor's office with thank you cards several weeks before the deadline. This will serve as a reminder to complete and send the letter.

- Include in the packet a single sheet of paper that states "The deadline for this letter is ___."

- Sending an e-mail about 10-14 days before the deadline saying "I'm just following up with you on the letter of recommendation you so kindly agreed to write for me. I wanted to see if I could provide you with any other information, or if you had any questions for me."

- Calling the student affairs office or visiting the Applicant Document Tracking System in MyERAS. Never assume that your letters of recommendation have been sent. Always verify.

The deadline you give the letter writer need not be the program's final deadline. Instead, it is acceptable to give the writers your own deadline, which you may arbitrarily decide is several weeks before the actual deadline. This extra cushion of time can be very useful if problems arise.

The above recommendations offer suggestions for how a student can offer letter writers gentle reminders of approaching deadlines. It is important not to harass or annoy your letter writers. Handle the situation with tact to avoid a less than stellar letter.

Tip # 39

There are some professors who always seem to be disorganized or running late. Clerkship directors, for example, will tell you that it can be very difficult to get certain faculty members to complete their evaluation forms on time. If you have ever had this experience with a professor, think twice before asking for a letter of recommendation. Every year, programs delay reviewing applications only because a single letter is missing. Should this happen, it may prevent you from landing an interview. If you must have a letter written by someone who has difficulty meeting deadlines, ask early and check in often with the writer.

Rule # 47   Say "Thank you."

When you're caught up in the stress and anxiety of completing applications, then interviewing, then making critical decisions about your future, it's easy to forget about the people who got you this far. You must convey your appreciation for all of their work, because they deserve to know. You must also provide them with follow up on your career plans, because faculty are always interested in their students' successes. And while you may think that once medical school is done, it's over, you may need the assistance of your mentors and letter writers in the future.

After the recommendation letters have been sent, send each of your letter writers a personal thank-you note. In your note, express your appreciation for their support. You should also provide your letter writers with follow up. Let them know how the application process is going, and ultimately, where you match.

Tip # 40

As you progress through residency, stay in touch with your letter writers. This doesn't involve tremendous effort or time on your part.
A short e-mail or postcard with a comment or two about your progress will suffice. Your letter writer has shown a desire to help you, and the time may come when his assistance will be needed again.

Chapter 8

Personal Statement

The most dreaded aspect of the residency application, for most students, is the personal statement. It's very frustrating trying to put into words your vision for your medical career.

Most students don't understand one basic fact about the personal statement, though. Unlike just about every other aspect of the application, you have complete control over the personal statement. You decide the content, the structure, and the form of the statement. This is a unique opportunity to impress the selection committee. In your statement you can showcase your strengths and those qualities that set you apart from other candidates. You can weave in evidence that confirms your qualities. You can use this opportunity to convince a faculty member that you would be an ideal candidate for their particular program. This is information that is not readily apparent to programs from their review of other application components.

With sufficient time and effort, you can create a personal statement that effectively sells yourself to the residency program. While a well-written statement can strengthen your application, a poorly written one can eliminate you from further consideration, even if you are at the top of your class.

Rule # 48   Recognize the importance of the personal statement to some specialties.

Individual specialties, residency programs, and application reviewers assign varying degrees of importance to the personal statement. In the screening phase, reviewers whittle down a large applicant pool to a select group that is ultimately extended interview invitations. Applicants often believe that the personal statement is used minimally, if at all, during this screening phase. While this is true at some programs, it is dangerous to assume that this is the case with all programs. For example, at the website for the University of Washington Family Medicine Residency, the "personal statement is the primary component that will be used to select applicants who are invited for an interview. Please write a careful and thoughtful document." In fact, a 1993 study of family practice residency program directors showed that the personal statement ranked second only to the Dean's letter for making decisions about whom to interview (Taylor). With regard to the ranking of applicants, it was third in importance, following only the interview and the Dean's letter.

Several studies have shown that competitive specialties give less weight to the personal statement. The study performed by Taylor showed that obstetrics and gynecology program directors differed from their family practice colleagues in the importance they attached to the personal statement, ranking it last in importance. The personal statement was also found to be least important in a survey of emergency medicine program directors (Crane).

It is important to realize, however, that within a competitive specialty, some programs will attach greater importance to the personal statement than others. At the Wake Forest University radiology residency program (Chew), readers use the personal statement along with the rest of the application to place candidates into one of five groups—interview (high priority), interview (normal priority), interview (low priority), hold for additional information, and do not interview (reject). The University of Texas-Houston Department of Orthopedic Surgery states that the "personal statement is read by each of our orthopedic faculty members, and is considered by our faculty to be a very important part of the application process. It is often used as a point of departure for interviewing the student" (www.uth.tmc.edu/med/administration/student/ms4/2003CCC.htm).

Otherwise excellent candidates have been ranked lower, or even rejected, because of a poorly written statement. In the words of the University of Alabama at Birmingham (UAB) department of obstetrics and gynecology, "poorly written personal statements may detract from an otherwise excellent application" (http://www.obgyn.uab.edu/medical-students/obgyn/uasom/documents/2005ResidencyGuidelines.pdf).

Tip # 41

Some specialties, programs, and application reviewers attach great importance to the personal statement, while others may only glance at it. You'll have no way of knowing how your personal statement will be read or weighted.

Did you know ...

Offering advice to the dermatology residency applicant, Dr. Heymann wrote that "assuming the consummate applicant has impeccable curriculum vitae, letters, and grades, the personal statement takes on immense importance. Who is this person? Is it someone I want to meet face-to-face? Tell me about yourself candidly. What do you want to contribute to the discipline in the course of your professional lifetime? In short, make me want to meet you" (Heymann).

Rule # 49 Programs don't always want a generic statement. Read the instructions.

While many programs give applicants complete control over the statement's content, some programs do ask the applicant to address specific questions or issues. At the website for the San Francisco General Hospital internal medicine residency (primary care track), applicants are asked to write "a personal statement specifically addressing why you want to work in a public hospital setting and care for a vulnerable and medically underserved population" (http://dgim.ucsf.edu/sfgh/Residency/residency.html). The dermatology residency program at the University of Utah informs applicants that the "personal statement should summarize how your qualifications and goals mesh with those of our Department" (http://uuhsc.utah.edu/derm/residency/residency.htm). At the website for the University of Oklahoma orthopedic surgery residency program (http://w3.ouhsc.edu/orthopedics/apply.asp), the following advice is given to applicants:

"It is desirable for the statement transmitted to our program to include information on:

1) Any involvement you have had with the State of Oklahoma or the surrounding region, the purpose being for you to consider and then translate to us why you believe you would be satisfied living and training in Oklahoma for five years.

2) Your class standing if your school ranks students.

3) An accounting for any breaks greater than three months in your education since high school."

Tip # 42

Before you write, carefully review any personal statement directions the program may have. While most programs leave the content of the statement completely up to you, others may make specific requests. Failure to follow the instructions may lead the program to assume you will have the same difficulty as a resident, removing your application from any further consideration.

Did you know ...

In their article "Crafting a Great Personal Statement," Drs. McGarry and Tammaro, program directors of the internal medicine residency at Brown Medical School wrote that "a great personal statement will make the program director eager to meet you and potentially work with you... A poorly written PS can cast doubt on your dedication and focus for a demanding profession like medicine...The PS that falls between these two extremes may be neutral in its overall effect, but represents a missed opportunity to add luster to your candidacy...While no personal statement can substitute for an excellent academic record throughout medical school, it may help you and your application stand out from the pack and win you an invitation to interview or gain a few points on a program's rank list." (McGarry)

Rule # 50   Know your audience. Convince them that you embody the qualities that they are seeking in a future resident.

Before drafting your personal statement, consider your audience. Your audience is the residency program director, your interviewers, and other members of the selection committee. An effective personal statement must focus on what the audience is seeking. In this case, the reviewers seek to learn more about you as an individual to help them determine if you have the qualities they are seeking in a future resident. What are they seeking in a future resident? How can you convince them that you embody these qualities?

There are several ways to make a convincing argument. Consider addressing the following questions in your personal statement:

● **Why did I choose this specialty?**

Programs seek deeply committed residents. Therefore, they are interested in learning about the factors that led you to pursue the specialty. What is it about the specialty that appeals to you? Is it the nature of the work? Is it the intellectual challenge? Were you motivated by a personal, family, or clinical experience, or a combination thereof? Give specific reasons why you are interested in the specialty. In answering this question, show them that you are deeply committed to the field. There should be no ambiguity. If you are unable to communicate a clear understanding of, or commitment to, the specialty, your application may be removed from further consideration.

We emphasize that you should be writing about the factors that led you to pursue the specialty, with the emphasis on *you*. As Dr. Oldham, the program director of the radiology program at the University of Texas Medical School at Houston, writes: "...please do not regale me with how much you like Radiology. I like it too and don't need convincing about how great a specialty it is-you would be preaching to the choir" (http://www.uth.tmc.edu/med/administration/student/ms4/2003CCC.htm).

- **What am I looking for in a residency program?**

  Programs seek out residents who will be a good "fit" for the program. Be specific about what you seek in a residency program. "Given my goals of providing health services to underserved communities, I'm seeking a residency program that..."

  Don't forget the corollary, which can be easy to do when you're applying to large numbers of programs. Don't confirm the fact that you would be a poor fit for the program. "I am very interested in continuing my basic science research on matrix metalloproteinases, and I hope to eventually make significant contributions in this field." You've successfully emphasized your research experience and highlighted your academic aspirations. You've also just made it clear that you're a poor fit for this clinically oriented program that has no time set aside for research endeavors.

- **What are my professional goals in the field I have chosen?**

  Some residency programs have institutional goals. They may aim to train doctors who will serve in primary care, who will serve underserved populations, who will serve as clinician-educators, who will advance research, or who will achieve any other number of goals. Therefore, career goals are often included in personal statements. Programs understand that these goals evolve with time, so you don't need to have absolute certainty. However, including your future goals in the statement gives the program some idea of your motivation and knowledge of the specialty.

- **What are my strengths?**

  Every specialty values certain qualities in their residents. Studies have outlined some of these qualities.

Skills and personal qualities frequently identified by residency program directors in defining an applicant's "fit"

Family Medicine	Good communicator Interpersonal skills Team player Lifelong learning skills Empathic Interested in community practice Non-judgmental Active in the program Experience with underserved populations
Internal Medicine	Good communicator Interpersonal skills Team player Hands-on patient care Potential positive impact upon program Reliable and stable· Warm and humane Demonstrated commitment to specific area (music, sports) Well-organized Able to get along with others Resourceful
Pediatrics	Good communicator Interpersonal skills Team player Well-organized Well-rounded Mature Independent Sense of professionalism Flexible (able to change) Enthusiastic Ability to cope with stress and change Positive attitude (views glass "half-full")
Surgery	Good communicator Compulsive Neat High energy Honest and straightforward Confident Hardworking Demonstrated commitment to specific area (music, sports)

From Villanueva AM, Kaye D, Abdelhak SS, Morahan PS. Comparing selection criteria for residency directors and physicians' employers. *Acad Med* 1995; 70(4): 261-271.

Study these lists. Determine which you can claim as your own strengths, and weave these into your personal statement. As always, naked statements don't mean much. Always include evidence in the form of personal anecdotes, clinical experiences, or other forms to back up your claims.

- **What accomplishments should I highlight?**

  Programs seek certain traits and qualities in their residents. Every program wants hard-working, enthusiastic, focused residents. They want individuals with proven skills of communication, perseverance towards a goal, and the ability to work with all types of people to achieve a common goal. The personal statement can be used to highlight different types of accomplishments that underscore your stellar qualities. You can highlight your commitment and dedication by discussing your long-term volunteer commitments. Areas such as occupational history and outside interests may be woven in. What did you accomplish in the two summers that you worked as an EMT? What type of qualities can you highlight from your one year working as an engineer?

- **What contributions can I make to the specialty?**

  In a very competitive field like dermatology, it is a given that applicants will all have extremely strong academic records. Since programs can pick and choose among so many academically stellar candidates, they have the luxury of looking for more. Programs seek out applicants who can actually contribute to the discipline as a whole. This becomes even more of an issue in the fields of dermatology, radiology, and ophthalmology, which have seen a rise in applications as lifestyle issues become more important to medical school graduates. Look at it from the program's standpoint. If you're interviewing so many outstanding applicants, why choose the ones who are going to graduate with the intention of working the least amount of hours for the most amount of money?

  Since programs seek out applicants who will contribute to the discipline as a whole, emphasize your own strengths, skills, and experiences and how these will aid you in contributing to the specialty. Do you have a background in research? What do you plan to do with that background? Have you done a fellowship and accumulated significant experience in clinical trials? What do you plan to do with those skills? Do you have significant volunteer experience in tutoring? Have you created educational materials or programs? Have you worked with cancer prevention programs or do you have an interest in preventive medicine strategies? Have you spent time working with underserved populations? Do you have additional skills, such as computer database management or graphic design experience that can be used to benefit the specialty in some way? Think long and hard about how you as an individual plan to contribute to your field when you finish residency training, and write about your individual skills and strengths that will help you accomplish those goals.

- **Why would I be a great fit for this particular residency program?**

  Most applicants write one statement that they then have ERAS forward to all programs. However, some students write several different statements. Students with research experience may choose to emphasize a different skill set for different programs. They may send a research-oriented statement to programs which place great emphasis on research, but send a statement that emphasizes their outstanding skills as a clinician to other programs.

  Some applicants will actually write a different statement for each program, tailoring their statement to each individual program. In doing so, they can successfully answer the question "Why am I interested in your program?" This approach demonstrates to program directors that you are genuinely interested in their program and are knowledgeable about the program's strengths.

- **What are my outside interests?**

  Again, your outside interests can be used to highlight desirable qualities, as in the marathon runner who is a focused, determined individual used to setting goals and working hard to achieve them. Your unique interests can also leave a memorable impression. Are you working on hiking all the state parks in Texas? Restore classic cars in your spare time? Do you specialize in cooking Thai cuisine? Tell a memorable story, and use it as a hook by which people will remember you.

Did you know ...

In a study evaluating the content of personal statements, members of the radiology residency selection committee at Wayne State University ranked eleven content areas from least to most important (Smith). Most important was a candidate's explanation as to why they chose to pursue a career in radiology. Personal attributes was second in importance while perception of radiology defined as the applicant's ability "to explicitly state what he/she feels are the most important characteristics of either radiologists or the practice of radiology" was third.

Did you know ...

At the website for the Wayne State University pathology residency, the program writes that "your personal statement should summarize your particular background and interests and depict you as a person. You should indicate in your personal statement why you are interested in Pathology, what kind of experience you have had with Pathology, and what career path you plan to follow after training" (http://www.med.wayne.edu/Pathology/residencytraining/FAQ.htm).

Did you know ...

In a survey of orthopedic residency program directors, 43% stated that "the most important aspect of a personal statement is to learn more about the candidate's personal interests and backgrounds" (Bernstein).

Rule # 51   Never exaggerate.

Students sometimes overstate their role in a research project. When asked about their work during the interview, they are unable to discuss the project in any depth, thus harming their credibility. Resist the temptation to exaggerate in your personal statement.

Under no circumstances should you lie in your personal statement. Unfortunately, some students will, and the following box demonstrates how surprisingly often this occurs. Although some lies escape detection, most don't. An application reviewer may note a discrepancy between the personal statement and other components of the application, such as the letter of recommendation. In other cases, the lie is discovered when an interviewer probes the applicant further.

Did you know ...

In a study of family practice residency program directors over a five year period, directors were asked about candidate deception (Grover). 339 cases of deception, accounting for 56% of all deception acts, involved the personal statement. Of the recognized incidents of deception, 89% were discovered before the Match, either during the interview or when programs made efforts to verify application information.

Rule # 52   Don't ever plagiarize.

Don't "borrow" any part of a personal statement for a starting point or for a framework, even if the rest of the personal statement is all yours. If you're not sure whether what you've done is sufficiently different from another's personal statement, then consider that a warning—a reader may also have concerns. In recent years, many examples of personal statements have been posted on different websites. While reading the statements of others can be useful, never copy part of another statement. Be careful about writing services which may recycle words, phrases, or text. ERAS has noted that personal statement plagiarism is an increasingly common issue. The list of sites that have been plagiarized includes www.medfools.com, www.usmleweb.com, www.medstudentcafe.com, and www.aipg.info.
(www.aamc.org/students/eras/policies/integritypromotioneducation.htm)

Did you know ...

Drs. Lehrmann and Walaszek, psychiatry faculty members at the Zablocki VA Medical Center and the University of Wisconsin School of Medicine in Milwaukee, wrote about finding a "personal statement development website for U.S. and international medical students which displayed example personal statements." They were shocked to see that they "actually recognized some of them. We had received several nearly identical personal statements that had been plagiarized" (Lehrmann).

Did you know ...

Drs. Speer and Khilnani of the internal medicine/pediatrics residency program at the University of Texas Medical Branch at Galveston wrote that "students can also use books or websites that offer advice when constructing personal statements. However, students are tempted to copy ideas, phrases, and paragraphs from sample statements and most programs can recognize these plagiarized statements" (Speer).

ERAS has a program (Integrity Promotion Investigation Program) in place to handle complaints of unethical behavior on the part of applicants. After a complaint is received, an investigation is launched to learn more about the alleged fraudulent activity. Applicants deemed to be in violation are added to a violator database and the final report generated from the investigation is sent to each residency program applied to, along with the applicant's medical school. Furthermore, ERAS states that the report will also be sent to programs applied to in future application cycles.

> **Did you know ...**
>
> In a review of 26 applications over a two-year period to the geriatric medicine fellowship at the Florida Hospital Family Medicine Residency Program, three statements were found to contain portions plagiarized from a particular website (Cole).

Rule # 53   Finish your personal statement early in the application cycle.

Some of your letter writers will request a copy of your personal statement, so plan your schedule accordingly. Your deadline will be the date that you provide information packets to your letter writers, and not the date for submission of applications.

It may not take that long to actually crank out a one-page statement. However, we recommend that you start the process a minimum of two months out. Brainstorming and outlining should be done in multiple sessions, especially since you need to provide multiple opportunities for inspiration to hit. You'll also need to give your reviewers sufficient time to complete their work, and to provide yourself enough time to process their comments and to make multiple revisions.

> **Tip # 43**
>
> Don't wait until the last minute to start your personal statement. Start early so that you give yourself enough time to develop a high quality personal statement. Many letter writers will ask for your personal statement before writing your letter of recommendation.

Rule # 54   Start the process by brainstorming.

Writing the personal statement is a daunting task, period. Most applicants have no idea where or how to start. Without a plan, you may be stuck waiting for random inspiration. A specific strategy can make this entire process easier by breaking a large task into smaller, more manageable components.

Your first step is to brainstorm. One goal is to pinpoint a unique or distinctive item about yourself that will pique the selection committee's interest. Take a piece of paper or sit in front of your computer, and plan to start writing down everything that you can think of, without any editing. It may even be better to record your answers to these questions on a tape recorder, since transcribing the text may provide further inspiration. Now ask yourself the following questions:

- When did I become interested in this specialty?
- What experiences, events, or factors led me to develop this interest?

- How did my interest in this specialty evolve? What specific turning points can I identify?
- What have I learned about the field and myself while exploring it?
- Was there a particular patient that I cannot forget? What was it about him or her that made such an impact?
- What are my professional goals and aspirations?
- What qualities do I possess that will enhance my chances for success in this specialty?
- What makes me stand out from the rest of the candidates?
- What are my strengths and skills?
- What is unique or distinctive about me or my life story (undergraduate, medical school, personal events, work experience, volunteer experience, teaching experience, research, hobbies, languages, travel, sports, etc.)?
- Why should the selection committee be interested in me?
- Was there a challenge or hardship that I had to overcome? How did this experience shape me?
- Are there any gaps or deficiencies in my record that need to be explained?

If you find it difficult to answer any of these questions, look over your CV. Discuss your accomplishments and experiences with a friend, family member, or advisor. Those close to you may be able to identify accomplishments which have escaped your attention. Consider polling those close to you while writing your personal statement. The following questions may be used as springboards for discussion:

- What is it about me that the residency selection committee absolutely needs to know?
- What is it about me or my background that you find distinctive?
- Are there any events or experiences in my background that would be of interest to a residency selection committee?
- Which of my qualities or skills should I showcase in my statement? How do you think these qualities or skills have helped me in the past? How might they help me be successful in residency and in my chosen field?

Responses to these questions can be used to help you outline your personal statement.

Tip # 44

Are you having difficulty coming up with a unique characteristic, experience, or subject to write about in your personal statement? Many students are anxious to complete their personal statement, and consider sitting around and "reflecting" to be a waste of time. Many therefore skip this critical step.

Tip # 45

Don't neglect any attribute that makes you extraordinary or unusual. If you are an accomplished musician, leader of a student organization, or top-level athlete, you should discuss this in your statement. Focus on the traits and lessons learned and how these relate in particular to your chosen specialty. Programs are interested in knowing how you differ from others.

Did you know ...

In a study designed to determine predictors of otolaryngology resident success, Daly found that candidates having an exceptional trait, such as leadership qualities, were not only ranked higher but were also found to be more successful during their residency training than those without exceptional traits (Daly).

Rule # 55   Plan on multiple drafts.

After you've completed your outline, you're ready to take on your first draft. This is only a draft, and should be approached as such. Creation of a high quality personal statement takes considerable time, and you can't expect a polished product after one draft. Qualified applicants often approach the first draft with the same perfectionist attitude that got them this far. In this case, though, just focus on getting something reasonable down on paper.

Tip # 46

The first draft is always the hardest. Do not approach this first draft with a perfectionist attitude. Instead, aim to get something reasonable down on paper, and plan on many revisions.

There are a million ways to start drafting your personal statement. Some applicants begin with the introduction, while others prefer to write the ending first, and others just attack the body of the statement. Start wherever you feel comfortable.

After you've written your first draft, set it aside for a few days. Then look at it again and ask yourself the following questions:

- Have I answered the questions that program directors ask?
- Does it flow logically?
- Is it too long? Is it too short?
- Do I need to add more details?
- Do I need to remove some details?

Now revise. With subsequent drafts, ask these questions once again. You will also start to deal with other issues such as sentence structure and transitions between paragraphs. Expect multiple drafts before you end with a product you like.

Tip # 47

Although you can type your personal statement directly into ERAS, it's more useful to complete your statement using your word processing software. This allows you to take advantage of editing features such as the spell checker. Once you have a polished product, save the statement as a text file, which you can then cut and paste into the ERAS personal statement section. Do not submit the statement to programs until you have printed a copy for your review. After you have carefully proofread it, you can send it to each program.

Tip # 48

You can solicit feedback from others at any point in the writing process; there is no need to wait until you have a polished product. Having others look over your first draft can be invaluable. One caveat: try to submit a polished product when seeking feedback from a faculty member.

Rule # 56   Submit a personal statement of the correct length.

Do whatever it takes to create a personal statement that is the "right" length. First, comply with all rules regarding the length of the personal statement. Second, don't go on and on. Your audience includes faculty members and residency program directors. These are busy individuals who have neither the time nor the patience to read through lengthy tomes.

Tip # 49

When you print your personal statement from the ERAS system, does it fit onto one page? If not, your statement is too long. Keep in mind that most program directors will spend just two to three minutes on average reading your statement.

Tip # 50

Application reviewers appreciate sentences that are concise and direct. Avoid using extraneous or unnecessary words. Choose your words carefully, using the right word rather than the longest word possible.

Don't submit a personal statement that is too short, either. A short statement suggests that you did not expend much time, energy, and effort in its creation. The natural assumption is that this would extend to your performance as a physician.

Rule # 57   Learn the art of effective self-promotion.

Some applicants downplay their successes in the personal statement. They hesitate to make strong statements about their strengths and skills for fear that it might be perceived as self-serving. While humility is an admirable quality, it shouldn't be the aim of your personal statement. You must be able to write about your accomplishments, skills, and strengths in a way that emphasizes that you are a desirable candidate. If you received numerous compliments during your surgery rotation about your manual dexterity, then you should find a way to include this in your personal statement for surgery residency. Applicants often don't realize that while exaggeration and overstatements can be damaging, so can understatements. The latter prevents the selection committee from getting a better sense of who you are, what you have done, and what you have to offer.

Tip # 51

The personal statement is no place to be modest. You have to be comfortable writing about your assets. If you don't, who will?

> **Did you know ...**
>
> In a study evaluating the content of personal statements, Smith and colleagues wrote that "although some candidates might hesitate to explicitly define their personal attributes for fear of seeming conceited, the fact that the members of the committee rated this category highly demonstrates that this is not the case. The committee members instead implied that they felt this type of self-promotion was an important part of the personal statement ..." (Smith).

Rule # 58   Leave out your entire life story.

In the one page that you have for your personal statement, you cannot, and should not, try to write your life story. Some applicants write about all the experiences and events that they consider significant. It is far better to describe a few events or accomplishments in some detail, and emphasize what these experiences meant to you, and how they reflect upon your individual strengths. A laundry list of experiences, events, and honors has no significance.

Rule # 59   Use your personal statement to highlight your outstanding communication skills.

Programs also use the personal statement to learn about your writing ability. Communication skills are of obvious importance in every specialty. A poorly written statement will raise concerns about your ability to care for patients, record the results of your patient evaluations, convey important and sometimes complicated information to other health care professionals, and educate patients about their illness.

> **Did you know ...**
>
> At the website for the psychiatry residency at the State University of New York in Stonybrook, the program states that "writing skills are an essential component of medical record keeping, particularly in psychiatry...The selection committee will evaluate the preparation of the application and in particular the personal statement for evidence of writing skills...Applicants with poorly written essays, e.g., multiple spelling and grammatical errors will not be invited for an interview" (www.hsc.stonybrook.edu/som/psychiatry/selection_procecess.cfm)

A poorly written personal statement is not hard to spot. Indicators include the following:

- Lack of flow (e.g., jumping from one tangent to another)

- Lack of structure. Remember that each paragraph should develop one idea or central point, and each sentence should build on the one before it.
- Spelling errors
- Grammatical errors
- Using clichés, tired analogies, and metaphors. These will bore your readers and make you appear lazy or lacking imagination. Instead, use original words to convey your intended meaning.
- Beginning every sentence with "I"
- The use of long or run-on sentences
- Using abbreviations. Don't assume that everyone recognizes your abbreviations.
- Not backing up descriptive comments about yourself. One classic example is writing that "I'm a very hard worker" without providing specific examples.

Tip # 52

Residency programs are looking for applicants who can communicate effectively. Speaking and writing English well is crucial to evaluating and managing patients, communicating with colleagues, and reading large volumes of detailed information. Your personal statement will be examined carefully for any deficiencies of written expression. Your writing ability and writing style count—in fact, they count a lot.

Did you know ...

In a survey of orthopedic residency program directors, 32% stated that "the most important aspect of a personal statement was to gain insight into an applicant's ability to write and to communicate effectively" (Bernstein).

Rule # 60   Do not permit even a single spelling or grammatical mistake.

Spelling and grammatical mistakes are glaring errors that can seriously damage your candidacy. Always seek out several reviewers to read your personal statement before submission.

One program director we know reads every personal statement with a red pen in hand. He then proceeds to circle all grammatical, spelling, and punctuation errors. At the end of the statement, if he has more than a few circles, he questions the applicant's ability to pay attention to detail. The obvious conclusion is that the applicant may approach the care of patients in the same manner.

Tip # 53

In reviewing your statement, program directors will look at the quality of your writing, not just its content. While the proper grammar and spelling will not impress them, errors will severely weaken your application. Program directors value precision and attention to detail.

To catch spelling errors, use the spell check function of your word processor. However, don't rely solely on the spell check. Proofread your work carefully, looking for both typographical and grammatical errors. It can be particularly useful to put aside your statement for a few days. Reading it with a fresh eye may help you spot these mistakes. Reading it out loud or backwards one word at a time are other useful techniques.

Did you know ...

In a study evaluating the content of personal statements, members of the radiology residency selection committee at Wayne State University ranked five elements of form from least to most important (Smith). Most important was a candidate's basic language skills. This was defined as the applicant's ability to "express his/her ideas in a way that is grammatically correct and free from major spelling and punctuation errors."

Did you know ...

Dr. Heymann, head of the dermatology department at Cooper Hospital of the UMDNJ—Robert Wood Johnson Medical School, wrote "I may eliminate an applicant because of too many typographical errors on the application (if the applicant does not care enough to proofread his own application, will he care enough to review the chart thoroughly?)" (Heymann).

Rule # 61   Customize your personal statement for each program.

You don't have to create a single generic personal statement that is sent to every program. You can customize your personal statements for individual programs. Applicants underutilize this technique, but it can and should be used in certain cases. Especially if you think you're a long shot to match into a particular specialty or program, take the time to tailor your statement to each school.

However, customizing your personal statement is only effective if you have specific points to make. "I am very interested in the residency program at Baylor due to the excellent clinical training available, and its location in the vibrant city of Houston." This is a generic statement, and lacks both impact and credibility.

When you refer to a specific program, you should talk about why it's perfect for you, and why you're perfect for the program. Why are you interested in becoming a resident there? Is there a particular aspect of the program that appeals to you? How will that benefit you? In return, what contributions will you be able to make to the program? Do you know what the program is looking for in a resident? If so, emphasize these aspects of your candidacy. Most applicants don't address these issues. The few that do, however, demonstrate that they've actively researched the program, and are able to show that they are a good fit for the program.

> "I'm very interested in pursuing nephrology as a subspecialty following my internal medicine residency, and your strong program is one of the reasons I'm so interested in training at your program. I also grew up in Columbus, and being able to return to my hometown would be wonderful."

> "I have a strong background in bench research, and my career goal is translational research. For my residency, I seek a program that would provide very strong clinical training. That's one of the reasons I'm so interested in the program at Strong University. The broad-based training, with coverage of all of the major facets of ophthalmology, along with the opportunity to work alongside faculty engaged in translational research, would be ideal."

Customizing your personal statement is a tricky process. Many applicants waste valuable space telling the selection committee about the fine reputation of their program and institution. There's no reason to do so. You're not telling them anything they don't already know. Another mistake made in this area is the discussion of geography. Certain points are important, and can be compelling reasons for seeking out a residency program. However, they should never be the entire focus of your interest in a particular program. "My husband's company has already expressed a willingness to transfer him to their branch here in Chicago." "I'm from Miami originally, and since I still have family in the area, I'd love to return here." These are of interest, and important, but such statements should always be preceded by a discussion of your professional interests in the program.

Applicants to competitive fields may apply to 50 or more programs. Is it possible to truthfully customize your approach for every program? No, but you must put in the hours to research each program to which you're applying. We recognize that the reason you're applying to fifty or more programs may be just to get in somewhere. We hope as you research various programs that you will find compelling reasons why certain programs would be perfect for you, and why you would be perfect for them.

Tip # 54

Selection committees don't expect to receive a personal statement tailored to their program. Not surprisingly, when they do receive such a statement, they tend to be impressed by the applicant's interest.

Tip # 55

If you do decide to tailor your statement for individual programs, triple check to make sure you don't mistakenly send the wrong personal statement. Sending personal statement for University X to University Y can lead to an immediate rejection. Likewise, if you are applying to multiple specialties, ensure that the right statement is sent.

Rule # 62   Your personal statement should be used to enhance your CV, not mirror it.

Your CV and personal statement should not be too similar. Students often receive the mistaken impression that the personal statement should simply be an expanded version of the CV. You should not simply repeat the information on your CV. Otherwise, your statement will essentially be a list of accomplishments and activities, revealing very little about you as an individual.

Instead, you should view the personal statement as an opportunity to elaborate on certain aspects of your CV. For example, you may have received the Michael L. Roberts Award during medical school and listed this under the honors/awards section of your CV. This award, which was given to you for exceptional leadership, deserves further elaboration. The personal statement would be an ideal place to provide the reader with details about the award.

Tip # 56

The personal statement provides a rare opportunity to differentiate yourself from other applicants. Although you may have attended similar medical schools or taken the same clerkships, no one has the same experiences. The events and experiences that have shaped you and your life are unique. If you can communicate this in a captivating fashion, your statement will stand out. In some cases, interviewers or program directors, after reading an applicant's statement, have found an area of common interest, establishing a connection.

Did you know ...

In advice for the dermatology residency applicant, Miller wrote that "many applicants look the same on paper, yet we know that each of you is unique and has something special to offer to our dermatology program...Your task is to bring who you are to life ... A good place to start is with your personal statement. Crafting a personal statement can be more difficult than writing a manuscript for publication. Thought and creativity are required to let the reader know who you are...The bottom line is to balance why you are interested in the field with who you are, weighing more heavily on 'who you are'"(Miller).

Rule # 63   Ask for help.

Developing a personal statement is a major source of frustration for most medical students. Students often have difficulties answering the following questions:

- What should I say?
- How should I say it?
- Where should I start?
- Does it flow?

If you are having difficulty developing your personal statement, don't be afraid to ask for help. You can turn to your advisor for valuable suggestions about the content of your personal statement. There is no rule that says you must wait to seek the assistance of your advisor until you have a finished product, although your statement should still be polished and free of any grammatical errors. Check to see if your medical school has a writing office. If so, it may be staffed with individuals able to help you. They may be able to help you get started, create an outline, revise and edit your draft, and proofread your finished product. Some writing offices also have examples of statements written by past students on file.

Rule # 64   Ask an experienced professional to review your statement.

When your personal statement is ready for submission, you should seek assistance from an experienced professional. Applicants often make the mistake of showing their statement only to a friend or family member. However, it is the rare friend who has both strong writing skills and an intimate knowledge of what makes a statement effective from a content standpoint. Therefore, they shouldn't be your only reviewers.

Seek the assistance of an individual with expertise in personal statements. This may include your advisor, the departmental program director at your institution, or other faculty members in the department, particularly those who sit on the residency selection committee. Ask if he or she would be willing to evaluate your statement and provide you with constructive criticism. Faculty such as program directors have probably seen hundreds of personal statements, making them an authority on reviewing personal statements.

When asking a faculty member to review a statement, avoid waiting until the last minute. Reviewers can make valuable suggestions, but only if they have sufficient time. Give them at least two to three weeks to read your statement. Anything less may be considered an imposition. You cannot expect a faculty member to drop everything and read your statement a few days before the deadline. Even if they agree to review your statement under the pressure of time, a hasty review may not be as thorough or helpful.

Tip # 57

Ideally, your personal statement should be reviewed by at least several people, including your advisor. If possible, have the residency program director at your own institution review it as well. Ask them to provide you with a detailed critique of your statement.

Your goal is to solicit detailed feedback from others. Note that you are seeking detailed feedback. Comments such as "it's great" are reassuring, but you really need to know how to improve your statement. Ask your reviewers if it holds their interest, if your main points are clear, if it flows smoothly, if it includes enough detail, and if it begins and ends in a compelling fashion.

Tip # 58

The ideal reviewer has extensive experience reading personal statements.

Tip # 59

Don't feel obliged to make every change that is recommended. However, if multiple reviewers make the same point, then give careful thought to their recommendation.

Utilize the following personal statement review form before submitting your statement for review.

Personal statement review form

	Yes	No
When held at arm's length, the statement looks pleasing to the eye		
Name and AAMC ID # at the top		
The font size and type allow for easy reading		
There is adequate space between paragraphs		
There is adequate space between the end of one sentence and the beginning of another		
There is at least a one-inch margin at the top, bottom, left, and right sides		
Statement begins with an attention-grabber		
Each paragraph revolves around an idea or theme		
The paragraphs are not too long		
The ideas flow logically		
Good transition between the ideas in each paragraph		
The word "I" is not overused		
Sentences are short and crisp rather than long and rambling		
Variety of sentence structures are used to keep the statement interesting		
Active rather than passive sentences are used		
Action verbs and words are used		
There are no unnecessary words		
Grammatical/spelling errors are not present		
Jargon and abbreviations are avoided		
Standard font size and type are used (Times New Roman or Arial, 10 to 12 point)		
Statement keeps interest throughout		
Statement revolves around a theme		
Statement is neither too long nor too short		
Written in a professional, confident, and upbeat tone		
Controversial topics are avoided		
There are no signs of arrogance		
Inappropriate material is avoided		
Negativity is avoided		
Printed on high quality paper (if applicable)		

Rule # 65 Start your statement with a hook.

Application reviewers may be reading hundreds of personal statements. It is imperative that you begin your essay with an attention-grabbing statement. You can capture your reader's attention by beginning with a story, question, quote, or even an anecdote. This will help your statement stand out. Does your opening draw the reader into the rest of your story?

Tip # 60

Begin your statement in a compelling manner. The program director has hundreds, perhaps thousands, of statements to read. Personal statements that hook the director from the start are more likely to be read in their entirety. Make sure your hook is relevant to your career interests.

No matter how you choose to hook your audience, make sure that the hook is relevant to the purpose of your statement. The purpose of your statement is to convince your audience that you embody the qualities that they are seeking in a resident. Telling a catchy story is only effective if you can tie it in to this point. Refer to the end of this chapter for some examples of personal statements that grab your attention.

Tip # 61

When leading your statement with a story, avoid writing about it in an overly dramatic manner. Be judicious in your use of language.

Rule # 66   Focus on your growth during the clinical years of medical school. Do not rehash your preclinical or undergraduate years.

The content of your personal statement should mainly focus on your growth during the clinical years of medical school, particularly as it relates to your chosen specialty. An extensive discussion of your high school, undergraduate, or even preclinical years is generally not appropriate subject matter for the personal statement. Focusing on your earlier years makes your statement seem sophomoric. One of your goals is to leave the selection committee with the impression that you are a mature, competent individual.

Exceptions to this rule include particularly noteworthy information pertaining to research experience, volunteer work, community service, or course work towards earning another degree (for example, a combined MD and PhD degree). If you include this information, you must tie it in with the specialty you have chosen.

Tip # 62

When preparing the personal statement for residency, many applicants refer back to their medical school statement. Some applicants then proceed to write about the factors that led them to pursue a career as a doctor. Residency programs are far more interested in knowing the reasons you chose the specialty. If you feel compelled to include your motivations for pursuing a career as a physician, don't waste too much space answering this question.

Rule # 67 Don't get overly creative. Your writing style should never overshadow your message.

Although creativity is encouraged, avoid getting overly creative with your personal statement. Highly unusual personal statements may be perceived in a negative fashion. Your goal is to present yourself as a mature and professional applicant. You don't want reviewers to remember your unusual style of writing to the exclusion of your qualifications.

In an attempt to be original, some applicants have taken creative approaches such as writing a poem or humorous statement. A reviewer may find these approaches appealing or refreshing. Some won't, and may even question your maturity and judgment.

Did you know ...

In a study evaluating the content of personal statements, members of the radiology residency selection committee at Wayne State University ranked five elements of form from least to most important (Smith). Creating a one-of-a-kind and inventive statement was the least important.

Rule # 68 Always provide evidence to back up your claims.

What distinguishes a memorable personal statement from a generic one? Your individual stories and examples make all the difference. Many applicants claim to be a team player or good communicator. Few, however, support these assertions with concrete stories and examples. Their personal statements start to sound like tired clichés. "I'm a team player, I work well with all sorts of people, and I have excellent communication skills." Applicants who are able to prove they have particular skills or traits leave the selection committee with a better sense of who they are, what they have done, and what they have the potential to do in the future. This is precisely the type of personal statement that reviewers find memorable.

Tip # 63

Personal statements that lack stories or examples to support the writers' claims often contain generalities and platitudes. How do you know if you have developed a generic statement? If what you have written could be written by someone else, then your statement is generic. If no one else could write what you have written, then you have succeeded in creating a unique statement.

Rule # 69   Provide an explanation of the negatives in your application.

Some applicants have a weakness or negative in their application and wonder if it should be addressed in the personal statement. Examples include taking five years to complete medical school or repeating a clerkship. Some advisors recommend using the statement as a vehicle to explain these problems. They argue that a selection committee may be hesitant or even decline to interview an applicant if a deficiency or negative is noted in the application. Addressing the problematic issue in the statement may convince the committee to consider the application further.

Tip # 64

If your record contains an issue that would be considered a red flag by a program, consider addressing it in your personal statement. Some applicants would rather wait until the interview to discuss it. However, your weakness or negative may prevent you from ever receiving an interview.

Tip # 65

Make sure you don't make a small problem look like a big one. If you are not sure whether the problem needs to be addressed in the statement, discuss it with the residency program director or dean at your institution.

If you decide to address a negative, follow these guidelines:

- Address the negative or weakness in a careful, matter-of-fact manner.
- Explain it positively, including the reasons (i.e., health issue, family issue, financial problem).
- Offer the explanation without making any excuses. Do not whine or complain.

- Explain what you learned from the experience, how it will help you in the future, and why it is unlikely to occur again.
- Avoid calling too much attention to the negative or alienating the reader by spending too much space or time on the issue. Be concise.

Since opinions regarding this matter vary widely, solicit the opinion of key individuals at your medical school, including the dean and the residency program director. Here are examples of how applicants might handle certain red flags:

Red flag	Explanation
Failed several basic science courses	During college, doing well in my course work came fairly easy to me. Many of my friends and classmates marveled at my grades. They often asked me how I managed to do so well, studying so little. I brought the same approach with me when I started medical school. My first-semester grades suffered as a consequence and I was suspended for the rest of the academic year. This gave me a considerable time to think. I had come to medical school to become the best physician I could possibly be. I realized that through my approach I was shortchanging myself of a good education. This led me to rethink my approach, and I resolved to change my ways. After reading books on study skills and taking courses on improving study habits, I resumed my medical education. Since then, I have consistently performed at a high level, earning As and Bs in my basic science and clinical rotations.
Failed USMLE Step 2 CK	My performance on the USMLE Step 1 and NBME end-of-clerkship shelf exams demonstrate my strong knowledge base and speak to my ability to handle the challenges of residency training. Unfortunately, I recently learned that I failed my USMLE Step 2 CK exam. Several weeks prior to the exam, a family member became quite ill and I was not able to devote as much time as I had planned for preparation. In retrospect, I should have delayed the exam until a better time. I believe, however, that the score is not reflective of my true abilities. In further support of this are my SAT, MCAT, and USMLE Step 1 scores, which have all been above the 95th percentile.

Contrast these two explanations with the following example:

I would like to use part of this space to elaborate further on some of the low grades I received during my third year of medical school. I do not feel that my performance is an adequate representation of my true abilities and my potential as a resident. In my internal medicine clerkship, my personality did not mesh well with the attending. I believe this colored his perception of me and the quality of my work, leading to a subpar evaluation. With regards to my failure in pediatrics, part of the grade was based on the submission of a write-up. My write-up was three days late because I had to take a week off to tend to my father who was very sick. Before the deadline, I e-mailed the clerkship director of my situation and informed him that my write-up might be late. I assumed that the clerkship would take this into account but, when I received the fail grade, it was too late for me to change the outcome. Despite talking with the student affairs dean, the grade stood as fail because, in the course syllabus, it was stated that the write-up needed to be turned in on time in order to receive at least a passing grade. Given the circumstances, I felt that the clerkship and school should have been more supportive.

The above explanation is lengthy, full of excuses, negative in its overall tone, and it fails to show what the applicant learned from the situation and how he would handle a similar situation in the future. More than likely this application would be rejected.

Did you know ...

In an article published online at the Alliance for Academic Internal Medicine website (http://www.im.org/AAIM/Pubs/Insight/ Winter2005/page10.htm), UTMB faculty members suggested "that students address weaknesses in their record, such as poor grades or leaves of absences, early in the personal statement. This is an opportunity to explain situations that may be seen as negative. For example, 'this experience helped me mature professionally and enhanced my learning in the following ways.'"

Did you know ...

During a workshop given by the Clerkship Directors of Medicine (CDIM), the following advice was given to internal medicine residency applicants:

"What do you do if you have significant weaknesses in your record? Address these up front. Program directors are more likely to overlook it if you bring it up. Similarly, a leave of absence will be assumed to be 'psychiatric if no comments are offered.'"

From "Giving advice to medical students applying for an IM residency position" - October 12, 2004 - CDIM workshop (gsm.tmck.edu/IM/FAQstudent_advice.htm)

Rule # 70   There is a fine line between self-confidence and arrogance.

Your personal statement should be written in a professional tone, conveying your self-confidence, maturity, determination, and your readiness for residency.

Tip # 66

Write in a tone that shows you have confidence in your abilities, skills, and accomplishments. If you don't express confidence in your own abilities, how can you expect the selection committee to do so?

However, there is a fine line between self-confidence and arrogance. We have actually read statements in which the applicant writes about how fortunate the program would be if it accepted him. We have also read statements in which the writers use overly elaborate words to show readers their high intelligence level and sophistication. Use of these words makes you appear pompous and arrogant. Lecturing the reader, or writing as if you know more about the specialty than those who are practicing it, are other turn-offs.

Tip # 67

Don't try to impress the selection committee with your vocabulary. Use simple rather than flowery language, and aim to explain your meaning precisely.

Rule # 71 Leave out taboo topics.

Certain items should be left out of the statement. When discussing your reasons for choosing your specialty, refrain from commenting on how you may have been influenced by financial or lifestyle issues. Yes, otherwise intelligent students actually bring up these issues. Avoid discussing subjects that are potentially controversial:

• Personal problems

• Religion

• Political beliefs

• Romantic relationships

• Opinions about sex, abortion, or other moral issues

Do not make inflammatory statements. These may include negative statements about a faculty member, patient, medical school, residency program, or medical specialty.

Finally, leave out anything you would rather not discuss at an interview. Remember that anything you include in the statement is fair game for an interviewer.

Tip # 68

In surveys of fourth-year medical students at the Brody School of Medicine at East Carolina University and New York Medical College done every year from 1998 to 2004, lifestyle and income became increasingly important factors in career choice during the period of study (Newton). While your specialty choice may have been largely based on these factors, refrain from including any mention of these factors in your personal statement. An obvious mistake? We have reviewed statements that discuss lifestyle as a motivating factor.

Did you know ...

The Association of Program Directors in Surgery consider the following to be red flags in a personal statement (www.apds.org):

"Strange personal statement"

"The word 'I' is used on almost every line"

"If the applicant had a leave of absence from medical school and does not address it any way"

Did you know ...

In their Power Point presentation "Make A Statement," the deans at Boston University School of Medicine warn their students to leave out "negative statements about other fields, statements that can be harmful or embarrassing to family or colleagues, political and religious opinions, anything about which you don't want to be questioned, general statements about the field (yawn), and cheesy generalizations ('medicine is an art as well as a science')..."

http://www.bumc.bu.edu/www/busm/osa/Residency_of_Choice_2008/
Personal_Statement_Workshop_2008.pdf

Rule # 72   Print your statement properly.

After you have finalized your personal statement, print it out on high quality 8.5" X 11" bond paper (e.g., 24 to 28 lb) using a laser printer. Select a white, off-white, natural, or cream colored paper. Give a professional copy of your personal statement to your letter writers. In fact, many letter writers will ask for a copy of your statement before they write your letter.

You will also need to carry copies of your personal statement with you to interviews. At some programs, you may be interviewed by a faculty member who is blinded to your application, including your personal statement. If you happen to learn this, you can always provide the interviewer with your statement if requested.

Sample Personal Statements

Radiology Residency Personal Statement

The coldness of the water startled me when it soaked through my clothing. I tightened my grip on our guide's head and repositioned myself more securely on his shoulders. As we waded across the river and Brazilian border, only the rippling of the water broke the silence. I could not see my parents nor my siblings in the dark. Images of lights shining down on us and voices telling us to stop haunted me. I was 8 years old.

My family first moved from Taiwan to Paraguay in 1976 in order to gain entrance into Brazil and join our relatives in Sao Miguel. Our aim was to circumvent the political sanctions which forbade our emigration. However, disillusioned with the political situation, we moved back to Paraguay after living in Brazil for one year. In search for better social and educational opportunities, we applied for permission to reside in the United States. During the five long years of waiting, my father worked 15-hour days at our restaurant while my mother walked door to door selling clothes and faux-jewelry. Since I was the oldest of three children, I was in charge of caring for my siblings while our parents were absent from home. At the age of 9, I cooked our meals and washed the dishes while my 8 year-old sister washed our clothes by hand and cleaned the house. We both acted as babysitters for our 6 year-old brother. I learned the meaning of responsibility, hard work, and self-reliance at an early age. These lessons helped me attain my dream of becoming a physician and will definitely be essential in my pursuit of a career in Diagnostic Radiology.

With all my might, I tightened the knob one last time. Bending over the gas tank, I placed my nose just millimeters away from the connection site and took in a deep breath. No smell of gas could be detected. With drops of water on my palms, I rubbed a bar of soap for a couple of minutes. I coated the soap suds over the connection site and waited for signs of bubbling but saw none. Gingerly, I turned on the stove and lit a match. What a sigh of relief! No explosion. I was 9 years old.

I am always systematic and detailed in my work. Whether the job is a routine replacement of the portable gas tank for the stove, preparing dinner for 20 guests, gathering data for my research projects, or taking care of my patients at the hospital, my performance has always been thorough. One cannot be an outstanding Radiologist without being detailed. No matter how much knowledge and experience a Radiologist has, she will undoubtedly miss the correct diagnosis if the subtle changes on the radiographic study are left undetected.

I sharpened my pencil and took another look at the model's face staring at me from the page of the magazine. Slowly, the expression in her eyes and the shape of her nose appeared on the white sheet of paper on which I had been drawing. I applied subtle shading around the cheekbones and nose in order to capture the lighting on her face. My art teacher entered my first attempt at a human portrait into the school-wide Art Contest. Surprise! I won Honorable Mention. I was 18 years old.

The ability to derive three-dimensional structures from two-dimensional pictures comes naturally to me. My grasp of the three dimensions combined with my eye for detail brought me recognition not only in the area of Fine Arts but also in other areas of my life. The wonderful taste and look of my Chinese cuisine are well-known to friends and family. They have also complimented me on my skill to bring to life a hairstyle off the pages of a magazine. I first discovered that I was such a "visual" person when I started attending school. I learned to read and write Chinese characters without difficulty because I was able to assemble and visualize every stroke in my mind. As a result, reading and writing Chinese now is no obstacle even though I received only two years of formal schooling in Taiwan. Diagnostic Radiology is a "visual" field, and the ability to extrapolate three dimensional structures from two-dimensional radiographs is indispensable.

The five year-old girl who had acute lymphocytic leukemia looked straight at me with her big brown eyes. "I am not going to cry," she said as she brought her knees onto her chest, in preparation for her usual prophylactic lumbar puncture. "I won't cry because I am a good girl...I am a good girl." She screamed as the needle entered her back but kept her body still. "I was a good girl, right? I didn't cry." She looked searchingly at me, dry-eyed. Tears welled up in my eyes, and I had to look away. I was 24 years old.

I have always been proud of the special relationship I share with my patients. Often I curse the painful procedures my patients have to experience, especially when I see innocent children suf-

fering from their terrible illnesses. Thankfully, several advancements in radiologic imaging have curtailed the need for invasive
diagnostic procedures. For example, disease staging for a number of malignancies can now be easily and painlessly obtained
through computed tomography instead of exploratory laparoto-
mies. Through my Pediatric Hematology-Oncology elective at
Caring Children's Hospital, I learned the important role Diagnostic
Radiology plays in the diagnosis, management, and treatment of
numerous oncologic diseases. I also had the chance to appreciate the value of different imaging modalities utilized in the diagnosis of malignancies while researching for my project in
gastrointestinal lymphomas. I have special interests in both Body
Imaging and Pediatric Radiology and would like to pursue further
studies in these areas at the completion of my residency.

*I feel I possess the qualities your program desires in a residency
candidate, and I look forward to my visit to your institution.*

Dermatology Residency Personal Statement

While I continued to pull through the heavy water, I heard the cox-
swain call out, "This is it!" My feelings of complete exhaustion and
loss of breath would have to wait. Months of getting up at five in
the morning for drills on the Strong River would come down to
one final moment. Rowing in college had meant working hard sur-
rounded by teammates who shared enthusiasm and drive.
Although my present goal is to train in dermatology, tenets in rowing continue to serve me today: hard work and perseverance
never go out of style.

As my fondness for rowing demonstrates, I love a good challenge. The opportunity for challenge and new discovery attracted
me to chemical engineering and medical research as an undergraduate. While working in a lab at Harvard, I became interested
in applying technology to the field of medicine. I was given many
hands-on tasks including learning tissue grafting. Surgery on animals allowed us to study tumor angiogenesis and directly visualize vessel growth and regression. My talents in engineering
proved to be of great use when I developed an algorithm to quantify blood flow. I had found research I truly enjoyed and this interest motivated me.

In medical school, I enjoyed the visual inspection of physical
diagnosis; clearly describing what I saw came naturally. I enjoyed
the focus of small, hands-on procedures. Dermatology captured

my interest and by early in my fourth year, I decided I needed more time to explore the field. Following medical school, I took a two-year position at Medical University where my engineering background allowed me to contribute to the creation of a survey tool for an outcomes research study where I gained critical skills in conducting clinical trials. I became expert in FDA and IRB regulatory issues and spent a great deal of time seeing dermatology patients. Gleaning clues from subtle distinguishing features required a true love of the diagnostic process; studying disease and following treatment outcomes continued to be satisfying. Together, these experiences confirmed my enthusiasm for dermatology was worth pursuing.

The field of dermatology appeals to me for many reasons. The relationship between doctor and patient is collaborative and often ongoing. Blistering and other diseases offer a spectrum of severities and clinical challenges. Our growing understanding of the skin's immune system makes this an especially exciting time to be in dermatology. Developing new therapies is tremendously rewarding—and the end results thrilling to see.

Since completing my medical internship in June, I have worked as a Clinical Fellow with the Department of Dermatology. I continue to add to my research skills guiding a Phase III melanoma vaccine trial. I have become expert in vaccine development, manufacturing, and testing. My experience has allowed me to collaborate with world-renowned dermatologists and researchers. Skills I develop here will surely serve me well throughout my career.

My goal is to utilize my unique background in engineering to one day design and test new dermatologic therapies of my own. I would consider myself lucky to return to My University for residency and my elective only strengthened this feeling. I believe My University can offer the ideal training environment for the type of career I have chosen. The diversity of clinical settings and spectrum of disease is appealing, and training with research leaders such as Skin Doctor would offer a great perspective on evolving therapies, as well as continued mentorship. I will continue to use hard work and determination to reach my goals in dermatology and like in rowing, look forward to new challenges and discoveries ahead.

From www.medfools.com (with permission)

Pathology Personal Statement

The woman lying in Bed 14 was totally disfigured. More than half of her body was covered by deep ulcers, foul-smelling pus and thick crusts. She had lost her hair and eyelids and her cheeks were penetrated deeply. Seven years ago I was a dermatology resident at a teaching hospital in Beijing. I had the opportunity to see a wide range of cases from across the nation where I met Mrs. Yao. From her husband I learned that her ordeal started with a coin-like macule on the forearm, which was first misdiagnosed as psoriasis at a local clinic. Believing the misdiagnosis, she treated herself with herbal medicine for several years until a full eruption of skin lesions occurred. She was later diagnosed as having mycosis fungoides, a cutaneous T-cell lymphoma, and sadly passed away on our ward despite an enormous effort to save her. The tragedy was reinforced by the fact that Mrs. Yao could have had a good chance of survival if treated early. During my residency I could not help but wonder: "How can we give every patient the correct diagnosis?" Personal experience has made me fascinated with Pathology as a science and as a career and although I started my medical career in dermatology, I have realized that my calling lies in pathology.

The person who correctly diagnosed Mrs. Yao is my mentor, Dr. Xavier, a brilliant dermatologist and dermatopathologist whom I deeply admire. My training in dermatopathology with Dr. Xavier turned out to be the most exciting time in my residency. Pathology is our most powerful weapon to reach a correct diagnosis. Dr. Xavier liked to say "Pathology is the third eye of the dermatologist." Indeed, in a specialty where cases tend to be diagnosed by a mere glance at the skin, Pathology has a dramatic impact on clinical decision making. I enjoyed sitting before a microscope, browsing through our collection of slides and making discoveries. Every slide, every cell tells a story. At that time I was convinced that Pathology would always be my passion.

I also chose Pathology because of enormous research opportunities. During my first residency, I studied p53 gene mutations in skin cancers and wrote a well received thesis while under the pressure of a tight residency curriculum. With great enthusiasm I performed most experiments at night in my spare time. This early adventure in science inspired me with great interest in scientific exploration. During the following years my adventure has gone further and deeper. It has moved from thermal cyclers to tissue culture rooms, to microarray chips, and even to supercomputers.

No matter what front I work on, my goal of applying science to furthering human health has never changed. Being a pathologist would give me an enormous opportunity to bridge basic science and clinical medicine, while applying the latest scientific advancements to solving the mystery of human disease.

No specialty attracts me more than Pathology. Making diagnoses is a complex task that requires gathering and integrating information, a great intellectual challenge that I always enjoy facing. As a pathologist, I will have the unique opportunity to work with physicians of every specialty, to deal with diseases of every organ system, and to combine clinical with morphological, biochemical, and even molecular findings. It will be intellectually rewarding and will be a continuous source of learning. Above all of these, Pathology will fuel the passion of all of us who have chosen Medicine as a career, because lives can be saved by correct diagnoses.

In the future I see myself pursuing a career in academic medicine. I will dedicate myself to providing the best diagnostic service to patients while exploring the nature of human diseases. I would love to educate young physicians and scientists. After residency I hope to pursue further training in a subspecialty. I believe a residency in pathology is a place where I can begin to fulfill my professional goals.

From www.medfools.com (with permission)

PM&R Residency Personal Statement

In the banquet room of an Italian restaurant in Northern Alaska, my high school track coach addressed his team and their families at the end of the season. Most senior athletes were complimented on either a winning season or a season of hard work. I had accomplished neither. In addressing me in front of the crowd he said: "Despite what the record books show, I know Karen is the best triple jumper to ever compete for this school." I was so proud to hear those words after a season which began with me favored to win the league title and break the school record, and ended without me having the chance. My senior season turned into months of physical therapy, sitting on the bench and hoping for a chance to get back to the form I once had. Although my injury kept me from breaking that record, the lessons I learned during that time have proven to guide me in my choice of careers.

Since then I have been drawn to a career where I am involved in helping people achieve optimum function and recover from similar experiences where dreams seem lost and rehabilitation can be difficult. I had my first hands-on experience with the field of rehabilitation during college when I volunteered at the first rehabilitation hospital to open in my hometown. I worked in the Transitional Care Unit leading activities including wheelchair aerobics, art therapy and pet therapy. The physicians and therapists I met there played a role in encouraging me to apply to medical school.

During my first two years of medical school I was able to work with three different Physiatrists who introduced me to a field where I witnessed the long-term relationships that developed between doctor and patient, as well as the opportunity to be the leader of a rehabilitation team. Both of these aspects of the specialty are important to me and coincide with my strengths, which include strong interpersonal skills and development of relationships as well as a love of organizing and motivating people. The ease with which I work with all types of people has always been one of the areas where I have been complimented most by others.

In my third year during my family medicine and internal medicine rotations I found my interest in the specialty confirmed by my enjoyment of my Workman's Compensation and orthopedic surgical recovery patients. I now look forward to broadening my exposure to the field of Physical Medicine and Rehabilitation during the two elective rotations I have in October and November.

In residency, I hope to attend a program that will provide a solid foundation in the pathophysiology as well as the clinical practice of rehabilitation medicine. I value structured training with diversity of exposure to patients and facilities. I would like to learn in an environment that encourages a close relationship with the patients as well as the other residents and faculty.

As far as my goals after residency, I would like to continue my education with fellowship training in either musculoskeletal or sports medicine. I aspire to a career in clinical medicine with opportunities to do clinical research and possibly supervise medical students and residents. I love the academic community environment and especially the constant learning that accompanies the field of medicine.

From www.medfools.com (with permission)

Emergency Medicine Personal Statement

The wind whipped through the airplane cabin as the door opened at 13,800 feet. As I sat waiting for my turn to jump, I felt more anxious and uncertain than I'd ever been in my life. "Ready?" the jump master yelled. I didn't have time to respond. My rotation in Emergency Medicine, as a fourth year medical student, had been going well. I never imagined it would lead me to this. I had accepted an invitation to go skydiving with a couple of the residents. Suddenly, I was flipping through the sky. Only moments before, my instructor and I had discussed why I wish to become an Emergency Medicine Physician. I told him about my experiences in the field and how intense, exhilarating, and rewarding I found Emergency Medicine. His response was, "Well, buddy, you are about to have one of the most exhilarating and intense experiences of your life!" He was right. For fifty seconds of free fall towards the Earth, I felt pure ecstasy. After pulling the rip cord, we smoothly glided down under the parachute. Everything became serene. Sailing down from the sky, the anxiety and uncertainty had disappeared. I found myself completely at peace and gratified with my decision to jump. I feel that same sense of peace about my dive into pursing Emergency Medicine.

Emergency Medicine appeals to me as a humanistic, challenging field, offering the opportunity to provide immediate help to people in the most vital aspect of their lives: their health. The emotional rewards of helping those during their greatest times of need are intangible. Twelve years ago, I encountered this first hand as knee surgery introduced me to medicine. It was an eye-opening experience to me; then, a 14-year-old kid who, before surgery, dreamed of playing professional football. As a result of the positive impression the entire experience had on me, the medical profession emerged as my newfound desire. My employment prior to and during medical school, working as an E.M.T. and a Scribe in the Emergency Department of Saint Elsewhere Regional Medical Center in Wyoming, introduced me to the field of Emergency Medicine. It was there, as well as my experiences with the Army National Guard, serving as a flight medic, that my interest blossomed. Being in the ED as a medical student has fortified my desire to enter the field.

Emergency Medicine offers me the opportunity to be at the forefront of medicine and to participate actively in making decisions right from the onset of patient care. I've learned that the ability to immediately establish rapport and make the patient feel better is not only a part of the Emergency Medicine Physician's responsibilities, but is also one of the most satisfying aspects of the specialty. The fast pace, community involvement, and the required broad knowledge base attract me to Emergency Medicine. The Emergency Medical System comes together to help all people, including those who have nowhere else to turn. I want to be an active part of that system.

I look forward to a career in Emergency Medicine involving clinical practice, education, and research. During my own medical education, spending time in a research lab studying the response to thermal injury in a rat model, I have become increasingly aware of the importance of research. I will seek out opportunities to participate in Emergency Medicine research that will promote advancement in the field. I also feel that teaching adds a gratifying and stimulating aspect to practice that can be incorporated into almost any situation. Having the opportunity to train residents and students is something I will weigh considerably when selecting a location to practice. I hope to be in an area that allows me to serve a diverse patient population, as well as providing an environment that supports my outside interests of mountain biking, golf, basketball, scuba diving, and skiing. Skydiving doesn't make the list just yet. These hobbies and my sense of humor allow me to keep a balance in my own life and increase my enthusiasm for practicing medicine. I'm ready to jump into residency training with this enthusiasm.

Emergency Medicine will endow me with a solid education and preparation for a profession in which I am able to deal with the entire spectrum of acute illness and injury in all age groups. I wish to enter a residency program that will provide a broad-based clinical education with a diverse patient population that emphasizes education, encourages mentoring, facilitates opportunities for research, and is intimately involved in Emergency Medical Services. I will bring to my residency program a hard working, mature individual who has a clear vision of a career in Emergency Medicine. My experiences and training have reinforced my dedication to this dynamic and exhilarating field of medicine.

From www.medfools.com (with permission)

Chapter 9

Dean's Letter (MSPE)

Applicants must submit a letter from the Dean as part of their application. Known previously as the Dean's letter, this letter is now formally termed the Medical Student Performance Evaluation (MSPE). The typical MSPE contains an assessment of both a student's academic performance and professional attributes. Residency programs find the MSPE an especially helpful tool to learn about your performance in medical school relative to your peers.

Rule # 73   Recognize the importance of the Dean's letter to some specialties.

The following table summarizes the studies on the importance of the Dean's letter in the residency selection process.

Importance of Dean's Letter to Selected Specialties	
Study	What was found
Survey of program directors in family medicine and obstetrics and gynecology inquiring about the importance of various application components (Taylor)	In deciding whether to invite an applicant for an interview, obstetric and gynecology program directors ranked the medical school transcript, Dean's letter, and USMLE score highest (in descending order). The Dean's letter was also among the top three factors used by family practice residency program directors for making decisions about interview invitations.
Survey of family practice residency program directors inquiring about the importance of various application components (Travis)	This study, done as a follow-up to the Taylor study, again showed that the Dean's letter continues to be one of the top three criteria used in the residency selection process.
Survey of program directors in internal medicine inquiring about the usefulness of various application components in making decisions about interview invitations and ranking applicants (Adams)	The Dean's letter was rated highly or moderately useful by 87% of respondents; 82% rated the Dean's letter as highly or moderately useful for making ranking decisions.

Questionnaire sent to PM & R program directors inquiring about the importance of various application components (DeLisa)	Most program directors used multiple criteria to complete their rank list, but the most important were the interview, letters of recommendation, medical school transcript, and the Dean's letter (in descending order of importance).
Questionnaire sent to radiology residency program directors to determine the importance of various application components (Otero)	Respondents were asked to assign a zero to ten score regarding the importance of variables related to extending interview invitations. The USMLE score was ranked highest with a score of 8.65 followed by the Dean's letter at 7.52.
Survey of orthopedic residency program directors to determine what program directors value most highly (Bernstein)	The Dean's letter was ranked 10th out of a group of 26 variables used in the resident selection process.
Survey of orthopedic residency program directors to determine the most important attributes to obtaining a residency (Bajaj)	The Dean's letter was ranked 7th in importance for resident selection.
Survey of program directors of American Osteopathic Association-approved primary care graduate training programs regarding the importance of 22 variables used in the residency selection process (Bates)	The Dean's letter was ranked 18th out of a group of 22 variables.
Study done to learn about characteristics of an applicant that might predict future success in an emergency medicine residency (Hayden)	It was found that the Dean's letter correlated fairly well with overall success in residency. In particular, the letter's categorical rating (outstanding, excellent, superior, very good, or good) was found to be a strong predictor of performance during residency training.
Study comparing Dean's letter categorical ranking (outstanding, excellent, very good, good) of University of Rochester students with program director ratings of these students nine months into their internship (Lurie)	The Dean's letter ranking was found to be a significant predictor of performance in internship.

As demonstrated in the literature, specialties attach varying degrees of importance to the Dean's letter. Even within a specialty, programs differ on the importance of the MSPE. Your ultimate goal with the MSPE is to provide assistance to the Dean's office in order to develop the best letter that can be written on your behalf. Fortunately, at most schools, students are involved in the preparation of this letter.

Rule # 74   Understanding the content of the Dean's letter is the first step in improving it.

Although the Dean's letter has been a standard part of the residency application for many years, there is considerable debate about its usefulness. Some schools produce letters containing highly useful, detailed and honest information about a student's medical school performance. Others are lacking in the key information that programs need to compare applicants.

Critics of the Dean's letter assert that these letters almost always contain positive information. They contend that significant information is often withheld or suppressed, including information about course or clerkship failure, leaves of absence, or lapses in professionalism. Supporters of the Dean's letter recognize these shortcomings, but maintain that the letter has value, especially in offering programs information about class rank and a comparison of students to their peers. Furthermore, they cite that schools often include an overall recommendation, usually at the end of the letter.

Because of variability in content and lack of standardization among letters from different schools, the AAMC convened several committees to make recommendations about the letter. These committees recommended that schools should not view the Dean's letter as a letter of recommendation predictive of future performance, but rather a letter of evaluation. As such, the letter should describe in a sequential manner a student's performance. In describing performance, the AAMC committee urged schools to include comparative performance information. In other words, how did the student perform relative to his peers?

The AAMC also recommended that the MSPE include six sections. These sections are described in the following table.

Sections of the MSPE	Description
Identifying information	Your legal name Name and location of medical school
Unique characteristics	Brief statement about your unique characteristics (e.g., leadership positions, research abilities, community service activities). May also include information about any significant challenges or hardships you encountered during medical school.
Academic history	Month and year of initial matriculation. Expected graduation date. Explanation of any extensions, leaves of absence, gaps, or breaks in your medical school education Information about courses or clerkships that you were required to repeat or remediate. Information about any disciplinary action you received from the medical school.

Sections of the MSPE	Description
Academic progress	Your academic performance and professional attributes during basic science and clinical years of medical school. Narrative information regarding your overall performance in basic sciences. Narrative information regarding your overall performance on each core clerkship and elective rotation.
Summary	A summative assessment of your performance in medical school relative to your peers.
Appendices	Graphic representation of your performance relative to your peers in each pre-clinical course and core clerkship. Graphic representation of your overall performance relative to your peers.

Rule # 75   You can influence the content of the MSPE.

Students may assume that the Dean's letter is written by the dean using information that the school has already obtained. However, students play a much larger role in influencing the content of the MSPE than they realize. Most schools ask students to complete a student information sheet, providing an opportunity for the student to highlight certain aspects of their education and activities. Deans may choose to emphasize certain aspects of a student's career if those aspects have been emphasized by the student. Prior work experience as a paramedic, a weekly commitment to volunteering in the children's education center of a homeless shelter, or an ongoing clinical research project are all activities that could be highlighted. Such items may also be emphasized when meeting with the dean in person.

The Dean's office provides students with a biographical information sheet that will be used to assist in the formulation of the MSPE. On this sheet, students are asked the following:

- Name
- Undergraduate institution (major, degree, dates attended, extracurricular activities)
- Graduate education (major, degree, dates attended)
- Awards (undergraduate, graduate)
- Notable or distinguished activities prior to medical school
- Extracurricular activities during medical school
- Publications/presentations
- Employment history before and during medical school
- Leaves of absence during medical school, including reasons
- Field/specialty of interest
- Additional information you would like included

Some schools will also ask for a CV and personal statement to help prepare the MSPE. This provides yet another compelling reason to begin working on these elements of your residency application early in the process.

Tip # 69

Per the University of Iowa College of Medicine:
"The more information you provide about your medical school activities, the more complete your Dean's letter draft will be."
From www.medicine.uiowa.edu.osac/programsrecords/DeansLetterProcess.htm

---

Just as in your CV, it's not enough to list certain accomplishments. You must highlight accomplishments that may be regarded by program directors as exceptional, such as leadership positions, athletic or artistic accomplishments, or significant volunteer work. As shown in the following box, these can be regarded as predictors of residency success.

Did you know ...

In a study done to determine the factors that predict success during an emergency medicine residency, having a "distinctive factor" such as being a top-level athlete, musician, or class officer was a significant factor that predicted future success (Hayden). The authors wrote that "it could be that an applicant who is capable of high-level performance in medical school and simultaneously capable of high-level achievement in sports, music, etc., is well organized and can prioritize and multitask well."

Rule # 76   Always preview your file in order to correct inaccuracies or identify red flags.

A preview of your file is critical. In the spring of your junior year, arrange to look through your file. Before the dean begins to draft your letter, it is your responsibility to ensure that everything in your file is accurate, including the official transcript.

You also need to search for any potential red flags. We review issues that are potential negatives later in this chapter. These types of issues are likely to be included in your letter. It is important that you note these well before you apply for residency. You will need to formulate a plan on how to address these issues in your application materials.

Rule # 77   The Dean doesn't always write the Dean's letter. If you can, choose your writer.

Since the writing of the Dean's letter is an enormous task for the Dean's office, schools have a number of administrators involved in the development of these letters. Some schools permit students to choose the author of their Dean's letter from this group.

Choose your writer carefully. Since the two of you will work together to develop your letter, choose a writer with whom you have good rapport. Slots with a popular writer may fill up quickly, so place your request as early as possible.

Rule # 78   Don't just assume that your final letter will be fine.

At some schools, students are able to read several drafts of the letter. More commonly, schools make only the final draft available to their students. Take advantage of any opportunity to review your letter, because it may be your only chance to make suggestions or corrections.

Tip # 70

If you will be at an away rotation when your letter is completed, make arrangements to receive this letter. Review it, make any suggestions or corrections, and return it by the date specified.

As you review the letter, pay particular attention to the ending paragraphs. Within the final paragraph or summary section of the letter is often a key word or phrase that provides program directors an idea of your overall performance relative to your peers. Schools will use different descriptors to convey this information, with "good," "very good," "excellent," and "outstanding" being among the more common scales. Make note of this final statement to ensure that the descriptor your school has used to describe your overall performance is indeed correct.

Schools will generally ask you to sign off on the final version. After signing off, you won't be able to make any further changes, and the letter will be sent to residency programs.

Did you know ...

The AAMC recommends that students be allowed to correct factual errors in MSPE but not be permitted to revise any evaluative statements. Despite this recommendation, schools often take student suggestions seriously. As far as negative comments are concerned, Deans may decide whether to exclude the comments based on the consistency of the problem and its severity.

Did you know...

In a 1992 survey, approximately 40% of deans reported that they did not always include ethical problems in their letters, 60% did not always include substance abuse, 70% did not always include emotional instability, and 75% did not always include physical illness (Hunt).

Rule # 79   Do not wait until the Dean's letter is sent before completing the rest of your application.

The uniform release date for the MSPE is November 1. Many applicants are under the assumption that programs won't invite applicants to interview until the application is complete. While some programs will wait until they've received the MSPE, many programs will extend interview invitations well before the uniform release date. For this reason, complete your residency application as early as possible.

Did you know...

In a survey of 73 interviewees to the emergency medicine residency program at the Oregon Health Sciences University, applicants were asked if they received any interviews from programs before November 1 and, if so, from whom (Delorio). 77% of respondents reported receiving interview invitations prior to November 1. At least 44% of emergency medicine residency programs were found to send early interview invitations. This study confirmed that many programs offer interview invitations prior to the MSPE uniform release date of November 1. Applicants should submit their applications as early as possible.

Rule # 80   Do extensive prep work before you meet with the Dean.

Following receipt of your student information sheet, some schools have their students meet with the Dean to discuss the letter. During this meeting, the Dean may ask you about the following:

- Your background
- Your medical school career
- Your career plans
- Programs to which you are applying
- Any events in your medical school career that require explanation (e.g., poor grade, leave of absence)

You may also be able to discuss your overall residency application strategy, an invaluable opportunity.

Tip # 71

A meeting with the Dean should be regarded as a valuable opportunity. Take advantage of this opportunity to discuss your chances of matching into a particular specialty or program. Having counseled many students in the past, the dean is in a unique position to help you. He or she may be able to offer valuable insight based on the medical school's experience with previous students of similar backgrounds and qualifications.

Rule # 81   Read the narratives section very carefully. Critical review of these comments will help you identify any potential areas of concern for program directors.

If your school follows the AAMC-recommended format, narrative information regarding your overall performance on each core clerkship and elective rotation will be included in the "Academic Progress" section of the MSPE. What is the source of this narrative information?

On clerkship evaluation forms, there is usually a section in which evaluators are asked to comment on a student's clinical performance. Comments about professionalism, knowledge, communication skills with other health care professionals, clinical reasoning, and clinical judgment are most common (Pulito). Often, the comments of the evaluators are taken and placed word for word in this section of the MSPE.

While comments are generally positive, evaluators may also include negative comments. Some schools have a policy to place all comments in their entirety within the MSPE, regardless of whether they are positive or negative. Other schools may edit out negative information, particularly if the comment reflects the thoughts of only a single evaluator.

As you review your MSPE, read the narratives section very carefully. Circle anything that might be viewed as a negative. Following is one example.

Third-year clinical clerkships

Comments regarding Mr. Ortiz's clinical performance are given below in chronological order:

Pediatrics: High pass; "Roberto was a very earnest student. His history taking skills were at a level that was expected for his training. He progressed nicely in the quality of his oral case presentations. He brought in articles to share with the team."

Family medicine: High pass; "Roberto has a good knowledge base. He tends to be quiet so it can sometimes be hard to realize this. He could be more involved in discussions. He worked well with team members and was always prompt at scheduled rounds."

Surgery: Pass; "Roberto was hard-working, motivated, and dedicated. Compared to other students on the service, Roberto was fairly quiet, often not being heard from for long stretches of time during rounds. He needs to work on participation during rounds. He will be a great student and physician once he develops more self-confidence."

In the previous example, a program director might be concerned about Roberto's level of participation in rounds and conferences, especially since similar comments were written by evaluators in two different clerkships. Does Roberto simply have a "quiet" personality, or does his lack of participation suggest indifference, inadequate knowledge, or lack of motivation?

Critical review of these comments will help you identify potential areas of concern for program directors. In some cases, negative information (i.e., failed clerkships) may have to be addressed in other areas of the application, such as the personal statement. Otherwise, the application may be rejected.

In other cases, the comment(s) may be relatively minor. With minor issues, you may not want to bring undue attention to them, because they may not have an effect on the strength of your application. However, you should still be ready to address these issues in the event that they come up during an interview.

Applicants often have a hard time deciding whether an issue raised in the MSPE requires addressing elsewhere in the application. Such issues should be discussed with your advisors.

Rule # 82   Identify and be prepared to address any red flags in your application.

Is there any other information in your file that would be considered a red flag to residency programs? Have you had any academic problems? Have you taken a leave of absence? Have you failed a preclinical course or clerkship? Have you received any disciplinary action for a lapse in professionalism?

These issues will need to be addressed with the dean. The following table outlines issues that would be considered a red flag to program directors.

Program directors' rankings of their concerns about selected academic and non-academic issues*	
Issue	Mean
Received disciplinary action in medical school	4.90
Treated for alcoholism	4.90
Received failure in a required clerkship	4.63
Took extended time to graduate for academic reasons	4.55
Has learning disability	4.47
Failed USMLE step I prior to passing	4.46
Passed USMLE with minimal scores	4.18
Graduated in the lower third of class	3.91
Received a failure in a preclinical course	3.73
Had mediocre preclinical grades but strong clinical evaluations	3.27
Had family responsibilities	3.00
Did not participate in extracurricular activities in medical school	2.91
*Responses from 794 residency program directors. Rating scale: 1 (no concern) to 5 (very concerned)	
From Wagoner NE, Suriano JR. Program directors' responses to a survey on variables used to select residents in a time of change. *Acad Med* 1999; 74 (1): 51-8.	

If your medical school experience includes any of the red flags listed in the above table, realize that the issue may be included in your Dean's letter. Keep in mind, however, that deans have been known to take liberties during the editing process in order to shine the best possible light on their students. In fact, several studies have shown that discrepancies between the Dean's letter and the official medical school transcript are common.

Did you know...

In a 1997 study looking at concordance between 532 Dean's letters and corresponding transcripts, Edmond found the following:

Among students who failed a pre-clinical course, there was no mention of this in 27% of letters.

Among students who failed a clinical rotation, there was no mention of this in 33% of letters.

Among students who took a leave of absence, there was no mention of this in 40% of letters.

Of the 4 students who had to repeat an entire year, there was no mention of this in two letters.

It was found that negative information was withheld one third of the time (Edmond).

There are several reasons as to why a dean would withhold negative information. First, some deans argue that an otherwise strong applicant's chances of matching into the specialty or program of his choice may be damaged by including negative information, especially if the issue was not characteristic of the student's overall performance. In this case, a dean may suppress negative comments from a single evaluator if all other evaluators were glowingly positive. In addition, deans would like their students to gain residency positions in highly reputed programs, and therefore may be hesitant to discuss their students' shortcomings. In some cases, there may be a fear of legal retribution.

If your transcript does contain a red flag such as a failed pre-clinical course, then do everything possible to make sure that the remainder of your transcript is impeccable. You can make a more convincing argument to the dean and in interviews if your failure is seen as an isolated incident that does not accurately reflect your abilities.

Chapter 10

The Audition Elective

An "audition" elective essentially serves as an extended interview, and should be regarded as such. Audition electives are valued by programs as a means to more reliably assess an applicant's cognitive and noncognitive skills and traits. For students applying to competitive specialties or programs, audition electives are considered a must by some advisors. These four- or eight-week rotations offer students the chance to highlight skills and qualities that aren't easily judged by the typical application materials. Students can showcase their clinical acumen, their skills in patient interaction, their abilities to work with colleagues and faculty, and their enthusiasm for the particular program and specialty. These electives also offer additional opportunities to highlight a student's qualifications for the program. Opportunities include deeper investigation of difficult cases, performing thorough literature searches, volunteering to give presentations, or seeking opportunities to publish in their chosen field.

Audition electives have increased in popularity as students increasingly try to gain a competitive advantage wherever possible. In response to this trend, some educators have criticized students and their medical schools for allowing applicants to do multiple audition electives. Some schools have adopted policies limiting the number of electives that students can complete in any given specialty. However, students continue to receive messages encouraging audition electives, and often these messages come directly from residency programs. Some make it clear that in order to be seriously considered, an applicant should rotate through the department. These conflicting messages confuse students. Should I do an audition elective? How many should I do? When is the best time to do one? How can I excel during the elective? Will it guarantee me an interview? We address these questions in this chapter.

Rule # 83   In some specialties, audition electives are considered a must.

In a survey of program directors representing multiple specialties, Wagoner found that 86% of program directors would give preference to students who had performed at a high level in an audition elective (Wagoner). This is not surprising, since an audition elective is essentially an extended interview, during which a program can more reliably assess an applicant's cognitive and noncognitive skills and traits. Some specialties attach great importance to the audition elective. In a survey of orthopedic surgery residency program directors, *the most important criterion in the resident selection process* was considered to be an applicant's performance during a rotation at the director's program (Bernstein). The authors of the study further stated that "60% of programs reported that 50% or more of their matching residents over the previous three years had performed medical student orthopedic surgery rotations at the program prior to matching for residency." Of note, applicants were also asked about their impressions regarding the importance of these selection factors, and the audition elective was not cited among their top three. In another survey of orthopedic surgery residency program directors, performance on a local rotation was considered *the most important attribute* in obtaining a residency. This was followed by class rank and the interview (Bajaj). Drs. Peabody and Manning, faculty members in the Department of Orthopedics at the University of Chicago, strongly recommend audition electives. "It's almost mandatory to do an away elective and shine."

In a survey of 2003 dermatology applicants, the audition elective was similarly important. A total of 53% of applicants matched at a program in which they had some prior experience. Of these, 29% matched at an institution affiliated with their own medical school, 18% matched with an institution where they had done an audition elective, and 6% matched with a program where they had done a research elective or fellowship (Clarke). In other specialties, by contrast, the audition elective may not have much of an effect. Following is a summary of the literature on the importance of this criterion to different specialties.

Importance of audition electives by specialty	
Survey	**Results**
Survey of orthopedic residency program directors inquiring about those factors considered most important in the resident selection process (Bernstein). Applicants were also asked about their impressions regarding the importance of these factors.	Most important criterion was an applicant's performance during a rotation at the director's program. Of note, applicants did not cite this factor among their top 3.

Survey of 2003 dermatology applicants (Clarke).	53% of applicants matched at a program where they had some prior experience, highlighting the importance of audition electives: • 29% matched at an institution affiliated with their medical school • 18% matched with an institution where they had done an audition elective • 6% matched with a program where they had done a research elective/fellowship
Survey of orthopedic residency program directors (Bajaj).	Performance on a local rotation was the most important attribute to obtaining a residency.
Survey of 41 PM&R program directors inquiring about the residency selection process (Garden).	While the interview was the most important overall factor, of the academic variables presented, an elective performed at the program director's hospital and the Dean's letter were rated highest.
Survey of 94 emergency medicine residency program directors inquiring about the criteria directors use to select residents (Crane).	Respondents were asked to rate each item on a scale of 1(least important) to 5 (most important). Performance at an elective at the program director's institution received a mean score of 3.76, making it a moderately important factor. Of note, it did have the largest standard deviations of all responses, suggesting that programs vary in the degree of importance attached to these electives.
Study reviewing the outcome of 99 students who completed audition electives in surgery (Fabri).	Results showed that while audition electives increase the probability of receiving an interview, these electives had no effect on the probability of matching with general surgery residency programs. However, authors noted that surgical specialties viewed audition electives differently, with some placing high priority on these electives.
Survey of 89 radiology residency program directors from 2005 (www.apdr.org).	31% rated an audition elective in their department as an extremely important criterion for selecting an applicant for interview, and 23% rated an elective as an extremely important criterion for ranking.

While the value of these electives varies considerably from specialty to specialty, as a general rule audition electives are less important in family medicine, internal medicine, pediatrics, neurology, and pathology. However, even within these less competitive specialties, an audition elective may be important to certain programs. This may be dependent upon other factors including the competitiveness of the program, the strength of your candidacy, and the program's familiarity with your medical school.

Rule # 84   Recognize the full advantages of an audition elective, and plan to maximize each one.

Audition electives provide many potential advantages in increasing the competitiveness of your application. However, applicants who have rotated with us and with our colleagues don't always realize the full roster of potential benefits. Before starting your elective, plan carefully so that you can take advantage of each of these potential benefits.

- An additional elective in your field can provide an unmatched clinical experience. It can allow you to work with and learn from some of the best faculty in the country. It can provide exposure to other facets of the specialty not available at your own institution.

- The audition elective serves as an extended interview. This is your chance to impress upon the program what an outstanding student you are, and what an outstanding resident you would be.

- The audition elective provides an ideal opportunity to impress upon the program how well you would fit in with their residency program. An outstanding student is not always a great fit for every program. You can use the opportunities presented by an audition elective to emphasize those factors that make you perfect for the program, and make the program perfect for you. If you have extensive experience in basic science research and your future plans include translational research, then discuss your desire to obtain complete and thorough clinical training in order to aid you in your future translational research. If you have spent all of your formative years and education in the city of Miami, make sure the program understands that you definitely want to experience a new part of the country. If you have an interest in pediatric gastroenterology, then discuss the specialized opportunities available at this referral center.

- The audition elective provides the chance for the chairman and faculty to recognize you as an individual. With over 400 applications received last year for a total of three residency positions at our dermatology program, it becomes very difficult for even outstanding applicants to stand out. Just rotating through a program is not sufficient, though. You need to meet key decision makers in the program, other faculty members, the residents, and the support staff. We discuss how to do so below.

- You've already set your application apart because of this personal experience with the program. With some applicants applying to 50 or more programs, it can be difficult for a program to gauge if a student is actually interested in the program, or if it was just one of many that a student targeted in order to increase their chances of matching. You have demonstrated a concrete interest in this particular program.

- You should plan to obtain a strong letter of recommendation from the experience. Particularly if you have chosen your elective well, you may have the support of a prominent, respected, well-known individual. Letters from such attendings can carry great weight nationally. In addition, a strong letter of recommendation from an attending within the program can be a stronger influence than a strong letter from an unknown letter writer. The section on letters of recommendation provides more guidance.

- An audition elective provides an unparalleled opportunity to directly impress your attending. Your outstanding work will hopefully impress an attending to the degree that they become your advocate in residency selection proceedings. Attendings will often argue for a certain applicant's candidacy, and often quite passionately, and that advocacy can be enough to tip the scales in your favor. Your work during the elective also provides exposure to other members of the department. Residents, nurses, and secretaries can also act as vocal advocates.

- An elective provides additional opportunities to work on a project. Seeking out case reports or review articles at the start of the elective signifies your enthusiasm and commitment to the field. Completing a project, and completing it well, signifies your skills and drive. Such work helps you stand out. It also provides additional material for your CV. It also gives your letter writer concrete information to discuss in the letter. "Soledad was a very enthusiastic student" doesn't carry all that much weight. However, this statement makes a reviewer take notice: "Soledad began the rotation by seeking out opportunities for articles. When we saw a case of actinic lichen planus together, she did an extensive literature search, presented her findings to me the next day, and asked if she could write up the case. I had a well-written case report on my desk three days later."

- It allows you to meet residents in your field. Residents are a great resource. Let them know on day one if you're interested in matching into this field, and if you're interested in this particular program. They can give you excellent advice on how to approach an attending, and which attendings would be best to approach, for letters or publications. They can introduce you to other faculty in the program. They can help you seek out interesting clinical cases that could serve as material for publication. They can, and often do, serve as vocal advocates for certain applicants with whom they would like to work in the future. They can sometimes be the most knowledgeable resources about programs around the country, having more recently completed the application process. Let the residents know on day 30 how you felt about the program and your experience there, particularly if it has become a top choice.

Caution...

Regardless of specialty, the practice of medicine requires a broad range of skills. In addition to being intellectually capable, physicians must have the noncognitive skills necessary to effectively interact with and relate to a wide variety of patients and healthcare professionals. Just because an individual can score at high levels on a standardized test, it does not mean that they have the skills of perception and communication required to excel in areas requiring interactions, which basically encompasses almost all of medical practice.

This is a difficult area in which to counsel students, and these are skills that are difficult to teach. Many students don't even realize that they excel in these areas, because they have acquired these skills intuitively. Other students don't even realize their lack of these skills. They may only start to realize it when they are evaluated in these areas, such as during clinical rotations. It may become more apparent when they receive feedback from patients on their bedside manner, from attendings on their communication skills, and from colleagues on their teamwork.

There's a fine line between many of the qualities that are important to residency selection, and many of the qualities that are perceived as negatives, as indicated in the following list.

Assertive / Aggressive

Enthusiastic / Playing the game

Confident / Arrogant

Friendly / A suck-up

Humble / Lacking in self-confidence

Quiet / Insecure

Polite and respectful of others' turns to speak / Disinterested or lacking in the knowledge required to speak

The first to volunteer to give a talk / A gunner

Meeting with decision-makers during the rotation / Too political

Obviously, we could go on and on. These negative labels may come from anyone—your colleagues, the residents, or the attendings.

How do you make sure that you're projecting the fact that you are enthusiastic about the specialty and the program without projecting an appearance of just trying to play the game? These are difficult skills to perfect, and entire books have been written about this subject in the business literature and in the career advancement genre.

Some of this is beyond your control, as with some attendings who think every other elective student is trying too hard to be political. Much of it is under your control, though, even though these skills are difficult to master. The process begins with self-evaluation and close attention to feedback throughout your career.

Rule # 85   An audition elective does not equate to an away elective. Your most important audition elective may in fact be the one at your own institution.

Away electives are important, and can be critical to your future career. Most students recognize this fact. However, a local elective can be just as critical to your career. In terms of matching into your field, some programs will give preference to a "known commodity." In the survey of dermatology applicants described above, 29% of applicants matched at an institution affiliated with their own medical school (Clarke).

As opposed to the snapshot of an applicant obtained from a 15-minute interview, faculty feel more confident in their impressions of a student after one month of working with that student and after hearing other attendings' personal knowledge of their qualities. Another important point is that faculty from your own institution, including your chairman, may be called or e-mailed by other programs for their candid opinion. The bottom line: recognize that the most important audition elective you take may be the first one you take.

Rule # 86   An outstanding audition elective can overcome shortcomings in your application.

We have witnessed the power of the audition elective. Residency selection committees often use screening criteria when reviewing applications. For example, a USMLE score under 200 may automatically exclude you from consideration, regardless of your transcript, Dean's letter, or letters of recommendation. However, students with such low scores can still match into competitive specialties, a fact we can attest to and a fact that is reflected in NRMP data. The audition elective is an ideal opportunity to impress upon the residency program that a low USMLE score will not prevent you from performing high-quality work and won't impact your ability to pass the specialty's board.

If you have average grades and an average USMLE score, your application won't stand out from the exceedingly strong applications under consideration at competitive programs. However, personal knowledge of your skills, qualities, and work ethic can provide a huge boost to your application.

Did you know ...

Dr. Terris, program director at the Medical College of Georgia, states that "participating in a urology rotation at an institution other than the student's home institution may be beneficial if it is a program at which the student is particularly interested in completing residency training. A visiting student rotation can give students the chance to impress the urology faculty at another institution if their clinical skills outweigh their academic record or who attend a medical school of lesser reputation."

(http://www.urologymatch.com/Program_Survey.htm).

Did you know ...

Some programs require applicants to do a rotation at their institution in order to be seriously considered. If you wish to match at one of these programs, you have no choice but to do an audition elective, even if you are a star applicant.

Did you know ...

The American College of Surgeons states that "the more they like you, the better your chance of being selected. When two candidates with similar credentials are being compared, the nod will likely go to the one who performed well on-site during a senior elective. However, we certainly do not recommend more than a total of two audition electives."

(http://www.facs.org/residencysearch/position/position.html).

Rule # 87   Choose the correct audition elective.

Audition electives provide many concrete benefits, as we've outlined. If you're going to actually receive any of these benefits, however, you need to choose your elective very carefully. Consider these factors:

- During an audition elective, you may be able to work with one of the top sub-specialists in the country. You may be able to work with one of the top interventional cardiologists in the country, or at one of the top clinical centers for juvenile rheumatoid arthritis. If you are interested in a particular area of medicine, this may be an unsurpassed experience.
- Some electives afford the opportunity to work with well-respected faculty members who are known to be good

advisors to students, and who have excellent potential as letter writers.

- Some electives are known to provide students with clinical material that is considered publishable. During certain electives, students are given the opportunity to participate in projects that are likely to be published, and likely to be published in prestigious journals.

Consider the negatives of certain programs as well:

- An obvious advantage to doing an audition elective is that you have the chance to make such a strong impression on a program that they will accept you as a resident. Don't waste this chance by doing an audition elective at a program where you have no chance of matching. Medical schools generally limit the number of away electives that students can do, so make sure your away electives are at institutions where you have a realistic chance of matching. If it's the top program in the country, they may be unlikely to accept a student with average grades and scores. If the program seeks out applicants with a strong basic science research background, then don't waste your time.

- Some electives are so popular that you may make no impression among a sea of other highly qualified applicants. With five applicants rotating during any given month, you may lose out on one of the main benefits of doing an audition elective, that of making a memorable impression.

- So many students rotate through some electives, that the program becomes unable to interview such a high number of applicants. In some programs, therefore, the elective becomes an "interview" and the student won't be invited back for a formal interview. This may be a negative if you had no opportunity to meet with the other faculty, and if the faculty member with whom you worked does not serve as a vocal advocate for your application.

Choose a program where you may benefit from all of the advantages of the audition elective. Look for programs where you have a chance of making a memorable impression, where you have a chance of publishing, where you can work with outstanding faculty, and hopefully come away with a strong letter of recommendation. Choose programs where you would like to match, from a clinical and geographic standpoint. Choose a program where you actually have a chance of matching.

Choosing such a program is difficult, and there is no easy answer on how to find the perfect elective. Some of the best have become so popular that it becomes a negative—in a sea of so many students, it is difficult to make a memorable impression. Start by seeking out advice from fellow students. Some schools ask their students to complete evaluations of their away elective experiences and store them in a file to aid future students. Check with your medical school to see if such a file exists. Seek out advice from residents in the specialty. Since they more recently have gone through the process, they are valuable resources. Also discuss the issue with your faculty advisor within the specialty. If you have a particular interest within the specialty, your advisor may be able to arrange for you to work with an attending who does not offer a formal elective.

Tip # 72

Before deciding whether to do an audition elective or where to do it, it is important that you speak with your advisor. Your specialty-specific advisor will have tremendous insight based upon his or her experience with previous students.

Most medical schools provide information about the electives available to visiting students at their website. An additional source of information is the Association of American Medical Colleges (AAMC). The AAMC publishes a list of extramural electives available at AAMC-member U.S. medical schools online at http://www.aamc.org/students/medstudents/electives/start.htm. This list, which is updated every January, contains a variety of information, including contact persons, application and other fees, and the earliest date at which application materials will be accepted.

Did you know ...

At a workshop conducted by the Clerkship Directors of Internal Medicine, the advice given to students included the importance of doing your research before applying for audition electives. "Ask around, don't just get one where you are doomed to fail. "

From CDIM workshop "Giving advice to medical students applying for an IM residency position (October 15, 2004) - gsm.utmck.edu/IM/FAQstudent_advice.htm.

Tip # 73

Among the disadvantages of audition electives are the costs incurred, including those related to travel, housing, food, and parking. Check with your school to determine if it offers any financial assistance. Some schools may have funds available to help students with these expenses. If you will be doing an away research elective, there may be outside funding sources you can turn to.

Rule # 88   Don't underestimate the risks of an audition elective.

Here's an unfortunate truth: applicants may sometimes end up looking worse in person than on paper. A review of discussion forums found that students are sometimes given the advice to avoid audition electives, especially if their application is particularly strong to begin with. Performing at a high level can be easier said than done when you are new to an institution. Unfamiliarity with your new environment may delay or even prevent you from performing at a high level.

Some factors may be beyond your control. You may be assigned to an attending known to be a hard grader, aka "a hawk," and the high quality of your work may not be recognized. Sometimes personality factors or misunderstandings may play a role. Unfortunately, we've seen these issues at play, and we are aware of cases in which an audition elective may have worked against a student. The bottom line is that you must recognize the risks associated with the audition elective, and act accordingly to minimize those risks.

Tip # 74

If you have a very strong application, to the point that you are likely to match into a program based on the strength of your application alone, then an audition elective at that program may not be the best use of your elective time. Discuss your list of potential away electives with your advisor before deciding where to apply.

Rule # 89   Take advantage of all the key opportunities during the elective.

An audition elective should never just be about showing up for work on time and doing a great job. This is where every skill you've learned about doing well in clerkships should come into play. You should be at every meeting and conference ten minutes early. You should have a handbook or textbook with you in the clinic, and you should refer to it often.

The types of patients you see in some specialty clinics or referral hospitals offer a wealth of clinical information that you may not see elsewhere, and you should take full advantage of these clinical opportunities. Search the literature after work hours and share your findings if appropriate. Actively seek out opportunities to highlight your skills and enthusiasm.

If the attending asks for a volunteer to give a talk on a subject or to research a clinical question, be the first to volunteer. If the attending is just pondering a difficult question out loud, offer to investigate further. If all elective students are expected to give a talk at the end of the rotation, then great; this is an excellent opportunity to make an impression. Talks are controlled situations in which you can research your issue, offer an excellent handout, and impress your attending and residents with your self-confidence, poise, and mastery of the material. All of this is absolutely basic third year rotation information, and yet so many elective students don't show mastery of these basics. Please see our companion book, *250 Biggest Mistakes 3rd Year Medical Students Make And How To Avoid Them*. The book outlines how to excel in clinical rotations and how to give an outstanding presentation.

In a highly competitive field such as dermatology, elective students who can perform at this level still don't stand out. It is expected by most attendings that a student applying to our program will also be seeking out additional material. Students should speak with the residents and the attending at the start of the rotation, and make clear their wish to work on a case report, review article, presentation, or any other opportunities that might be available, during their time in the elective. For further information on locating opportunities to publish in your field or participate in a research project, see the chapter, "The Competitive Edge" starting on page 253.

Rule # 90   Make it a point to meet the key faculty members.

You have the best chance of matching into the program if you directly impress key faculty in the department. Key faculty include the chairman, program director, and other members of the selection committee. As you schedule your elective, ask if you can be assigned to one of these individuals. In some programs, particularly smaller programs, the selection committee may consist of every faculty member. In this case, every faculty member becomes key faculty, with equal ability to affect your chances.

Even if you can't work directly with key faculty, there are still many opportunities for interaction. Learn how to introduce yourself appropriately. If you're in clinic working with one faculty member, you should introduce yourself to any other faculty members that you encounter. If you're putting away your bag in the staff room and Dr. Shell arrives at the same time, then take that opportunity. "Good morning, Dr. Shell. I wanted to introduce myself. My name is Grace Donald. I'm a visiting student from Wayne State working with Dr. Pelsky this month."

If you've attended an interesting lecture and learned useful information, then feel free to impart that information as well. Such an introduction must be done carefully, so keep it short and not too over the top. "Thank you for that lecture, Dr. Wells. I'm a visiting student from Wayne State, and we just saw a patient last week with a herald bleed, so your lecture was very helpful."

Attend all departmental conferences and journal clubs. The non-required conferences are excellent opportunities to distinguish yourself, since students taking a required rotation won't attend. If you're interested in the program, then schedule appointments with the chairman and program director to introduce yourself and express your interest in their program. These meetings should be used to ask if there are any projects that you would be able to work on during your elective.

Tip # 75

Don't ignore other faculty. You never know who may have input into the residency selection process. Also note that residents often have significant input. Take every opportunity to meet and interact with as many faculty and residents as you can.

Rule # 91   To obtain an away elective, you first have to apply for one.

The steps involved in the application process for an away elective are summarized here.

How to apply for an away elective

- Contact the appropriate person or office at the away institution for an application. In many cases, a visiting student application can be downloaded from the institution's website.

- Complete the student portion of the application and gather any supporting documents. While there are differences from one application to another, commonly requested are the medical school transcript, immunization record, certificate of student standing, application/processing fees, documentation of health/malpractice insurance, HIPAA certificate, criminal background check, board scores, and photo ID. Make arrangements to obtain these documents through the appropriate office at your school. You may also be asked to complete your school's away rotation approval form.

- Your school may require some time to process their portion of your application. Take this into consideration to avoid any delay in the submission of your application.

- Once the application is completed and the necessary documents are obtained, schools will generally send the application materials to the other institution.

- Once the institution informs you that you have been accepted as a visiting student, notify your school.
- Provide the away elective director with the elective evaluation form. Your school may not consider your transcript to be complete until they receive all evaluation forms from away electives.

Rule # 92 Apply early for the chance to do an audition elective.

Some of the best electives are the most competitive. Some programs are so competitive that you have to apply just to do an away elective. The earlier you apply, the better your chances. Check the institution's website and www.aamc.org to learn about the earliest date at which applications are accepted. Generally, visiting student applications are not acted upon until the schedules of the institution's own students are finalized. This typically takes place some time in the spring. To maximize your chances of securing preferred away electives, apply for these positions in the spring of your third year of medical school.

Tip # 76
Apply *early.* Some away elective slots fill quickly.

Rule # 93 Complete your local elective before taking an away elective.

Always complete your own school's rotation before you do any audition electives. The experience that you gain will help your performance. As per the words of the Saint Louis University School of Medicine, "Conventional wisdom says that if you are going to do audition externships, you would first want to do the senior year floor service or other appropriate senior year clerkship in that same discipline … to raise your skill levels up to those expected of someone who has already completed that clerkship" (oca.slu.edu).

Tip # 77
As you prepare for an audition elective, analyze the elective that you completed at your own school. How did you do? What specifically did you do well? What could you have done better? Read your faculty and resident evaluations. An analysis of your previous clerkship experience can be invaluable.

Rule # 94 Time your audition elective so that you can obtain a letter of recommendation.

A major advantage of the audition elective is the chance to secure a strong letter of recommendation. If you have any chance of sending this letter to all of your programs, then you must schedule the rotation as early as possible. Letter writers may need considerable time to write and send a strong letter.

Tip # 78

The ideal time to do an away elective is as early as possible. If it is possible to do a rotation in your third year, after completing the rotation at your home school, then do so. Most applicants will do audition electives in July through September of their senior year due to the requirements of their medical school.

Rule # 95 Avoid any audition electives during nterview season.

While you can do an audition elective during interview season, you should never schedule interviews during the rotation. Demonstrating your sense of responsibility and commitment to hard work is difficult to do when you're away interviewing at another program.

Rule # 96 An audition elective is a great chance to impress a program. It's also a great chance to evaluate a program.

Audition electives offer multiple benefits beyond increasing your chances of matching with a program in your chosen specialty.

- Greater exposure to the residency program allows you to make a more informed decision about your rank list.

  An audition elective provides you the opportunity to see the ins and outs of a program. How do the faculty relate to the residents? How do the residents get along with one another? What is the quality of the educational conferences? There is no better way to assess your fit for a particular program than by doing an audition elective. Among students who had done an audition elective in pediatrics, approximately 45% found the elective experience helpful in delineating the program's strengths and weaknesses, and 25% noted negatives that steered them away from the program (Englander).

- The elective provides the chance to learn about the geographic area in which you will be training and quite possibly practicing for many years.

Residency graduates often remain in the area to practice. An audition elective will allow you to explore the area to determine if you would enjoy living there.

• The elective may provide exposure to a specialty not available at your own medical school.

Medical schools are not created equal. Some offer rotations in all specialties, while others don't. If you attend a school that doesn't offer a rotation in your chosen specialty, you will have to arrange an away elective. You obviously need the experience to confirm that you have chosen the right specialty.

Rule # 97   The audition elective does not guarantee an interview.

You may hear that an audition elective will guarantee you an interview. At many programs, all students who perform audition electives will receive an invitation to interview. However, the number of programs that do so is far from 100%. Some programs make it quite clear on their websites that they do not interview all applicants who complete an audition elective. For example, at the website for the diagnostic radiology program at the Oregon Health Sciences University (http://www.ohsu.edu/radiology/med/index.html), it is clearly stated: "We do not automatically interview all applicants who do an audition elective here."

Chapter 11

The Competitive Edge

If you plan to apply to a competitive program or a competitive specialty, you'll need to bring into play all of the recommendations throughout this book. In this chapter, we go further and review in detail how to add an extra competitive edge to your application. To begin with, you should make every effort to be published in your field. Such opportunities are available to every student, although they can be difficult to locate. We review how to find these opportunities and the process of writing for the medical literature. We also review the topic of research. If you're applying to a competitive field, NRMP data indicate that the vast majority of your competition will have participated in research. We review how to locate research opportunities and how to excel.

Rule # 98   **If you're applying to competitive programs, you should make every effort to be published in your field.**

In every academic medical center, there are ample opportunities to publish. We meet many medical students who would choose to describe themselves as "self-starters." Opportunities to publish only go to those students who truly are self-starters.

Locating these opportunities is often the hardest step, because there are no hard and fast rules. Different types of opportunities to publish exist at the medical school level, even if you've never been involved in formal basic science or clinical research. A few include:

1. The case report of a classic case
2. The case report of an interesting case
3. A case series
4. A review article

The case reportscase report is typically the entry point for medical students who lack experience in research. Even if you've researched and published extensively, it can be important to have additional scientific study in your chosen field. This confirms your interest in the specialty and your ongoing commitment to scientific pursuits.

How can a case report strengthen your application?

- By seeking out the opportunity, you've demonstrated your drive and enthusiasm.

- You've confirmed your interest in the specialty.
- You've confirmed your thirst for additional knowledge.
- Just the act of seeking out the opportunity demonstrates your commitment to the field.
- Seeking out opportunities to publish provides a professional way in which to speak with or meet residents, faculty, and program directors in the institution.
- On a basic level, you've added to, or at least started, the publication section of your CV.
- By writing the case report, you have become an expert in one specific area.
- Your expertise becomes a potential topic of discussion in interviews.
- Your publication may also act as a point of commonality in interviews that can build rapport. "I'm very pleased to meet you, Dr. Lo. I referenced your work on …when writing my review article on…"
- Writing provides an ideal opportunity to showcase your work ethic, your drive, and your skills.
- By writing the case report in record time and by producing outstanding results, you'll be able to highlight your skills to your attending, an individual who can influence your acceptance to the residency program.
- Faculty members with concrete knowledge of your skills may use this specific example in their rotation evaluation, and in their letter of recommendation.
- Such faculty members can also act as vocal advocates for your candidacy for their own program.

Students who produce outstanding case reports in record time are also more likely to be considered for more substantial research projects or publications. More substantial projects are difficult to locate on the medical student level, but obviously are much more valuable in strengthening your application. An attending who has been asked to write a book chapter for the new edition of a well-respected textbook will only collaborate with individuals of known merit. By showcasing your skills, you've increased your chances of being awarded such valuable opportunities.

Rule # 99   Possibilities for publishing abound.

In general, medical students can be involved in publishing two types of case reports. The first type is what we term "classic" cases. These are typical examples of certain diagnoses, and may be published in a variety of journals in sections entitled "diagnostic puzzles," "clinical pearls," "grand rounds," or others.

The other type of case report describes rare or distinctive clinical findings. "This represents the first case of pseudoporphyria due to the medication sulindac."

If an opportunity to publish has been presented to you by your attending, then they will typically advise you on journal selection. Certain types of clinical material are appropriate for different journals. However, as we discuss the process of publishing on the medical student level, we'll start with a discussion of opportunities in different journals.

Peer-reviewed and indexed journals are preferred, as they signal a higher level of scientific scrutiny. This information will typically be found in the journal's front pages, or under the instructions for authors. Indexed journals will be listed on Pubmed. If the journal is found when searching on www.pubmed.com, it is indexed.

Many options are available within this category of peer-reviewed and indexed journals. However, on a medical student level, an opportunity to publish in any medical journal is significant. Publication in a non-peer reviewed, non-indexed medical journal is still quite an accomplishment, and will be regarded as such.

Your residents and faculty advisors are the best source of suggestions for appropriate sections of journals to which to submit. These may include specialty-specific or non-specialty specific journals. For example, in the field of dermatology alone, we can list a dozen journals that accept classic cases that are published for the education of the reader. These types of classic cases are often seen in a typical week at an academic dermatology outpatient clinic. A case of epidermolysis bullosa acquisita, for example, may not be all that interesting to the dermatology attending, but may prove to be an interesting case for submission to the Photo Quiz section of *American Family Physician.*

We could list many examples of medical journals that students may wish to investigate further. *Medscape General Medicine,* www.medgenmed.com, is a general medical journal, available online without a subscription, and is indexed and peer-reviewed. The journal includes a number of different types of publications, including case reports. "The Learning Curve" is a section of the journal in which submissions are limited to medical students and residents, with faculty co-authors encouraged. The guidelines state that submissions may be case reports, original research or reviews, or editorial content. *Postgraduate Medicine* (www.postgradmed.com), a peer-reviewed journal published for primary care physicians, invites submission of articles, including case reports. It also has a section called "Puzzles in Practice" which offers a brief report of a patient's symptoms for the readers to reach a diagnosis. Journals such as *Patient Care, Consultant,* and *Cortlandt Forum* are examples of non-indexed journals that publish classic cases. These are simply a few of the many journals that accept case reports of classic or interesting cases. Again, your faculty advisor is the best source for suggestions, particularly for specialty-specific journals.

Residents and faculty are very helpful in suggesting clinical material that is appropriate for publication. However, with both the case report of an interesting case and the discussion of a classic case, students can take the lead in suggesting a publication. You may see an interesting case, perform a thorough literature search in order to learn more about the disease, and recognize its potential for publication. You can then suggest the case and ask your resident and attending for their thoughts about its potential acceptance.

Case series are more substantial publications, but will require a faculty member asking you to collaborate using their clinical material. Review articles are also typically identified by the faculty member. Clinical and basic science research projects require a more formal and in-depth commitment. While there are some one-month clinical and basic science research electives, many research projects require much more of a commitment. In order to participate in research, you'll need to identify a faculty mentor who can support and educate you about the process. We review research later in this chapter.

Note that we've only focused on opportunities to publish. Many of these opportunities, however, can also translate into opportunities to present a poster at a national meeting, or to make a presentation at a local, regional, or national meeting. Can this case be presented at the monthly meeting of the Atlanta Pediatric Society? Can it be submitted as a clinical vignette for the national American College of Physicians meeting? Your faculty advisor can advise you of any potential opportunities.

Rule # 100 In order to publish, you need to locate an opportunity.

In some departments, students are frequently involved in publishing case reports, case series, review articles, and book chapters, even if they have not formally participated in basic science or clinical research. In such departments, students will find it easier to locate opportunities to publish, because the path to doing so is relatively clear-cut. They can often locate opportunities just by discussing the situation with their classmates or upperclassmen.

In other departments, it may be uncommon for students to be involved on such a level. While there may not be a track record at your program of students authoring publications, ample opportunities to do so can still be found. Students can easily be involved in publishing case reports, which simply describe a clinical case. There are ample cases of interest in any academic medical center. You need to be extremely motivated and ready to work independently, but you can still successfully publish in your field.

How can you identify opportunities to publish? As we mentioned, there are no hard and fast rules, and you really need to exhibit the skills of a self-starter to even be given the opportunity to start writing. Speak to other students, especially in the class ahead of you. They can relay their own experiences, and how they found their opportunities to publish. Speak to the residents, and let them know your interest in strengthening your application. They can identify clinical material that is interesting and appropriate for the medical literature. They can also, most importantly, direct you to the appropriate faculty members.

Certain faculty are prolific writers, and have an interest in adding to the medical literature. Such faculty may be willing to work with you on case reports. They may have clinical material in their files that is awaiting an eager medical student to perform a literature search and prepare it for publication. Alternately, they may ask you to keep an eye out for interesting clinical cases during your time on the elective. Such faculty are often asked to collaborate with colleagues in their field. They may have been asked to write a book chapter, or a review article. Such opportunities are ideal for medical student collaboration, and many faculty welcome interest by medical students.

In some institutions, it would be appropriate to send an e-mail to the faculty in your department highlighting your interest in working on a paper. Depending on your circumstances, you may seek to work on a paper during your elective or at any time during your third year. Many motivated students complete papers during their time on other rotations. Some students arrange time for a research elective, and then search for a faculty member to work with. In these cases, it is also appropriate to schedule a meeting with the chairman or program director to seek their advice.

Another ideal way to locate opportunities to publish is by participating in an away elective. Certain programs are well-known to provide ample opportunities for student participation in such projects, and your away elective can be chosen with this goal in mind. As with much of this section, there's no single best method to locate such programs. You can speak to the residents, your faculty advisor, and the program director. You can participate in online forums, or even scan journals to note which programs publish work with student authors.

Locating an opportunity to write is an accomplishment in and of itself. Congratulations. Now do everything in your power to maximize this opportunity.

Rule # 101 Finish what you've started.

The first and most important point about identifying opportunities to be published in your field is a simple one. Once you've identified an opportunity to write, you need to submit a finished product.

The reason we choose to discuss such an obvious rule is that somehow, despite its obvious nature, students just don't always finish projects. We've witnessed for ourselves many cases in which students don't complete a project. We've heard many negative comments from our colleagues about students who don't complete a project. We've sat in faculty meetings where the inability to complete a project is used as evidence of a student's poor fit for a residency program.

It's not just that you'll have lost out on an incredible opportunity to impress your attending and strengthen your application. Unfortunately, your inability to complete the project will convey a lack of commitment, a lack of dedication, and a poor work ethic.

It's rare that students in this situation actually have a poor work ethic and lack commitment. In many cases, students become paralyzed by their own perfectionism. They're not sure what they're doing, are insecure about the results they've produced, and can't bear to turn in a final product that's not perfect. As a student, though, hardly anyone has experience with preparing cases for publication. You need to read extensively, plan to work hard, and move forward. We've outlined the process in more detail here.

Rule # 102 Before you write, you need to read.

A great deal of literature exists on designing and conducting medical research, but not so much when it comes to writing a straightforward case report or review of the literature. We've outlined the process in more detail below.

Learning how to write medical papers starts with reading medical papers. Read the articles in your targeted journal. If you'll be writing a case report, pay close attention to that section. Get a feel for format, sentence structure, and word usage. Move on to articles written in prestigious medical journals. Review articles written in specialty-specific journals. This type of reading provides the foundation for your medical writing.

Rule # 103 It may be one of the most important papers you've ever written, but it's not easy to write an outstanding case report.

Arrange to meet with your attending before you start. You need to obtain several key pieces of information. To which journal will you be submitting the paper? Which section in that journal? What is the anticipated timeline for submission of the paper? How would your attending prefer that you communicate with her? Would an e-mailed first draft be acceptable? If submitting a case report, what makes your case unique and compelling to the readers? Can your attending provide you more information on what makes the case worthwhile for publication? These are all critical to the creation of a compelling, publishable report, and we review each of these points in further detail.

Rule # 104 Your publication must include a "hook."

What important point are you trying to convey to your readers? What makes this case unique or compelling to the readers? What is the point of publishing this case?

If you're submitting the case of a patient who presented with the classic features of Wegener's granulomatosis, you are presenting the case for the further education of your readers, so that they can recognize such cases in the future. As we discussed, many journals have sections in which they present examples of classic cases for their readers.

If your case is the first reported case of pseudoporphyria due to sulindac, then your hook is this: "We present this case of pseudoporphyria due to sulindac. While pseudoporphyria often occurs due to NSAIDS, this is the first reported case due to the medication sulindac. Therefore, this medication must be added to the possible causes."

If you're presenting a syndrome or disease that is well-described in the medical literature, then you need to search more deeply for what makes your case either unique or worth publishing. This can be difficult. It may be a fascinating syndrome, but if there's not a compelling point to make, then many journals won't see what use the information will have for their readers.

The insight and extensive clinical experience of your advisor will be critical in this situation. Was the last reported case of this syndrome 20 years ago? Then a reminder of its features may be useful. Does this case demonstrate a new association? Did the patient respond to a previously undescribed therapeutic measure? Did you note an interesting clinical finding that may serve as a clue to the diagnosis? "This case illustrates a complication of systemic amyloidosis and emphasizes its utility in reaching a timely diagnosis." Your point is that this information has educational or clinical significance for the readers.

Another option is to write a case report and review of the literature. "We present a case of Dowling-Degos disease and review and summarize the medical literature, with an emphasis on clinical and histologic presentations." What is the point of this type of publication? You describe an interesting case and summarize the medical literature to date, so that your readers will be fully educated on all aspects of this condition.

Rule # 105 For extensive projects, you need to establish a timeline.

"What timeline did you have in mind for this project?" If you'll be working on an extensive project, this question becomes very important. In your mind, a review article with over 200 references may take at least eight weeks. Your advisor may expect it in four, especially if she herself was given a deadline for submission. If you have a prior commitment, such as Step 2 in four weeks, then it's important to let your advisor know that you won't be able to meet that deadline. Be specific about your reasons, offer an alternate timeline, and ask if that would be acceptable.

We're going to emphasize an important point here. The date you're given is NOT a deadline. Some students will delay, then work feverishly for the week before, and then turn in a first draft on that date. That represents a wasted opportunity. The date you're given is actually an indication of your advisor's expectations, and is really an opportunity to exceed those expectations. Once you've heard the expected timeline, plan to cut it significantly. Turning in an outstanding finished product that exceeds expectations in terms of both quality and timeliness is an impressive accomplishment.

As a final note, a lack of a timeline is not an excuse to delay. Many attendings won't have a timeline in mind. "Just do your best, and we'll work with it." Other attendings will say the same, but are in actuality judging your work ethic.

Note that we specified asking for an expected timeline in the case of extensive projects. Case reports are a different situation, because they should be completed and submitted promptly. Realistically, many case reports can be completed in one very lengthy weekend spent at the library and at your computer. This is particularly true for presentations of a classic case, which take less time to research and write. Submitting a high-quality case report at that speed will get you talked about.

Rule # 106 Model your report on others in your targeted journal.

Find the right journal for your submission. This is easier when your attending has a concrete idea of where your article should be submitted. Find out what journal you'll be submitting to. Seek out the instructions for authors. Seek out prior examples of publications for that section. Model yours using that format.

Rule # 107 You cannot write a strong case report without becoming an expert on your topic.

Perform a thorough literature search. You cannot write a strong case report without becoming an expert on the topic. You should begin by reading the textbooks. You can then move on to online sources such as emedicine (www.emedicine.com), which are regularly updated textbooks. You should then seek out review articles that summarize the literature on the subject. Lastly, you should review prior case reports on the topic.

Some students, when first writing a case report, heavily reference the major textbooks. However, such references are not ideal. For general information on the topic, it would be better to reference a review article, ideally one which is more recent, up to date, and in-depth. Including such a review article is helpful to your readers, as they can use that reference to obtain more information on the topic. However, review articles should never be used as a substitution for the primary source of a piece of information. "Pseudoporphyria has been described as occurring due to ibuprofen, naproxen, and diclofenac.[1]" While it would be easier to include one reference that summarizes this information, such as a review article, it would be more appropriate, and in some cases more helpful for your readers, to include examples of publications that described each of these cases. "Pseudoporphyria has been described as occurring due to ibuprofen[1], naproxen[2] and diclofenac.[3]"

We assume that by this point in your career you've learned to navigate Pubmed. You may find it helpful, however, to further maximize your knowledge of Pubmed and the various search options available. Our own medical library offers multiple classes on maximizing the use of Pubmed, and online tutorials are available as well.

Rule # 108 Write the case.

Once you pinpoint why your case would be compelling to readers, the work of writing the case report becomes more straightforward. For a case report, you'll typically write an introduction, a description of the case, and a discussion. The introduction will be brief, but should capture the reader's attention. Why would they care to read about your case?

In summarizing the clinical features of the case, make sure you review other cases previously published in your target journal. Your description of the clinical features of the case, including the depth of detail included, should be modeled after that type of case report.

In the discussion, just as in a typical college review paper, you will summarize and present the existing literature on this subject, with an emphasis on the important take home points learned from the case. Learning the appropriate focus and level of detail in the report is a skill that can take years to develop. "Should I focus on the clinical features of pseudoporphyria in general, and how to make the diagnosis, or should I just limit myself to a discussion on the prior reports of the NSAIDS that have triggered pseudoporphyria? Do I need to go into the pharmacological details of the different NSAIDS?"

The level of detail included will depend, in large part, on the goals of your advisor and the limitations of the journal. The instructions to authors specify a range of word counts, and it's very important to adhere to these guidelines. Hopefully the meeting with your advisor will have clarified the focus of the report. If in writing the discussion, though, you sense that you can go in two directions with your focus, you should contact your advisor for further guidance.

Rule # 109 Even your first draft should conform to the journal's exact specifications.

The first draft that you turn in to your attending must be perfect. As always, every aspect of your performance is up for scrutiny, and you need to be sending a consistent message throughout the application process. And yes, without a doubt, writing a paper is part of that process. Your message is that you bring excellence to whatever task you perform, and that your attention to detail is impeccable. Proof your paper for grammatical and spelling mistakes, especially with medical terms for which neither you nor your spell-checker are familiar. Submit a title page that adheres to the journal's specifications. Ensure that the format of your paper adheres to these specifications as well. If the journal requires an abstract for case reports, then submit an abstract of the specified length. Instructions for clinical photos, radiologic or other images, tables, and graphs should all be studied closely. Journals vary in their requirements for listing of references. Follow these requirements exactly.

Since this is a first draft, your content will be revised. Therefore, you should maintain two versions of your first draft. In the draft submitted to your advisor, the references should be formatted according to the instructions of the journal. In many cases, this means that references would be numbered and superscripted as directed, and the references section would include the numbered references in order of their inclusion in the body of the report. In the other draft version, you would note the author after the sentence, and avoid numbering your references at all. The references section would then list the authors in alphabetical order. This way, if your advisor suggests a change in the order of the content, then the work required for significant renumbering of your references won't be as difficult. The second version would be for your use only.

Sulindac has been described as a cause of many different types of cutaneous reactions (Smith, Jensen).

Rule # 110 The follow through is just as important.

Most students feel a tremendous sense of relief when they can finally turn in a paper and say they're done. However, follow through is just as important. Always offer to make any necessary revisions. Provide explicit instructions on how to reach you in the months to come. "I'll be doing an away elective in the month of February, but please feel free to contact me by e-mail, because I'd like to make whatever revisions are necessary without delay."

Sometimes the revisions suggested by your advisor can be lengthy and painful. Your ability to complete suggested revisions, and to do so promptly, will be noted. If a paper is submitted and subsequently accepted, there are almost always required revisions to be completed before the paper will be published. Be available for these revisions as well.

While your revisions should be submitted promptly, the converse won't always be true. Some attendings may take a great deal of time to respond to your first or second draft of an article. While you should have made it clear that you are available to work on any suggested changes, you cannot do much more than that to speed up the process. Some students, after working so hard on a paper, are understandably impatient for the paper to be submitted, accepted, and published in time to help their application. However, it's easy to annoy an attending when you check in too often on the status of your paper.

Research

In the last section, we focused on being published in your field. Opportunities to publish case reports are easily available to motivated, driven students, and as we outlined, simply publishing a case report can boost your application. In this section, we focus on research opportunities. These can more significantly strengthen your application, but opportunities to participate in research projects are more difficult to locate and complete.

Rule # 111 Many applicants who apply to competitive programs or a competitive specialty will have participated in research. Those applicants are your competition.

Participation in research can significantly strengthen your application. However, it is not a requirement. A survey of program directors in 14 specialties found that in most fields, published medical school research was not among the top three academic criteria important to the residency selection process (Wagoner). A review of the data in the following table highlights this point. In most fields, many applicants without publications or research experience will still match. In radiology, for example, only 38 of the 338 applicants lacking publications failed to match. (http://www.nrmp.org/data/chartingoutcomes2007.pdf).

However, there are several important caveats. If the majority of students applying to your field have research experience, your lack of experience will make you stand out. While it may be ranked behind factors such as class rank and strength of letters of recommendation, research experience will still carry great weight with certain programs. In the fields of pathology and radiation oncology, published medical school research was among the top three academic criteria important to the residency selection process. In psychiatry and PM&R, it was fourth in importance among 12 academic criteria.

In many fields, including both the highly competitive fields and those considered not as competitive, your competition will have participated in research. In 2007, the NRMP published data on how applicant qualifications affect match success. Included among the data were the percentage of U.S. seniors who had participated in research projects and the percentage with publications. In each of the fields below, over 75% of U.S. seniors applying to the field had participated in research projects. In highly competitive fields such as dermatology, orthopedic surgery, otolaryngology, plastic surgery, and radiation oncology, over 90% of U.S. seniors had participated in research projects. Even in the fields that are not the most competitive, including the fields of anesthesiology, pathology, and general surgery, over 80% of U.S. seniors had participated in research projects.

Percentage of U.S. seniors in the 2007 Match participating in research and reporting publications			
Specialty	% of U.S. seniors having participated in research projects	% of U.S. seniors with publications	Of note …
Anesthesiology	80%	51%	82/84 applicants with > 5 publications matched. Over 90% of applicants with no publications or research experience matched
Dermatology	93%	86%	Most applicants participate in research. Only 26 applicants had no research experience. Of this group, 16 did not match. Of the 136 applicants with > 5 publications, 35 did not match; 35 of 59 with no publications did not match.
Emergency medicine	77%	50%	All applicants with > 5 pubs matched. Nearly 90% of applicants with no publications or research experience matched
Obstetrics and gynecology	77%	46%	7/59 with > 5 pubs did not match 59/509 with no pubs did not match 196/220 with no research experience matched

Percentage of U.S. seniors in the 2007 Match participating in research and reporting publications			
Orthopedic surgery	93%	65%	19/117 with > 5 pubs did not match 62/244 with no pubs did not match 34/53 with no research participation matched
Otolaryngology	95%	78%	6/65 with > 5 pubs did not match 17/68 with no pubs did not match 10/14 with no research participation matched
Pathology	80%	54%	Only 2/56 with > 5 pubs did not match 12/143 with no pubs did not match 58/64 with no research participation matched
Physical medicine and rehabilitation	75%	46%	All applicants with > 5 pubs matched 15/111 with no pubs did not match 43/52 with no research participation matched
Plastic surgery	93%	76%	7/40 with > 5 pubs did not match 28/63 with 1-5 pubs did not match 16 of 33 with no pubs did not match 5/10 with no research participation matched
Radiology	88%	63%	11/136 with > 5 pubs did not match 38/336 with no pubs did not match 101/114 with no research participation matched
Radiation oncology	97%	89%	4/62 with > 5 pubs did not match 7/16 with no pubs did not match 3/4 with no research participation matched
General surgery	84%	57%	9/100 with > 5 pubs did not match 48/385 with no pubs did not match 129/147 with no research experience matched
Data from http://www.nrmp.org/data/chartingoutcomes2007.pdf			

Rule # 112 Participate in a research project for the right reasons.

We've emphasized that your competition will have participated in research projects. We've emphasized that such projects can significantly enhance the strength of your application. However, you should never participate in a research project for those reasons alone. If buffing up your CV is your only motivation, this will be transparently obvious to your colleagues and preceptor. Your project can then become detrimental to your chances of matching successfully.

Your main motivation for participation in a research project should be that it can help you become a better doctor. Upon completion of a research project, students often report an increased ability to formulate a hypothesis, conduct a literature search, critically appraise the literature, collect data, analyze results, and prepare a manuscript. Some students find the experience so intellectually satisfying that it leads them into a career with a heavy emphasis in research.

Others find that the experience provides them with the foundation to practice evidence-based medicine. Since research is the foundation of evidence-based medicine, exposure to research and scientific methods will strengthen your critical thinking skills. You will be in a better position to critically analyze and interpret scientific advances, and then translate those findings into improved patient care.

Rule # 113 Participation in a research project provides a number of distinct benefits.

Some students who participate in a research project will focus on the advantages to their CV. A research project can be listed under research experience. Publications or presentations may also result, further enhancing a student's CV. However, there are a number of other distinct advantages.

- Participation in a research project provides invaluable experience, as we've already discussed. Many accomplished investigators credit research experience in medical school as the impetus for their present careers. Even physicians who ultimately decide not to make research a focus of their career still speak highly of their experience. These clinicians report an enhanced ability to search the literature, answer clinical questions, and analyze and interpret scientific data.

- Students who perform research through a research elective in their third or fourth year of medical school will receive credit for the course. Your research preceptor will assign a final grade, which will appear on your medical school transcript. The formal evaluation with written comments and the transcript itself can all strengthen your application.

- Working closely with your research preceptor presents a unique opportunity to highlight your abilities. Your preceptor can become familiar with the quality of your work, your communication skills, and your skills in research. Such close interaction can lead to a strong letter of recommendation.

- Your research preceptor may become a career advisor or mentor. In one survey of third- and fourth-year medical students at one medical school, UCSF, 96% of all participants rated mentors as important or very important (Aagard). Mentors provide invaluable guidance and advice, and their recommendations alone can significantly strengthen your application.

- Your research preceptor's connections at other programs may open doors for you, as in opportunities to participate in audition electives or other research projects. In some cases, research preceptors who have advocated on behalf of their students have been able to increase the chances of a successful match in a particular specialty or program.

Rule # 114   Research involves a number of different processes. You may be involved in any or all of these.

What do we mean when we use the term "research?" Taber's *Cyclopedic Medical Dictionary* defines research as "scientific and diligent study, investigation, or experimentation in order to establish facts and analyze their significance."

In a more general sense, research involves answering a question. The scientific process involved in answering that question can be quite complex, and consists of a number of different processes.

Steps in the process of research

Review of literature
Hypothesis generation
Study design
Requesting approval from the institutional review board
Data collection
Data tabulation
Data analysis
Manuscript preparation and revision
Manuscript submission/resubmission

Years ago I saw a child with cutaneous mucormycosis at the site of an intravenous catheter. I had never seen a case before in a child. Despite a thorough literature search, I was left with a number of questions. How often did such cases occur in children? What were the risk factors involved? What was the ideal therapy, and what was the usual outcome? I designed a simple (relatively speaking) study to try to answer some of these questions, which consisted of a retrospective chart review. I obtained Institutional Review Board (IRB) approval to do a chart review at Texas Children's Hospital. Obtaining IRB approval can be an in-depth, complicated process in and of itself, as the IRB ensures that the study is safe and effective for human participation. IRB approval is necessary even for a chart review.

Once I obtained IRB approval, I had to locate and contact the point person who could perform a computerized search of the pathology records. We limited our search to ten years' worth of data, and searched for biopsies of skin that carried a diagnosis of "fungal" or "mold." We read each of these biopsy reports, and only included those that demonstrated hyphae extending into the dermis. We then contacted the medical records department, and asked for the complete chart on each of these cases. A review of these charts excluded some of these patients from our series. For the remainder of the cases, we created a data collection form.

What information were we seeking on the cases? Our data collection form included demographic information (gender, age) in addition to the clinical factors that we wished to study, including clinical appearance, underlying medical conditions and medications, other predisposing factors, treatment, and outcome.

Once the medical records were reviewed, we collected all of this clinical information. We created tables that summarized the information. We analyzed the data, and in doing so came to several conclusions about cutaneous mold infections in children, the risk factors involved, and the outcomes. We prepared the manuscript, submitted the manuscript, made the requested revisions, and our study was ultimately published (Katta).

As a medical student, you may find yourself involved in any of these aspects of research. While this is an example of clinical research, you may have the opportunity to participate in either clinical or basic science research. While you may be able to work on a project from inception to publication, as described above, that is unusual on the medical student level.

The typical entry point to medical student research is the identification of a faculty member who is willing to involve you in a study of their design. The type of involvement may vary quite a bit. You may be involved in the literature search and IRB approval process. Your involvement may be a relatively simple, one-time involvement in data collection. For example, during your one month research elective, you may participate in reviewing medical charts and collecting information from those charts. You may even be involved in analyzing the results, drawing conclusions, and preparing a manuscript. Whatever aspects of the research process you ultimately participate in, you should make every effort to understand all aspects of the research process and all aspects of your particular project.

Rule # 115 If you are to participate in a research project, it's not enough to understand the background literature on your particular subject. You must be able to describe the question that you are attempting to answer, the specific methodology used, the results, the weaknesses of the study, and the ultimate relevance of the research.

Students are often asked about their research at interviews. Some are unable to describe the relevance of their research, let alone the specific methodology used. While the reasons for this are many, chief among these reasons is not having a solid understanding of the project. According to Dr. Michelle Biros, editor-in-chief of *Academic Emergency Medicine,* there are certain questions every student should be able to answer when embarking on a project (Biros).

Important questions to answer about your research project

Why was this research topic chosen?

What is the background that makes this question important?

What is the specific study hypothesis?

What is the study design?

Why was it designed this way?

What are the methods that will be used to answer the question?

Why was this method developed for this research question?

How is the data to be collected and managed?

If the data is collected and managed properly, will the study hypothesis really be answered?

What are the unanswered questions?

From Biros M, Adams J. Medical students and research: getting started in emergency medicine research (www.saem.org).

If you will be participating in any type of basic science or clinical research, you should be reading more extensively on scientific methods. Even a simple chart review or questionnaire study entails a great deal of work, from study design, to IRB approval, to data analysis. Although many decisions will be made by your advisor, you should be able to understand the basis for those decisions and offer your own input. You can start by reading introductory texts on the subject. Further study would include formal courses and more advanced textbooks. This is in addition to asking questions of your advisor.

As we mentioned previously, participation in a research project should not be limited to the one aspect of the project in which you are directly involved. While you may participate only in the chart review, you should read and ask questions in order to develop a full understanding of the research question, the study design, the results, and the relevance of those results. You should understand and be able to intelligently discuss your research.

Rule # 116 Locating a research project can be a significant project in and of itself.

Locating opportunities to participate in a research project can be difficult. The advice in this section is very similar to that for locating opportunities to publish. You can't just look up job postings on medstudentresearch.com. You will need to be motivated and persistent in order to locate these types of opportunities. While projects may be difficult to locate, in many schools there are ample opportunities to participate in research on the medical student level.

Start by seeking information and advice from your peers. Your classmates may already be involved in research. Upperclassmen at your school may have participated in projects, and can provide additional information. The residents in your program may also be involved in, or aware of, different research projects.

Your institution will often have resources available. Many schools keep an updated database in which faculty members are listed, along with their projects. Most schools have a research office, and the members there may be able to offer additional information and insight.

You may also schedule an appointment with the clerkship director, program director, or chairman of your own program. Ask them for advice about potential research opportunities. Be prepared to provide your CV, and be prepared to respond to questions about your anticipated time frame for research and prior experience. In some institutions, it may also be considered appropriate to e-mail all of the faculty members in the department to let them know of your interest in participating in a research project. In this case, you would attach your CV.

As we discussed in the section on case reports, the best opportunities may not be available for the asking. However, once you have demonstrated your skills and abilities during a rotation or with a case report, faculty members may be more willing to work with you. If you've worked with any faculty members during a clerkship or on an outside project such as a case report, you should approach them for additional guidance. You can ask if they have any ideas for research projects that you could work on, or if they know of any potential opportunities within the department.

Rule # 117 If you plan to participate in research in a meaningful way, you'll need advance planning.

Starting and finishing a research project takes considerable time. Students who are new to research often believe that two or three months are sufficient. In reality, while a several month block of time is helpful, research projects usually require a much greater commitment of time.

Students who are sure of their specialty choice when entering medical school have the advantage of being able to start a project early in their education. However, while many students have an idea of the specialty they wish to pursue, surveys have shown that this specialty choice often changes. In AAMC surveys of students graduating in 1991 and 1994, 80% chose to pursue a career in a different specialty from what they had declared at the time of medical school matriculation (Kassebaum).

Most advisors will suggest that you dedicate a block of time to devote to research, rather than trying to find time for a project during busy rotations. While you may schedule a research elective during your fourth year, it would be to your advantage to do so earlier. While the research itself may be completed at an earlier date, preparing for presentation and publication can add significantly to the length of the project, and much of the follow up work will be done past the completion of your elective. If your school allows flexible scheduling, you may consider breaking up your core clerkships with a research elective in your third year.

Rule # 118 Maintain realistic expectations about your chances for publication.

Many students who participate in research have the expectation that their work will lead to publication. However, research is a difficult and complex process, and you need to maintain realistic expectations. If you're planning to participate in a research project and are purely focused on completing that project so that you can add a publication to your CV, you are likely to be disappointed. Students may sign up for a one month, or even a two month, research elective, and hope to complete a project in that time. However, that depends greatly on the nature of the question you hope to answer.

Even one year of full-time research may not be sufficient. The Clinical Research Training Program at the National Institutes of Health (NIH) and the Doris Duke Clinical Research Fellowship are prestigious programs that immerse students into one year of full-time experience in clinical research. In a recent study, only 23% of fellows in either program had publications in print by 6 months post-fellowship (Cohen). This date was chosen to indicate publications that could be included in residency applications, as fellows usually participated between their third and fourth year of medical school. While a variety of factors may account for this, in an anonymous survey of the Doris Duke Clinical Research fellows, 18% felt that their research question was not well suited to the time available (Gallin).

The conclusion is that not all research experience will result in a publication to add to your CV. However, research experience can be an invaluable addition to your application. It demonstrates your dedication to the field, may result in stronger letters of recommendation, and provides a topic of discussion in interviews. Most importantly, the value of research experience extends far beyond what it can do for your application.

Rule # 119 Hard work and follow through are critical.

Once you commit to working on a research project, your preceptor will expect a full-time commitment. Research often requires long days and work on weekends. As a student free of other responsibilities, you need to be willing and able to work the long hours that are required.

Follow-up is critical as well. A month or two of research is rarely a sufficient period of time to complete a project, although this depends on the nature of the project. Once the research itself is completed, significant work is still required to bring the study to publication. Therefore, it will be important to remain involved in the project, even after your research block has ended. If you have participated in a research elective, make it quite clear to your preceptor that you would like to be involved in further stages of the project. Provide explicit directions on how you can be reached.

Rule # 120 Finish what you start.

Finish what you start. The same rule that we listed for publications applies to research projects. If you hear of an opportunity to participate in a research project, make sure you fully understand what is required. Before committing to a project, make sure you clearly understand the time frame and degree of work involved. If you can't get the project done in the eight week period of time before you start your surgery rotation, you can't commit to the project. Let your potential advisor know your schedule.

Estimating the time frame on a project can be difficult in some cases. If the project in question is a chart review that involves extracting clinical information, then it will be easier to estimate the investment of time. Other projects may require a year of intermittent work to complete. You may have to wait until specific goals and objectives are defined, the methodology to perform the research is established, funding is secured, and approval from the institutional review board is granted. Some projects, especially laboratory-based projects, require the acquisition and development of specialized skills. Acquiring these skills may take a considerable investment of time.

Rule # 121 Be prepared for your initial meeting with a potential research preceptor.

During an initial meeting about a potential research project, the following issues will be discussed:

- ## Previous research experience

  You may be asked about your background and previous research experience, particularly if you will be involved in bench research or in a clinical research project from inception that would involve IRB approval. Have you done research before? If so, are you grounded in the basic research concepts?

- ## Your timetable

  Issues related to scheduling should be discussed before the project begins. Inform your advisor when you would be able to start, the time you have to devote to the project, and when your research block will end. Discuss any potential interruptions, such as vacation, exams, or clerkships. Your timetable will help your advisor determine the most suitable project for you.

- ## Questions

  Be ready to ask questions and take notes. What aspects of the project will you be involved with? What will be your duties and responsibilities? How often and in what fashion would your advisor like to be kept apprised of your progress? What is their anticipated timetable for the completion of your portion of the project?

Rule # 122 You should make it explicitly clear that you are willing and hoping to participate fully in all aspects of the project.

When embarking on a research project, you will discuss with your advisor the aspects of the project in which you will participate. For example, it's relatively easy to involve an inexperienced student in data collection for a chart review. However, you should always attempt to participate more fully in a project. At the very least, you should work on data tabulation, after asking how your advisor would like the data to be presented. You should also let your advisor know that you are willing and hoping to participate fully in all aspects of the project. Ideally, you would play a role in all aspects of the project, including data collection, analysis of the results, and development of the manuscript. This won't be possible with all research projects, particularly those that are more complex or large in scope, but your willingness to be involved in further aspects of the project should be clearly conveyed.

Some students participate in a research project in a very limited fashion. They may perform the chart review, collect the data, and then hand it to their advisor. However, if you seek additional participation in a research project, such as inclusion as an author or participation as a presenter, then you need to be fully involved in the project. If you did the grunt work, but didn't analyze or interpret data, present results, or write the paper, you can't expect to receive the honor of first authorship.

Chapter 12

Before the Interview

An invitation to interview is a significant honor. During the screening process, the residency program has worked hard to whittle down a large applicant pool into an elite group. Contrary to commonly held belief, the purpose of the interview is *not* to determine if you have the qualifications needed to be a resident at their institution. By granting you an interview, the program has already made that determination. Rather, the purpose of the interview is to assess fit. Are you the right fit for the program? Is the program the right fit for you?

Fortunately, or unfortunately, your work has just increased exponentially. Although the CV, personal statement, letters of recommendation, and other aspects of the application are all of great importance, there is no disputing the fact that the interview is possibly the most critical step of the residency application process. While the other elements of the application will help you get an interview, your interview performance will strongly influence your ranking. Surveys of program directors have shown that success in the interview is critical towards securing a position in the residency program.

Unfortunately, many otherwise qualified applicants lose any chance of matching into the residency program of their choice because of a poor interview. In a study of internal medicine residency applicants, one third of the applicants were ranked less favorably following an interview (Gong). In a study of emergency medicine residency programs, with data obtained from 3,800 individual interviews, a total of 14% of interviews resulted in unranked applicants (Martin-Lee). The conclusion here is that the interview has the potential to destroy your chances. Preparation is critical.

A successful interview is one that moves you higher on the program's rank list. Successful interviewing requires a considerable amount of preparation. You need to know what to research before the interview, what to wear, what to say, how to conduct yourself, and what to do after the interview. In this chapter, we outline the steps to ensure that every one of your interviews will be a success.

Rule # 123 The interview is a critical factor in ranking applicants.

In 1979, Wagoner and Gray surveyed program directors in internal medicine, family medicine, surgery, and pediatrics (Wagoner). Survey participants were asked to consider the importance of 31 variables in the selection of residents. Interpersonal skills, as demonstrated in the interview, were found to be the number one criterion. In 1999, Wagoner and Suriano again surveyed program directors (Wagoner). They wrote that "the interview continues to be the most important part of the selection process for both directors and students."

In fact, over the years, many surveys of program directors have inquired about the importance of the interview in the selection process. These surveys have consistently found the interview to be a major factor used to rank applicants. In fact, the results of multiple studies indicate that the interview is *the most* valuable factor used in the ranking of applicants. Following is a summary of the results of these surveys.

Surveys of residency program directors regarding the importance of the interview

Study	What was found ...
Survey of program directors of family practice and obstetrics/gynecology investigating the value directors place on various selection criteria (Taylor)	Directors in both specialties ranked the interview as most valuable in the ranking of applicants.
Study done at The Children's Hospital of Philadelphia to better understand the impact of interview on the ranking of applicants (Swanson)	Interview scores were found to be the most important tool for the ranking of applicants.
Survey of 282 family practice residency program directors to determine the strategies used by programs to select residents (Galazka)	The interview was the most important element in the resident selection process.
Survey of program directors of osteopathic rotating internships and residency programs in internal medicine, obstetrics-gynecology, general surgery, orthopedic surgery, and pediatrics to determine the relative importance of academic and nonacademic variables in the selection process (Bates)	The interview was most highly valued in the resident selection process.
Survey of 94 emergency medicine residency program directors to determine the importance of various residency selection criteria (Crane)	The interview was the second most important selection criterion, following the emergency medicine rotation grade.
Survey of 96 residency program directors in Ontario, inquiring about the importance of various selection factors (Provan)	84% of the program directors considered the personal interview to be the most important selection criterion.

Surveys of residency program directors regarding the importance of the interview	
Survey of orthopedic residency program directors and applicants (Bajaj)	According to faculty, the interview was the third most important attribute to obtaining a residency, following performance on a local rotation and class rank. Of note, applicants did not give interviews the same level of importance, citing performance on a local rotation, USMLE Step 1 score, and recommendation letters as the three most important criteria.
Survey of 24 faculty members at a University of Minnesota primary care internal medicine residency program to determine the importance of various selection criteria (Leonard)	Personal and interpersonal qualities were given the greatest weight and were considered to be more important than academic success.

Applicants are often surprised to learn about the importance that programs attach to the interview. However, several studies have shown poor correlation between academic performance during medical school and later performance during residency training. In one study of radiology residents, while honors or A grades in clinical rotations (medicine, surgery, pediatrics) and high USMLE scores were predictive of performance on the American Board of Radiology exam, they were not predictive of clinical performance as a resident (Boyse). In a study of obstetrics and gynecology residents, Bell found similar results (Bell). USMLE scores did not correlate with faculty evaluations of resident performance.

Therefore, programs can't rely solely on objective data such as class rank and USMLE scores to make resident selection decisions. Behavioral and noncognitive skills have significant value in predicting resident performance, and programs recognize this fact. However, they are limited in how they can assess these skills, and therefore the interview takes on greater importance. The interview becomes the chief means by which programs can evaluate these noncognitive skills.

Did you know ...

In a prospective study, Wood interviewed thirty radiology resident applicants. These residents were interviewed again four years later during their radiology residency. Wood found that noncognitive and cognitive factors were equally important in predicting residents' performance (Wood).

Did you know …

In a survey of junior medical students and residency program directors at the Medical College of Wisconsin, researchers sought to learn the importance of different residency selection criteria. Program directors and students were asked to rank these criteria in terms of importance. Program directors seemed to place more emphasis on personal characteristics, whereas knowledge and skills were rated most important by students (Zagumny). Swanson wrote that "social skills and the level of development of professional behavior are more important than the sophistication of clinical skills and knowledge gained in medical school" (Swanson).

The interview is never just a formality. It can absolutely make or break your chances of matching. In support of this is a study performed by Gong and colleagues, who determined the importance of the interview on the ranking of internal medicine residency applicants (Gong). They found that following an interview:

- 1/3 of applicants were ranked more favorably
- 1/3 of applicants were ranked less favorably
- 1/3 of applicants had no change in their ranking

Another study found that "final student rankings correlated well with interview scores and poorly with initial applicant scores based solely on pre-interview information" (Curtis).

Did you know …

A poor interview can destroy your chances. In a survey of emergency medicine residency programs, data was obtained from 3800 individual interviews taking place at 44 programs (Martin-Lee). It was learned that 14% of these interviews resulted in unranked applicants.

Rule # 124 What are the goals of the interviewer? A successful interview involves understanding these goals and responding to them.

In order to interview successfully, you need to understand the goals of the interviewer. The primary goal is to determine if you would be an outstanding resident at their program. An AOA applicant with a 250 USMLE score does not equate to an outstanding radiology resident. Interview questions are asked to learn more about noncognitive factors, including your communication skills, your interpersonal skills, your strengths, and your drive. Interview questions are also asked to determine "fit" with the program. Depending on the goals of the particular residency program, interview questions may also seek to determine your commitment to community service, your interest in translational research, or your commitment to a career in academic medicine.

Did you know ...

In describing the results of a survey of emergency medicine program directors, Crane wrote that "much concrete and personal information about the applicant's interactive skills and mannerisms can be obtained from the interview. Similarly, the interview provides the opportunity to obtain more information or clarify deficiencies in the interviewee's application. Some interviewers also use this time to test the interviewee's composure, asking a nontraditional question, or offering a simple clinical scenario. Finally, the interview affords the applicant the opportunity to express items not specifically mentioned in the application, including hobbies, interests, volunteer activities, and previous exposure to the medical field" (Crane).

Did you know ...

Contrary to commonly held belief, the purpose of the interview is not to determine if you have the qualifications needed to be a resident. By granting you an interview, the program has already made that determination. The purpose of the interview is to assess fit. Is the program the right fit for you? Are you the right fit for the program? In a survey of radiology residency program directors, 15 directors stated that the 'fit' of the candidates in the program and a 'gut feeling' were the most important criteria for deciding admission (Otero). In another survey, program directors wrote that they sought to find applicants who were "people like us" (Villanueva).

An interviewer can't learn about your interpersonal skills from your application alone. He can't learn about your strengths or weaknesses. He can't find out what drives or motivates you. He can't discover how well you handle pressure. Do you have the qualities that make someone a valued team member? Will you fit in and work well with others in the department? The only way an interviewer can learn any of these things is by speaking with you and asking questions. While the personal statement and letters of recommendation provide some information, the interview is the chief means by which programs can directly assess these noncognitive factors.

Did you know ...

Having the cognitive skills needed to succeed during residency is important, but is not enough. Program directors also want residents who are socially competent. Social competence is defined as "someone who knows how to manage his/her emotions and responds to others' emotions in a mature manner" (Carson). Socially competent individuals are said to be emotionally intelligent. Emotional intelligence has been widely researched in business, but less so in medicine. Since many of the skills required for success in the workplace are also the skills needed for success as a resident, many have hypothesized that emotional intelligence would correlate with residency performance. In one study looking at the relationship between patient satisfaction and physicians' emotional intelligence, a relationship, albeit limited, was found (Wagner). Future studies will likely shed additional light on this issue.

In a survey of program directors in multiple specialties, published in 1986, Wagoner, Suriano, and Stoner found that the following applicant characteristics were most important (Wagoner):

- Compatibility with the program
- Ability to grow in knowledge
- Maturity
- Commitment to hard work

In a survey of physical medicine and rehabilitation program directors, DeLisa and colleagues found that compatibility with the program was one of the three most important candidate traits, along with the ability to articulate thoughts and work with others (DeLisa).

Programs are also interested in assessing an applicant's communication skills. The interview is considered a reliable way to assess this skill (Villanueva).

In a survey of program directors of American Osteopathic Association-approved primary care graduate training programs, the authors determined the relative importance of academic and nonacademic variables related to resident selection. Work habits were rated highest, followed by the ability to work with others and maturity (Bates). The following table lists personal qualities that are valued by residency programs, and therefore are important qualities to convey during an interview.

Personal qualities you should aim to convey during an interview		
Ability to work with a team	Recognition of limits	Responsibility
Ability to solve problems	Willingness to admit error	Poise
Ability to manage stress	Perseverance	Positive attitude
Enthusiasm	Initiative	Reliability
Energy	Intelligence	Honesty
Flexibility	Maturity	Dedication
Effective time management	Motivation	Compassion
Efficient problem-solving	Communication skills	Curiosity
Confidence without	Conscientiousness	Determination
arrogance	Listening skills	Work ethic
	Professional competence	Sense of humor

Rule # 125 Research the program in advance. Always.

As interviewers, we continue to be amazed by how many applicants come to interviews unprepared, having done little research about the program or the faculty. Consider the recent following exchange:

"Welcome to Baylor. How has your visit with us been?"

"Great. The Texas Medical Center is so amazing. I had always heard that, but you don't really get an idea of its size until you see it firsthand. I think it's great that Baylor residents have the chance to rotate through such well-regarded hospitals. When do residents rotate through MD Anderson?"

"Our residents don't spend any time at MD Anderson since it's affiliated with the University of Texas-Houston Medical School."

"Oh, that's right. Do residents do research?"

"Yes, our residents are required to pursue a scholarly project."

Not only did this applicant reveal his lack of knowledge about affiliated institutions; he also asked a very basic question about research which was clearly addressed in the program website. By choosing this particular question, he came across as uninformed.

Another example:

"What are you looking for in a residency program?" asked Dr. Smart.

"I loved spending time in the operating room during my general surgery rotation, so I'm looking for a program that will allow me a great deal of time in the OR right from the get-go," replied Gwyn.

"You do realize, though, that our surgical interns are required to spend most of their time on the floors and in the clinics taking care of patients on the surgical service. We believe that it's important, early on, for interns to be comfortable evaluating patients preoperatively and managing their care postoperatively. Then, in the second year, we have our residents scrub in on cases..."

Prior to your visit, familiarize yourself with all information received from the residency program. Become familiar with both the institution and program, so that you can get the most out of your visit. Gathering information about the program before, during, and after your visit will help you make an informed decision about where you should place the program on your rank list.

Ask thoughtful and specific questions, the type that demonstrate your interest in the training program. This is one of the easiest ways to create a favorable impression. Utilize the following sources of information when researching the program:

- Printed materials sent from the program
- Fellowship and Residency Interactive Database (FREIDA)
- Websites for the program and its affiliated hospitals
- Other residency applicants
- Residents and faculty from your own institution who have trained at the institution where you will be interviewing
- Graduates of your medical school who are currently training at the program you will be visiting
- Program director, chairman, and faculty advisors at your own medical school's residency program
- Internet search using the name of the program and its affiliated hospitals
- Internet and literature search (www.pubmed.com) to learn about the faculty's recent publications

Utilize these sources to learn about the program's history, mission, philosophy, focus, areas of excellence, and key faculty. Programs and departments often post their latest news on their website. Print key information to read and reread before the interview.

Tip # 79

Have you researched the residency program before your visit? If not, you are doing yourself a great disservice. Without proper research, you won't be able to ask thoughtful and insightful questions. These are the questions that impress interviewers.

Tip # 80

In addition to knowing basic information, try to obtain information about the financial health and other aspects of the program. Did you know that approximately 40 family medicine residency programs have shut down in the past five years, including university programs such as the one at Duke University School of Medicine (which has since reopened)? Knowledge of a program's financial condition is important. If you highly rank a program that is in poor financial health, what will you do if the program closes?

Reading information about the program may also enlighten you about the type of house officer the program seeks. This is essential information that you can use to demonstrate to the program that you are precisely that type of person. For example, at the website for the Phoenix Integrated Residency in Obstetrics and Gynecology (http://www.mihs.org/mededucation/graduate/pirog.html), "factors important in the resident selection process include the following:

Academic qualifications
Interpersonal and communication skills
Dependability, responsibility, maturity, courtesy, confidence
Leadership skills
Dedication to women's health
Sense of humor and work ethic"

An applicant to this program would be best served by highlighting her skills and qualities in these areas. In doing so, she would be seen as a "good fit" for the program.

Rule # 126 Learn about the faculty who will be interviewing you.

Try to learn your interviewers' names prior to your visit. If any have names that are difficult to pronounce, master the correct pronunciation. With names in hand, you can start your research. Who are these individuals? Are they purely clinicians, researchers, or both? What are their areas of interest? Do their interests overlap in any way with yours? For example, have you referenced their work in one of your projects? Where did they train?

It takes time and effort to perform this research, but it is well worth it. Advance knowledge of your interviewers may help you feel more comfortable. You may establish a connection. For example, if you learn that you and your interviewer are graduates of the same university, you might mention this during the interview. This may establish an immediate connection, as long as you don't overdo it.

Tip # 81

Learn all you can about the interviewers by exploring the program's website. Websites often have faculty bios. Read about their areas of interest and background. Perform an internet and literature search (www.pubmed.com) using the interviewer's name. Look for anything you might share in common (e.g., attended the same university, research interests, etc.). Gathering this information is an important part of preparation. This knowledge may help you establish rapport during the interview.

Tip # 82

Faculty from your home institution may know your interviewers. They may be able to fill you in on some background information.

Did you know ...

According to the 2005 Association of Program Directors in Radiology survey, "42% of programs replied that the chair interviews each applicant, and 99% of programs stated that the program director interviews each applicant."

Rule # 127 Prepare for the standard questions.

It is the fear of many applicants: Will the interview be a grueling grill session in which the interviewer asks questions to gauge the applicant's knowledge base? Highly unlikely. Grill session interviewing is a thing of the past. Interviews today are mainly an exchange of information, usually starting off with the interviewer asking some basic questions. Questions to assess your medical competence are rare, and most questions are asked in an effort to learn more about you as an individual. The interviewer is trying to ascertain your personal qualities to determine how you will function as a resident.

Tip # 83

If asked a yes-or-no question, always elaborate on your yes or no. This is especially true of questions such as "Do you have research interests?" "Do you plan to pursue fellowship training?"

Tip # 84

Among the most common questions that applicants are asked is "Why did you choose to apply to our program?" Too often, applicants first mention their attraction to the city, weather, or family in the area, rather than using the question as an opportunity to discuss appealing aspects of the program. A far better answer would focus on factors such as the program's reputation, unique training opportunities, areas of research emphasis, and other program attributes.

In most cases, you should be able to predict the questions and prepare for them accordingly. If you think you can wing it when it comes to answering these questions, you are mistaken. To be at your best, you should anticipate the questions and think about your responses. Begin by jotting down the key points you would like to convey for each interview question. Then rehearse your answers to these questions. In rehearsing your responses, your goal is not to deliver a canned response, but rather to ensure that your responses convey the correct message. Unfortunately, some applicants choose to memorize their answers, which we don't recommend. Your responses will sound canned, and if you forget a point, you can easily become flustered.

Questions interviewers (faculty) may ask

Tell me about yourself.
Why are you going into this specialty?
What have you done to inform yourself about a career in this specialty?
What do you see as the positive features of this specialty?
What do you see as the negative features of this specialty?
What problems do you think the specialty faces?
What are your future plans?
What are your practice plans after finishing residency?
Do you have plans to pursue fellowship training?
Do you have research experience?
Do you have any interest in research?
Tell me about your research.
Where do you see yourself ten years from now?
What do you consider to be important in a training program?
What are you avoiding in a training program?
What are you looking for in a program?
What is your ideal program?
Why have you applied to this residency program?
What is your perception of the strengths of this program?
What is your perception of the weaknesses of this program?
What qualifications do you have that set you apart from other applicants?
Why should we choose you over the other highly qualified applicants?
How would you contribute to our residency?
Tell me three things that would make you especially valuable to our residency.
Where else have you interviewed?

How have you done in medical school?
What is the best experience you had in medical school?
What is the worst experience you had in medical school?
What were the major deficiencies in your medical school training?
What rotation gave you the most difficulty and why?
What was your most difficult situation in medical school?
Are you prepared for the rigors of residency?
What was the most interesting case you were involved in?
What are your strengths?
What are your weaknesses?
How would your friends describe you?
Have you always done the best work which you are capable of?
Of which accomplishments are you most proud?
How do you best deal with conflict?
Whom do you depend on for support?
What do you do with your free time?
What are your interests and hobbies?
With what kinds of people do you have difficulties working?
With what types of patients do you have trouble dealing?
What is your most memorable patient encounter?
What other programs have you applied to?
Can you explain your grades/board scores/leave of absence?
What if you don't match?
Why have you chosen to interview in this part of the country?
Are you applying to any other specialty?
How will you rank us?
What do you think about what is happening in ...? (current event question)
How do you see the delivery of health care evolving?
What was the last book you read?
From your CV, I see that you are an international medical graduate. Why did you
    leave your country?
As an IMG, you are familiar with the health care delivery system in your country.
    How does this system differ from the one here in the United States?
From your CV, I see that you are an IMG. What have you done to familiarize
    yourself with medicine as it is practiced in the United States? Have you done
    any observerships or rotations?
Do you have an ECFMG certificate? What ECFMG requirements remain for you
    to complete?
From your CV, I see that you are an IMG. How would you rate your oral
    communication skills? How would you rate your written communication skills?
From your CV, I see that you are an IMG. How well do you see yourself adapting
    to the American health system?
In your CV, there is a gap of one year. What did you do during this time?
Why are your USMLE scores so low?
Do you have any questions for us?
Can you think of anything else you would like to add?

Rule # 128 Prepare for both the traditional and behavioral interview.

The most common interview format is the traditional one-on-one interview. With this format, you will find yourself face to face with your
interviewer. Typically, the interviewer will ask questions about your
education, activities, and goals. Examples include the following:

- Tell me about yourself.
- What are your strengths and weaknesses?
- Why are you interested in our residency program?

Note that these are broadly based questions, as are the questions listed previously in Rule #127. Contrast these with the following questions:

- Tell me about a time when you had to deal with a difficult attending physician.
- Tell me about a time when you showed initiative.
- Describe a situation in which you had to deal with an angry or upset patient.

These more specific questions, which ask for an example, are a feature of behavioral interviews. By learning how an applicant handled or reacted to the situation in the past, the interviewer is able to determine how he might handle the situation in the future. Behavioral interviewing is based on the premise that future behavior is best predicted by past behavior.

The behavioral interview was introduced and developed by Dr. Tom Janz, an industrial psychologist. Research looking into its validity and accuracy has shown that behavioral interviewing is more accurate than traditional interviewing in predicting who will succeed (Motowidlo) (McDaniel). While more popular in the business community, residency programs may also conduct behavioral interviews. Since each question calls for a specific example, those who best answer these questions have prepared in advance by recalling specific past experiences and scenarios.

In answering these questions, begin by describing what happened, what you then did, what was the result of your actions, and what you learned from the experience. Use the acronym STAR to help you answer these questions:

S - Situation (Describe the situation in detail.)
T - Task (What was the task or obstacle?)
A - Action (What action did you take?)
R - Result (What was the result?)

Following is a list of behavioral questions.

Examples of behavioral questions

Tell me about a time when you worked effectively under a great deal of pressure.
Tell me about a particularly stressful situation you encountered in medical school and how you handled it.

Tell me about a time when you made a mistake and had to admit it to your resident or attending.

How would you deal with a fellow resident who is not doing his share of the work?

Tell me about a negative interaction you had with an attending or resident. How did the two of you deal with it?

Tell me about a time when you were really upset by the words or actions of an attending or resident.

Tell me about a patient from whom you learned something. How will this experience help you as a physician?

Describe a relationship with a patient that had a significant effect on you.

Tell me about a time when you had a personality conflict with another team member. How did you deal with it?

Your attending physician asks you a question and you are not sure of the answer. What do you say or do?

Your colleague is abusing alcohol or drugs. How would you handle this situation?

Tell me about a time when you were disappointed in your performance.

Tell me about a time when you disagreed with how an ethical situation was being handled.

Tell me about a situation in which you overcame adversity.

Describe a clinical situation you handled well.

Tell me about a clinical situation that didn't go as well as you would have liked.

Give me an example of a time when you had a difficult communication problem.

Tell me about a time you had to build a relationship with someone you didn't like.

Tell me about a problem you had with a classmate, faculty member, or patient. How did you handle it?

Tell me about a time when you handled a stressful situation poorly.

Tell me about a time when you became really angry over a situation at work.

Discuss a particularly meaningful experience in your medical training.

Discuss a particularly difficult experience in your medical training.

Describe to me a situation in which you had to break someone's confidence.

Was there a time during rotations in which you didn't feel like part of the team? How did you handle the situation?

Tell me about a time when you witnessed unprofessional or unethical behavior on the part of a resident or attending. How did you handle it?

Tell me about a time when you had to build rapport quickly with someone under difficult conditions.

Tell me about the major challenges you have faced in your medical school career.

Tell me about a time you were able to successfully work with another person even when that person may not have personally liked you.

Tell me about a time when you were able to successfully work with another person even when you did not personally like that person.

Tell me about a time during rotations in which you went above and beyond.

Describe to me a time when you received an evaluation with which you disagreed.

Your senior resident insists on a treatment plan you feel may harm the patient. What do you do?

Rule # 129 Remember that you do have a fair amount of control over the interview.

Most applicants feel that in an interview session, all of the power is in the hands of the interviewer. This assumption is wrong. The interview is essentially an exchange of information during which two parties are learning more about one another. As long as you remain an active participant during the interview, you will have a fair amount of control over the direction of the interview.

As the interviewee, you control the content of the discussion. You control the message that is conveyed. Because of this fact, you should enter the interview knowing full well the items that you wish to convey about yourself. Only with this knowledge, and some degree of assertiveness, will you be able to sell yourself effectively.

"What have you enjoyed most about your medical school education?"

"Spending time with my patients and educating them about their illness has been most enjoyable for me. I really enjoy teaching. I've also had the chance to tutor freshman and sophomore students in the basic sciences. During clinical rotations, as a senior student, I've had opportunities to mentor and teach junior students. These experiences have been very rewarding and I would like to make teaching a major part of what I do as a physician. I know that, in your program, residents have tremendous opportunities to teach. I am particularly excited about the workshops your program offers to help residents improve their teaching skills. After interviewing at a number of programs, I must tell you that your program is unique."

The question asked what the *applicant* enjoyed most about their medical school education. Instead of focusing on the education, as some applicants might have done—"Our medical school was great"—this applicant was able to effectively convey a message about her own strengths and abilities, and how these fit well with the program's strengths.

Rule # 130 Have a case ready to present.

On occasion, you may be asked to present an interesting case. "Tell me about the patient you learned the most from."

As is the case with all interview questions, the goal of the question is to learn more about the applicant and not the case itself. You need not and probably should not choose the most difficult or challenging case you have encountered.

Choose a patient who made an impact on you. What challenges did the care of this patient present? What did you learn from the patient? Did your involvement in the patient's care change the way you practice? Did it lead you to see things differently, or help in your career choice, or highlight certain goals for you as a physician?

In asking this question, your interviewer is also hoping to learn how well you present clinical information. Without good communication skills, patient care suffers. Therefore, you must be able to present patient information clearly and concisely.

Prepare an approximately two-minute case presentation. Your goal is to be able to intelligently discuss all aspects of the case. You may want to consider preparing two cases. These cases should deal with topics in two different subspecialties. It is usually preferable to present a case that is outside of the interviewer's discipline. If your interviewer is a cardiologist, you may wish to avoid your cardiology case and instead present your endocrinology case. If you choose to, or must, present a case in the interviewer's discipline, make sure that you are well read on the current literature, as you may just be presenting to the world's foremost expert.

Rule # 131   Panel interviews may be used to gauge your composure and ability to deal with a stressful situation.

In a panel interview, you will be interviewed by two or more interviewers simultaneously. Panel interviews allow the program to assess your composure, your ability to deal with stressful situations, and your interactions with different people. Through the use of panel interviews, programs can expose more members of their selection committee to applicants. This provides the program additional judgments on each interviewee. This can allow for a more productive discussion of each candidate at the resident selection committee meeting.

Although panel interviews may seem more intimidating, your preparation will essentially be the same as it would for a one-on-one interview. Don't let the fact that you are outnumbered affect your poise, confidence, and your ability to sell yourself.

The following suggestions are helpful when facing a panel interview:

- Be clear on the interviewers' names and, from time to time, use them during the interview.
- Direct your response initially to the interviewer who asked the question.
- Try to position yourself so that you can see all members of the panel without having to move your head from one side to another. Constant head movement can be stressful, and will appear distracting.
- As you delve further into your answer, make eye contact with the other interviewers.
- Do not dart your eyes from one interviewer to another. Instead, make eye contact, pause briefly on each, and then move on to the next panel member.

- As you conclude your response, make eye contact once again with the interviewer who asked the question.
- Don't be alarmed if one or more interviewers show little to no expression or enthusiasm. Continue your efforts to sell yourself, and don't let their lack of emotion dampen the enthusiasm of your responses.
- Often, one of the panel members will take the lead in asking questions. The natural response may be to focus on this individual. However, your goal is to establish rapport with all interviewers.
- Sometimes, a panel interview may turn into a conversation between the interviewers themselves. With this scenario, an applicant loses the chance to make an impression. Should this happen, don't hesitate to insert yourself into the conversation in a tactful manner. "Would this be a good time for me to talk about ..."

Did you know ...

In a survey of radiology residency program directors, it was learned that 6.5% of programs utilize panel interviews (Otero).

Tip # 85

Do not treat resident interviewers any differently than faculty interviewers. It's best to assume that both have equal input into the resident selection process.

Rule # 132 The conversational interview can be quite dangerous.

"That didn't feel like an interview. It was just a normal conversation."

We've heard many applicants say something to this effect following an interview. If you leave an interview feeling this way, you have taken part in what is termed a conversational interview. In this type of interview, the interviewer does not have a list of prepared questions. The next question is often based on a point you just made.

Conversational interviews may be conducted by both trained and untrained interviewers. The goal of the former is to put you at ease and build rapport in an effort to learn more about you as a person. The trained interviewer has a certain agenda in mind, knows what information he seeks, and has decided that a conversational interview is the best way to elicit this information. The interview quickly becomes a chat, akin to two friends speaking with one another. With this type of interview, you can't become too relaxed, or you may reveal things you wouldn't have in a traditional interview.

By contrast, the untrained interviewer has no plan. Direction and focus are lacking. The danger here is that, if you are not proactive, you may leave the interview without sharing key experiences and strengths that show the interviewer that you are a good fit for the program. If you sense that the interview is lacking focus, we recommend that you make efforts to redirect the conversation.

Tip # 86

While you can't control the type of interview you will experience, you do have control over the content of your responses. Always enter an interview with an agenda. In advance of the interview, ask yourself what are the key experiences, skills, and strengths that you need to convey to the interviewer.

Tip # 87

If an interviewer runs out of questions well before the allotted time is over, you may wish to take some initiative. "Perhaps this would be a good time for me to share with you ..." If the interviewer seems receptive, you can proceed from there.

Rule # 133 There are always two major goals of all interviews. Don't forget the second one.

You must have a clear understanding of your goals for the interview. All of your goals can be summed up by the major two:

1. You must have a successful interview so that the program will rank you highly.
2. You must gather enough information about the program to make an informed decision regarding its place on your rank list.

In your desire to demonstrate compatibility with the program, you may lose sight of the second goal. While it may not always feel that way, remember that the interview process involves two parties selling themselves. While the program is trying to ascertain your strengths and weaknesses, you should be doing the same with respect to the program. You must use the short time that you have during your visit to learn as much as possible about the program. With every program you visit, ask yourself the following questions:

- How compatible am I with this program?
- Can I see myself working well with the program's faculty and residents?
- Will this program provide me with an environment in which I can thrive?
- How well will this program help me meet my future goals?

Rule # 134   Always prepare with a mock interview.

Practice, practice, practice. We cannot emphasize this rule enough. Unfortunately, we've sat through too many residency selection meetings in which strong applicants are unranked due to their interview. The message they sent during the interview was that they absolutely did not belong in this residency program. We believe that most of these applicants are completely unaware of the messages they send during the interview. Be it the inappropriate answers to interview questions, the mannerisms that overshadow the message, the affect that hides their true qualities, or the subtle findings that send a negative message, we believe that most of these applicants just didn't realize what message they were actually sending.

Interviewing is not a skill where you can just wing it. Too many students are overly confident about their abilities to convey their individuality, their strengths, and their fit for the program in one fifteen-minute session. Too often applicants prepare minimally or not at all for interviews. Such overconfidence has the potential to inflict serious damage. To interview successfully, you must anticipate the questions that will be asked, prepare your responses, and deliver them confidently.

In preparing for interviews, practicing both alone and with others is a must. With adequate practice, you can become comfortable with the interview process. Practice improves self-confidence. It also helps pinpoint deficiencies in your interviewing skills. You may not recognize your own tendency to twirl your hair, but an interviewer will find it distracting. Nervous habits, distracting mannerisms, poor grammar, a blunted affect, or a tendency to speak too softly may all be features that you're not likely to recognize in yourself.

Rehearsing your interview in front of a mirror may help you identify some problems. Note body language, as it sends a significant message. Do you smile? Do you keep your arms folded across your chest? Do you clench your hands tightly?

Practice with a friend. Have him ask you interview questions, and respond as you would if you were at a real interview. Consider videotaping your performance. Together, you can review the interview, critique your performance, and use this information to make improvements in your verbal and nonverbal impressions.

One of the most useful methods of preparation, and one of the most underutilized, is to ask your advisor if they would feel comfortable helping you prepare by participating in a mock interview. Many advisors are members of residency selection committees, and they often have considerable experience in interviewing applicants.

The mock interview with your advisor can be designed to simulate the real interview. Ask your advisor to assume that he knows nothing about you but that which is found on your CV and personal statement. After the mock interview, you should meet with your advisor to evaluate your performance. Ask for specific feedback on the following:

- Content of your responses
- Your body language
- Your poise and level of confidence
- Whether he would select you based upon your performance

This type of feedback is invaluable, and should be utilized. Make any necessary adjustments prior to your first actual interview. If you are unable to set up a mock interview, check with your medical school. Some schools have developed workshops to help students with these skills.

Rule # 135 Every element of your residency application is up for discussion. Know it cold.

Prior to each interview, review each element of your residency application. Anything in your application is fair game for an interviewer. As you review each line of your CV, determine if an interviewer might ask you about an item, why he might ask, what he might ask, and how you might respond. Do the same for the rest of your application. Such an approach will help avoid this unfortunate real-life scenario:

> Jordana spoke eloquently about her research during her interview for internal medicine residency at a major university institution. She had performed this research between the first and second years of medical school. In describing her role in the project, she spoke with great enthusiasm and energy. The interviewer asked, "Which journal was your work published in?" Jordana couldn't remember, stammering "I'm blanking on the journal but I believe I have it here somewhere." She fumbled through her portfolio, finally saying, "I think it was in *Vaccine*."

Did you know ...

Dr. Amorosa, a faculty member in the radiology department at UMDNJ/Robert Wood Johnson Medical School, reminds applicants that they may be asked about anything in their application. "Make sure that whatever research or other experience you have had, you know it cold—otherwise you lose your credibility. Be prepared to answer questions about yourself and your experiences."

Tip # 88

Are there any areas of concern that might come up during the interview? A failing grade? A low USMLE score? Unfavorable clerkship evaluation comments in the Dean's letter? A leave of absence? If so, determine how you will handle these queries well in advance of your interview.

Did you know ...

In the article, "USMLE Scores, matching formulas, and more," Dr. Paul Jones, associate provost of student affairs at Rush Medical College, wrote that "in his experience, students who are unsuccessful in the residency match are unaware of how they measure up against other applicants. Students who have a red flag, but who also realize it and address it in their interviews, seem to do better" (www.medscape.com).

Rule # 136 Meet with residents or faculty in your own institution who trained at the institution where you will interview.

Before you visit a program, seek out all house officers and faculty at your own institution who have received any of their training at the institution where you will be interviewing. These individuals will be able to give you important information about the program. They can often talk to you about how the program compares to the one at your own institution.

Tip # 89

Some medical schools ask their students to complete forms describing their interview experiences at other institutions. If so, you should read about their experience at the program you will be visiting. Check with your student affairs office to see if your school does this.

Information obtained from someone "in the know" is often the most useful knowledge. Using this information, you can make powerful statements about your desire to become a resident in that program.

> "I've had a chance to speak with Dr. Lisa Sanders, who is a faculty member at my medical school. She is a graduate of your training program and had wonderful things to say about her residency experience. In particular, she spoke glowingly about morning report and how it..."

"Our internal medicine chairman at Strong University, Dr. Grant, was invited by your program to be a visiting professor several years ago. Dr. Grant has always spoken very highly about your program. He was especially impressed with how your program encourages and supports residents to participate in research and scholarly activity..."

"While attending the ACP conference, I had the opportunity to meet with Dr. Chen, one of the faculty members in your department. We spoke at length about the residency program. From him, I learned a great deal about your program's strengths. What particularly piqued my interest was the unique mentorship program ..."

Rule # 137 Consider your first interviews practice sessions. Save your most valued programs for later.

If at all possible, avoid scheduling your first interviews with programs you highly covet. Your first interviews should be with programs that are lower on your list. The pressure won't be as intense, and you can ease into the process somewhat. You're likely to make mistakes early on, so get them out of the way here. With each successful interview, you will gain confidence.

Tip # 90

If you have many interviews, consider placing interviews at your top choices somewhere in the middle. Don't save them for the end because you may find that by then you are tired of interviewing. This may affect your performance.

Rule # 138 In our opinion, interviewing early or late in the season does not have a significant impact on your ranking.

Applicants often wonder if it is better to interview early or late in the season. There has never been a clear answer, and opinions vary. Those who favor interviewing late maintain the following:

- You may be better remembered and, therefore, more highly regarded.
- You'll have had lots of practice.
- Your application will be compared with the true applicant pool, since the rest of the pool has already interviewed. If your application is of higher quality when compared to the rest of the applicant pool, this could be of great benefit.

- Interviewers have a tendency to downgrade applicants who interview early because they have not yet developed a good feel for the applicant pool.

Proponents of early interviewing maintain the following:

- You will have more energy and enthusiasm, as will your interviewers. Neither one of you is likely to be tired of the interview process.

- Interviewing early is better because interviewers tend to choose as they go along. These interviewers may have already made their decisions by the time the later interview season arrives.

For years, there was no data on this issue. However, in 2000, Martin-Lee published the results of a study involving 44 emergency medicine residency programs (Martin-Lee). In this study, the date of an interview (early, middle, or late in the interview season) had no bearing on the ranking of candidates. In another study from the department of anesthesiology at New York University, the authors determined the interview dates for each of the applicants that matched at the program during a three year period (Wajda). They found no significant association between the interview date and likelihood of matching. Since there is no evidence to suggest that interview timing has an effect on how a program ranks applicants, our recommendation is to not worry about it.

Tip # 91

When scheduling interviews, do not make any special requests such as asking for an interview on days the program does not interview. While the program may grant your request, it will require busy faculty to rearrange their schedules.

Rule # 139 Arrange for maximum flexibility during interview season.

Residency interviews are generally conducted from October through late January. However, some programs, particularly those that participate in an early match, may begin interviewing earlier.

While the policy on absences differs from school to school and from clerkship to clerkship, schools generally ask their fourth year students to schedule interviews not during clerkship time, but rather during vacation time, breaks, or off months. Students often take a month or two off during the interview season, particularly if they are planning to interview around the country.

Despite your best efforts to schedule interviews that won't conflict with clinical work, you will find that some programs offer little or no choice in scheduling. If you are unable to schedule an interview during vacation time, you must contact the clerkship director for permission to attend the interview. Do so as early as possible. Be professional and courteous in your interactions with the clerkship director. Offer to make up any time that you will be away, and be ready to provide documentation of the interview invitation. Once the clerkship director has granted an approved absence, inform all team members, including the attending physician, resident, and interns.

Tip # 92

Some rotations prohibit students from taking any absences at all. Plan to schedule flexible rotations that will allow you to be absent for interviews. However, even with flexible rotations, time off is generally limited to a handful of days.

Tip # 93

Follow the absence policy at your school and clerkship. Failure to follow these guidelines may result in the submission of unfavorable clerkship evaluations.

Did you know ...

In a survey of 2006 urology applicants, 54% of applicants reported that skipping medical school clerkships and classes was detrimental to some extent (Kerfoot), and 1% of all applicants reported that it was "greatly detrimental."

Rule # 140 Don't cluster your interviews too closely.

The interview season can be a long one, which is why it is important to schedule your interviews at a reasonable pace. If you crowd too many interviews into a short period of time, you will become fatigued and stressed. This may affect your interview performance. One of the keys to successful interviewing is to interview when you are well rested. You are more apt to come across as attentive, enthusiastic, and relaxed, which are precisely some of the personal qualities residency programs are seeking in their future residents.

Rule # 141 Convey your utmost respect to the administrative staff.

Prior to your interview, you will have to contact the residency program's administrative staff. You may have a question or you may simply need to contact the staff to schedule your interview. Convey your utmost respect to the administrative staff, and convey your appreciation of their help. Don't be too demanding as you try to agree on a day and time for the interview visit.

Tip # 94

When does your interview start? It starts with the first phone call you make to the residency program. When speaking with members of the administrative staff, remember to be courteous and appreciative of their help. Displaying good manners won't increase your chances of securing a position in the program. However, poor manners can sink your chances. Reports of surly behavior or a poor attitude will most certainly be conveyed to the program director.

The program director and the administrative staff work together closely. Don't give any member of the administrative staff a reason to speak poorly of you. You never know which individuals may impact resident selection.

Tip # 95

Try to arrange interviews in a specific geographic region during a single trip. While this won't always be possible, it will save you time, energy, and money. As you are planning the trip, if you haven't heard from a program in the same region, then consider contacting them. Let the program know of your upcoming trip. This may spur the program to review your application and offer an interview invitation. They may even be able to accommodate you during the trip.

Did you know ...

In a survey of 2006 urology match applicants, respondents reported a median of 12 interviews with total costs at a median level of $4,000. The median expense per interview was $330, with travel expenses and lodging accounting for 60% and 25% of total costs, respectively (Kerfoot).

Tip # 96

During the application process, programs become deluged with applicant e-mails and phone calls. There are typically some applicants every season who call or e-mail repeatedly to check on the status of their application. These applicants quickly become annoyances. Be patient, let the process unfold, and contact the program only if you must.

Rule # 142 Respond quickly when invited to interview.

While most programs will inform you of interview invitations by e-mail, some prefer to contact applicants by phone or mail. No matter how you are notified, respond to the invitation as quickly as possible. Interview slots are limited and a delay on your part may leave you with less than desirable dates.

When responding to an interview request, always thank the program for the invitation. If you contact the program by phone, it's a good idea to send a thank you note by e-mail as well to the program coordinator.

Dear Ms. Jones,

Thank you for inviting me to interview at your residency program. I consider it an honor to be selected for an interview, and I look forward to visiting your program.

After looking over the list of possible interview dates, any of the following dates, if available, would be suitable for me:

November 14
November 18
November 23

Thank you once again.

Sincerely,

Rebecca Conley

After a date has been agreed upon, you will generally receive another e-mail from the program with further instructions, including when to arrive, where to stay, directions, and the day's events. Note the following:

- Place and time of the interview
- Directions
- Where to park
- Where to stay

- Whether you are required to bring any additional documents with you
- Whom you will be meeting, including the names, titles, and pronunciation of all interviewers. Pay special attention to the positions of those whom you will be meeting.
- Interview itinerary (schedule of events)
- Type of interview (one-on-one versus panel, blinded versus open, number)

Tip # 97

Applicants often schedule their flight home or to another interview destination without taking into account when the interview day ends. Leaving early can inconvenience administrative staff, other applicants, and faculty, all of whom may have to rearrange their schedule. If you're going to interview at a program, then do so properly.

Rule # 143 Always confirm.

Approximately one to two weeks prior to your interview, call the residency secretary to confirm your scheduled interview. Confirming each interview can help you avoid the following scenario, as described by one applicant:

> "At a few places, the coordinator did not communicate a change in the schedules for the interview day that was sent out prior to the visit. This was particularly distressing for applicants who had made travel plans based on the original itinerary" (Nawotniak).

Tip # 98

Don't just ask for directions to the program's physical address. You also need directions to guide you to the department's office once you reach the hospital or medical center. Applicants have been late because they lost their way in the hospital.

Rule # 144 Never be a no-show.

If you accept an invitation to interview, but later decide not to visit that program, inform the program immediately. Notify the program first by phone, then in writing. Always thank the program for the opportunity. Notifying the program in advance allows the program to offer the interview slot to another applicant.

The community of program directors can be a small world. Program directors do speak with one another, especially in smaller, more competitive specialties. Program directors have also been known to contact the Dean's office about students who were no shows for their interviews.

Rule # 145 Prepare for a typical interview day.

The typical day will begin with the program director welcoming applicants, introducing the program, and providing an overview of the program, usually via slide show or PowerPoint presentation. Following this, applicants are often invited to morning report, another conference, or rounds. One or more interviews will then take place with faculty and possibly residents. A tour of the institution and lunch with the residents are also common. The day may conclude with a wrap-up session, which at some places is one-on-one with the program director.

With so many programs, this schedule will understandably vary. For this reason, you should review the interview materials to learn about the interview day. How will your day be structured? Knowing what to expect may allow you to feel more at ease and less stressed. It may also help you prepare better for the interview. For example, if you'll be attending a conference, what will be the topic? While you won't be asked to participate, advance reading may allow you to ask insightful questions or participate in a meaningful discussion.

Rule # 146 Not all of your interviewers will have access to your file. Always arrive prepared with your own materials.

Applicants generally believe that interviewers will have read their applications prior to the interview. However, some programs do not allow interviewers to view a candidate's application. These interviews are called closed file interviews because the interviewer knows nothing about you. Interviewers may also be given some application information, but quantitative information such as grades and USMLE scores may be absent from the file (i.e., partially open file interviews). In other cases, interviewers have full access to your application, but haven't reviewed it yet, or haven't reviewed it thoroughly.

Programs that limit access to the full application file feel that an interviewer who has quantitative information at his disposal may develop preconceived notions about the strength of an applicant. For example, an interviewer may be quite impressed with an applicant's grades and USMLE scores. Colored by this information, the interviewer may approach the interview differently than he would have had he been blinded to this information. In fact, Robin and colleagues demonstrated that bias does occur when interviewers have full access to an applicant's file (unblinded or open file interview) versus when files are not reviewed (Robin).

Did you know ...

In one study, Smilen found "a strong, striking, and statistically significant correlation between interview scores and board scores when their interviewers knew these grades, with no correlation when they did not. This finding should not be particularly surprising. The halo effect is a well-known phenomenon ... in which a conclusion is reached about a job applicant within the first half minute of an encounter. After that point and during the remainder of the interview, the interviewer will subconsciously discount anything that does not fit the predetermined image of the candidate. By providing interviewers with the available performance markers, this effect can be established even in advance of interview" (Smilen).

Tip # 99

If you have strong grades, good board scores, or have been elected to AOA, you should convey this information to an interviewer who lacks access to your file in order to benefit from the halo effect. At the beginning of a closed file interview, you may offer the interviewer a copy of your CV and transcript. Make sure that your honors grades and board scores are on your CV.

Rule # 147 Don't ever be remembered for what you're wearing.

I've interviewed a few applicants that I can still, to this day, remember distinctly what they were wearing. I can't remember what their scores or strengths were, but I can remember the dangling, hypnotic ear-rings, the too-short skirt with the high heels, the long pinky nail, and so many more. In an interview, you never want to be remembered for what you were wearing. You want to be remembered for your strengths, your communication skills, your great scores, and your out-standing letters of recommendation, or any or all of these.

You should dress conservatively, with the goal of presenting your-self neatly and professionally. In choosing interview attire, select clothing in which you feel comfortable. Your clothing should not inter-fere with your ability to give a successful interview.

Interview Attire		
	Yes	No
Men	Suit, well-fitting, dark blue or gray Shirt, ironed, long-sleeved, typically white Tie, long, conservative Shoes, clean, polished Well-groomed hairstyle (neat and trimmed beard and mustache) Nails, clean, trimmed	Earrings Visible body piercings Strongly scented cologne Strongly scented aftershave
Women	Suit, dark blue or gray, or tailored dress Shoes—clean, closed toe, dark or neutral color, low to moderate heels Hosiery, conservative, at or near skin color Well-groomed hairstyle Nails, clean, trimmed (if nail polish, clear or conservative color)	Low neckline Excessive or distracting jewelry Strongly scented perfume Distracting hair or make-up

Your appearance is of the utmost importance, since the way you look is one of the first factors that telegraphs a message during an interview. If you are sloppily dressed or poorly groomed, your message is that you are not the highly professional, mature physician with compulsive attention to detail that the residency program seeks. Highly qualified applicants are sometimes remembered more for their attire than for their qualifications.

Did you know …

In a survey of orthopedic residency program directors, directors were asked to rank the importance of 26 residency selection criteria. Personal appearance was ranked fifth (Bernstein). In another study involving 54 residency applicants, ratings of neatness and grooming correlated positively with final interview ratings for women (Boor).

Tip # 100
If you are flying to the interview, keep your interview outfit in your carry-on luggage.

Rule # 148   The informal restaurant "get-together" is absolutely part of your interview.

During the interview season, you may be invited to interview at restaurants, usually the evening before or on the actual day of the interview. Programs don't ever call these meetings "interviews." They'll tell you about the informal get-togethers that allow you to interact with residents and/or faculty. While these are generally optional, you should make every effort to attend. These get-togethers are a rich source of information about the residents, faculty, and program. Even more importantly, they give you another opportunity to highlight your sparkling personality and scintillating wit.

While these get-togethers tend to be more relaxed than the actual interview, never forget that you are being judged. Even if faculty members are absent, any representative of the program, including residents and support staff, may be asked for their impressions of you. Remain alert and don't ever let your guard down. Be cordial, friendly, and polite. Engage in conversation freely with residents and faculty. Just take care in what you reveal. For (a true life) example: "This is one of my favorite restaurants in Houston. How do you like Vietnamese food?" "I've never had Vietnamese food. I always thought it smelled funny." The message: this applicant may not be ready or open to the big city experience.

Did you know ...

Dr. Lee, professor of ophthalmology at the University of Iowa, wrote that "we include a resident in our residency selection process and have found anecdotally that resident input can provide valuable information that might not be revealed in an asymmetric hierarchical faculty-applicant interview. In addition, informal feedback obtained from the residents during the social activities associated with the interview process can reach the selection committee through the resident liaison" (Lee).

Tip # 101

Make every effort to attend these get-togethers, because your opportunities to interact with residents on the day of your interview may be limited. These get-togethers are an ideal setting in which you can learn more about the program, and in which the residents can have a better chance to be impressed by you. They provide an ideal opportunity to discuss the program with the residents, gauge their level of happiness, and determine whether they would make the same choice if they had to do it all over. Try to obtain the names and e-mail addresses of several residents in case you need questions answered later.

Chapter 13

Interview Questions

How are you today?

Did you have any trouble getting here?
How do you like the weather?
Did you have any trouble finding a place to park?
How do you like [our city]?Have you ever visited [our city] before?
Was there a lot of traffic on your way here from the airport (or hotel)?

The above questions, known as icebreaker or "small talk" questions, are usually asked at the beginning of an interview. While this portion of the interview may only last several minutes, its importance can't be overemphasized. If icebreaker questions are answered well, they can set a positive tone for the rest of the interview, and put both you and the interviewer at ease.

While these questions appear simple, many applicants handle them improperly. Generally, applicants prepare well for the deeper questions, but give no thought to these types of icebreaker questions. Savvy interviewers recognize this and purposefully engage applicants in small talk. In doing so, they hope to learn more about an applicant's true personality.

The key with this type of interaction is to reinforce your overall message, and therefore respond in a confident and positive manner. Answer "How are you today?" with an answer like "I'm doing great. I'm really happy to be here today" rather than "OK," or "Tired." Unfortunately, we've interviewed many applicants who end up whining or complaining about one thing or another. You may hate the weather or dislike the city. You may have had difficulty finding the office or struggled with the commute. There's no reason to share this with your interviewer.

Do you have any questions?

Applicants expect this question will be asked at the end of the interview. However, this isn't always the case. Occasionally, an interviewer will open with this question. She may wish to test your composure and initiative. Or you may be dealing with an inexperienced interviewer. Have a list of questions ready.

Regardless of when asked, this is a very important question. In fact, some would argue that it is the most important question. Some interviewers consider the quality of the questions asked to be more important than answers given.

Many interviewers consider it a red flag when an applicant has no questions. The worst thing you can say is "No, I don't have any questions" or "My questions have already been answered." This is akin to saying that you have no interest in the program. Your interviewer may also wonder if you've actually prepared for the interview. Answering "no" also robs you of the opportunity to gain valuable knowledge about the program, the type of knowledge that would help you make an informed ranking decision.

Too often, applicants ask standard or basic questions that have been answered at the program's website or in their brochure; such questions imply poor preparation. Ask informed questions to learn more about the program. You should convey the fact that you are knowledgeable about the specialty, and your questions should convey the fact that you were interested enough in the program to research it in advance.

To ask the "right" questions, begin by researching the program in great depth. Learn all that you can about the program by using a variety of sources—the program's website, an internet search, the program brochure, your advisors and faculty, and so on. Savvy applicants begin their question with a reference to what they have learned. "On your website I learned about the importance the program places on developing resident teaching skills. I was excited to read about this because I've really enjoyed my teaching experiences as a medical student tutor. I understand that teaching workshops are offered several times a year. Can you tell me more about these workshops?" Note that in this example, the applicant starts by making a reference to the program's website. He then proceeds to ask a thoughtful and specific question tailored to the residency program. In doing so, he clearly conveys his experiences teaching as a medical student, his passion for it, and his desire to continue it as a resident. If the program is seeking dedicated teachers, this applicant has succeeded in matching his skills to the needs of the program.

Often the best questions are those derived from something the interviewer said earlier. "You mentioned that the program offers a unique lecture series to train residents as researchers. What topics are covered in this series?"

We've provided a full table of possible questions to ask faculty members in Chapter 14 "During the Interview" (see Rule # 164).

Some other tips:

- After making a list of questions, prioritize them. You usually won't have the chance to ask all of your questions. If you could only ask a single question, which one would it be?

- Use your best judgment regarding the number of questions to ask and when to ask them.
- Ask open-ended rather than yes/no questions.
- Keep the questions short.
- Avoid "Why" questions. These can sound critical.
- Be aware of the manner in which you ask your questions. If you are not careful with the language you choose or the tone of voice you use, your interviewer may feel that you are grilling, challenging, or confronting her.
- Take care in how you phrase a question. Avoid asking questions that suggest biases, such as "Will I have to work with a lot of private attendings?"
- Allow the interviewer to finish replying; avoid interrupting.
- Never ask a faculty interviewer about salary, vacation, or benefits.

Tell me about yourself

This question is typically asked at the start of an interview, either as the first question or the question that immediately follows icebreaker questions. Given its common use, you should prepare for this question in advance. Script and rehearse your response.

In developing your response, include the type of information that the program wants to know about you. What is impressive about your qualities or achievements? What sets you apart from other candidates? Why should the program select you as a resident?

Too often, applicants give their entire life stories, beginning with when and where they were born. Don't interpret this question as one that is focused purely on your personal background. Rather, regard it as an opportunity for you to share your most important skills, experiences, and accomplishments. In developing your response, focus on what qualifies you to be a resident at their institution.

Think of your response as a positioning statement. The questions from the interviewer that follow will often be based on the information you provide.

Summarize your background in sixty to ninety seconds. Time yourself to make sure you don't exceed this amount of time. Avoid providing irrelevant details, since we can state from personal experience that many candidates tend to ramble needlessly.

Because this question can be interpreted in different ways, interviewers are also eager to learn about the approach that you take in answering it. What do you focus on? How do you organize the information? Your content and delivery provides the interviewer information about your composure and communication skills.

What are your weaknesses?
> What is your worst quality?
> If you could change one thing about your personality, what would
> it be?
> What are your pet peeves?
> What would your friends say is your biggest weakness?
> What might your last resident or attending physician want to
> change about your work habits?

Above all, don't respond by saying you have no weaknesses. Some interviewers actually ask for several, so you should prepare three weaknesses to discuss.

You are not obliged to share your worst qualities with the interviewer. Unfortunately, many applicants do just that, usually because they're taken off guard. When choosing a weakness to discuss, avoid stating one that is damaging. If your weakness would interfere with your ability to function as a resident, then present a different one. Stating that you are often late or have trouble working with other people would be presenting damaging weaknesses. Avoid sharing a character flaw or a negative personality trait. These can be difficult, if not impossible, to change.

Classically, applicants have been advised to relate a potential strength as a weakness. One example of this approach is the classic "People tell me I'm a workaholic." Who wouldn't want a resident with a strong work ethic? Equally common is the "perfectionist" example. Who wouldn't want a resident who pays close attention to detail? "I expect too much of others" is another commonly used example. This suggests that you set high standards. Yet another example is "I try to be friends with everyone." This suggests that you would be a good team player. We caution you on these four examples. Because many applicants have used these weaknesses over the years, they have become trite and unoriginal, and interviewers are tired of hearing them.

One approach would be to present an area that needs improvement, preferably something that can be acquired through training. For example, you could discuss how you would like to become fluent in Spanish and how that would be beneficial to you as a resident physician. With this type of response, you would always include the steps taken to correct this weakness.

What are your strengths?
> What sets you apart from the crowd?
> What do you think your fellow medical students would say about
> you?
> How would your friends describe you?
> How would your teammates describe you?
> How would you describe yourself?

Name three adjectives that describe you.

What are your key skills?

What attributes will make you a valued presence at our program?

Why are you a more attractive candidate than others?

What personal quality makes you perfect for a position in our residency program?

What are your greatest assets?

While these may seem like easy questions, too often applicants deliver a response that isn't as strong as it could have been. Your choice of which strengths to share should not be taken lightly. Too often, applicants choose to mention strengths that have little or no relevance to one's ability to excel as a resident. You should research and determine the qualities that are highly valued in your chosen specialty and at the specific program. Think about work strengths (e.g., organizational skills, problem solving) and personality traits. Cite those strengths that you have in common and that are most relevant to the position you are seeking. For example, the American Society of Anesthesiologists states that "an anesthesiologist has to be incredibly detailed-oriented, skillful at procedures, calm in stressful situations, and warm and caring to ease patient's anxiety" (http://www.asahq.org/career/faq.htm).

Rather than providing a long list of strengths, pick three of your top strengths. Too many applicants end up rambling. Keep your response concise. Many applicants will name their strengths and then stop. The responses that make the deepest impressions are those that use examples to support the strengths. One example: "My ability to persevere has been central to my success. The pathology interest club that I wanted to set up at my medical school was initially applauded, but my cofounder and I hit many obstacles. Even though I started during first year, the club didn't come into existence until my third year, and it was my perseverance that kept me going and dealing with all the roadblocks."

Be careful when you answer the questions, "What sets you apart from the crowd?" and "Why are you a more attractive candidate than others?" Don't speak negatively about the rest of the applicant field, as is easy to do. Respond by stating that you realize the other applicants are qualified, but that you are confident that your abilities and qualifications will make you an excellent resident. There's a fine line between self-confidence and arrogance, so tread carefully.

Why have you chosen this specialty?

How can you be sure that this specialty is the right career for you?

Why would you be particularly good in this specialty?

Be prepared to discuss the factors or reasons that led you to select the specialty. One approach would be to begin with whatever piqued your initial interest in the specialty. Was it a personal experience, a course, or an inspiring professor or mentor? From there, consider discussing how your interest was further solidified through rotation experiences, discussions with residents and faculty in the field, and the knowledge you've gained through your own research and reading.

In asking this question, your interviewer is trying to determine your interests and motivations, and your fit with the specialty and the program. Avoid discussing lifestyle or financial issues as motivating factors. Don't say that a family member in the field encouraged you to consider the specialty; you need to emphasize your own enthusiasm for the specialty. Your interviewer is also interested in learning the steps that you took to make this important decision. The way you describe your decision-making process will give the interviewer an idea of how you might approach other important decisions.

As you progress through the interview season, you will become tired of answering this question. Avoid giving the impression that you are bored and lacking in enthusiasm for the field. It is essential that you remain passionate about your chosen field.

Why did you apply to this program?
   What qualities are you looking for in a program?
   What are you looking for in a residency program?
   Describe your ideal residency program.
   What do you believe our program would give you that another
      program would not?
   What interests you the most about this program?
   Tell me what you know about this program.
   What have you learned about our program from others?
   Why do you want to be a resident here?
   How do you view our program?
   What two or three items are most important to you in a residency
      program?

Questions like these are often asked in interviews. Be prepared with an outstanding response. The best response is one that demonstrates that you are perfect for the program, and that the program is perfect for you. After answering this question, your interviewer should be convinced that you really want to be a resident in their program.

Begin by researching the program thoroughly. What makes the program unique? What do you find particularly attractive about the program? This information will allow you to tailor your response to the program. In other words, if the program values research highly, you should discuss your interest in research.

If a faculty member recommended the program, then by all means say so. Programs like to know that they are well regarded. Taking the time to speak with someone who has firsthand knowledge of the program also demonstrates that you have taken the time and initiative to learn as much as you can about the program. It demonstrates the seriousness of your interest in their program.

Be specific as possible to confirm that your selection of their program as a possible residency choice was based on some thought and effort. Too often, applicants give a general answer. If you could give the exact same answer at another program, then your answer isn't good enough. "I first learned about your program through my faculty mentor. Dr. Garcia is a graduate of your program and she has always spoken glowingly of the training she received. As I researched your program, I learned about how many of your graduates have gone on to become academicians at medical schools across the country. As I look to the future, I too see myself as an academician and would like to go to a residency program that will prepare me for a career in academics. I have also developed an interest in healthcare management and was quite excited to learn that you offer residents the ability to obtain the MBA degree during residency. I know of no other program that can say that."

There are certain responses that you need to avoid at all costs. Avoid answers that confirm a disconnect between what you're seeking and what the program offers. Never put down another program. Lastly, while the geographic location of the program may be a major factor in your interest, avoid offering program location as the only or initial reason for applying to the program.

What will you contribute to this program?

In what specific ways will our program benefit from selecting you?

Make a list of your attributes and skills. Which of these would be highly valued by the program? While the skill set that programs value is, in general, going to be very similar, programs will often describe what they are specifically seeking in a resident. This information is typically available at the program's website. If it is, determine which skills or qualities you possess. Then prepare your response accordingly.

For example, at the website for the Department of Surgery at the Temple University School of Medicine, Dr. Dempsey, the chairman, writes that "we achieve excellence in patient care and resident education by adhering to our departmental core values...They are quality, respect, safety, teamwork, trust, and integrity. These are the core values that our faculty, residents, and support staff will not compromise...We are looking for people who share our department's core values" (http://www.temple.edu/medicine/departments_centers/clinical_departments/surgery.htm).

Having read this, an applicant preparing for an interview at Temple may respond, "I know that your program highly values professionalism. In me, you'll find someone who shares the same values. I have been fortunate to work with many attendings who have demonstrated compassion, respect, and sensitivity in their interactions with patients and colleagues. These faculty members have been my role models. Recently, I was selected for membership in the Gold Humanism Honor Society chapter of my medical school. As a resident, I will continue to make this a top priority."

Why are you interested in training in this city/area?

Programs recognize that the geographic location of a program is a major factor influencing how candidates rank a residency program. In a survey of applicants to one emergency medicine residency program during the 2004 match, program location was one of five factors rated most important (DeSantis). In a larger survey of over 7000 applicants applying to a variety of surgical and nonsurgical specialties, geographic location again was cited as a top factor influencing residency selection (Nuthalapaty).

Express your sincere interest in the city or area (and if you're applying there, you should have a sincere interest in living there for the next several years). If you're dealing with an unfamiliar geographic region, you'll have to do some research. What does the city have to offer? If you have family or friends in the area, feel free to mention that fact.

What do you do outside of medical school?
What is your favorite hobby?
What extracurricular activities do you participate in?
What are your leisure-time activities?

Programs are looking for applicants with outside interests, not those who are all work and no play. While the degree to which programs value outside interests and hobbies varies considerably, it's important to emphasize that you're interested in more than just work.

Stating that you have no time for hobbies or extracurricular activities may be viewed as a red flag. It would be better to state that although your free time is limited, you do enjoy _____. Another option would be to state that whenever you have free time, you spend it with your family.

Consider what your hobbies or interests reveal. Do they demonstrate your attention to detail or your ability to work as part of a team? These are qualities that are valued by residency programs. Savvy applicants use this question as an opportunity to highlight these types of qualities.

Avoid the obvious negatives, such as activities or interests that are controversial or may be viewed negatively.

Where do you see yourself in 5 or 10 years?
What are your long-term goals?
How much thought have you given to your future plans?
Are you planning to pursue a fellowship?
What are your plans after residency?

While these may seem to be innocent questions, the interviewer's intent may be to learn whether your professional goals are compatible with the overall philosophy of the program and the opportunities avail- able there.

In answering this question, think about the program's mission. How does the mission align with your future plans? Does the program pride itself on the development of academicians? If so, telling the interviewer that you wish to enter private practice will clearly demon- strate that your goals are incompatible or unrelated to the program's mission.

Never lie about your future goals and plans. The pressure that many applicants feel to do so is real, and we acknowledge this fact. We discuss the issue further in Chapter 15. However, you do need to research and determine a program's mission before you start the application process. If their mission differs markedly from yours, then the program won't be the best place for you to reach your own goals.

There are several points we emphasize to applicants when pre- paring for this question. First, many students just aren't sure of their future plans at this stage in their career. Faculty recognize this fact. Therefore, avoid giving the impression that your plans are rigid. You may state that you are considering… as a future professional goal. While you may not be sure of your eventual goals, however, you should always provide evidence that substantiates your interest in and potential for achieving that goal. For example, if you state an interest in international health, then you should use this question as an opportunity to highlight your past experiences in the area.

Second, your answer should emphasize those aspects of your own application that would dovetail with the program's mission. If the program or specialty values the development of clinician-educators, then you should emphasize how much you enjoy teaching, how that is reflected in your prior employment and volunteer commitments, and how you plan to incorporate that goal in your future professional career.

Lastly, this question almost always refers to professional goals. We've had many applicants respond with the classic "I see myself as married and with children." Who doesn't? Your goal is to distinguish yourself with your answer, and to emphasize your personal and pro- fessional attributes that will lead to the development of an outstanding clinician.

What happens if you don't match?

Applicants applying to highly competitive specialties are most likely to be asked this question. International medical graduates applying to any field may also be asked about their future if they don't match. Don't be unnerved by this question. Some candidates mistakenly assume that if the interviewer asks this question, they are not a com- petitive candidate.

The interviewer asks this question hoping to learn about the depth of your commitment to the specialty. If you don't match, will you abandon your desire to enter the field? Or do you have a back-up plan that will allow you to reapply in one year? What does your back-up plan consist of? Will you do a transitional or preliminary year with the intent to reapply? Will you pursue a research fellowship in an effort to strengthen your application? A well thought out back-up plan that allows reapplication implies a deeper commitment to the specialty.

Where else are you interviewing? Where have you applied other than here?

These questions should be answered in a straightforward and honest fashion. You may have applied to or interviewed at twenty programs, but you don't need to provide the entire list. It is acceptable to state, "I've applied to over twenty programs, including..."

In choosing which programs to name, consider your current interview location. Try to offer programs that are similar in caliber, philosophy, geographical location, and so forth. We've seen applicants try to impress interviewers by naming two or three top tier academic programs. This may not resonate well with an interviewer at a community-based program.

While you may not see the need to be honest in answering this question, remember that the community of program directors is a small one. Once you respond, your interviewer may ask for your impressions about other programs. Respond, but avoid negative comments.

Close your response effectively. After providing the names of some programs, restate your interest in the current program.

Tell me about your research.
Tell me about _____.

Everything in your application is fair game, including your research experience. Prepare in advance to discuss your research experience succinctly and eloquently. Review your projects and rehearse your response. Be prepared to discuss your research at any possible level, since you may be discussing it with an expert in the field. This is more important if your project was done several years ago. A poor response to this question may suggest that you embellished or exaggerated your involvement in the work.

I see that you had some difficulty in ___ course/clerkship. Could you tell me what happened?

I understand that you passed your USMLE Step 1 exam on the second attempt. Can you tell me what happened?
What explains this D on your transcript?

No one has a perfect application. Some applicants have a blemish on their record that requires explanation. Since interviewers will often bring up these issues, you need to have a plan in place to field these difficult questions. We recommend that you discuss your approach with your advisors.

Of major concern to the interviewer is the possibility that your poor performance was related to a lack of commitment, dedication, or intellectual ability. The concern is that these problems may resurface during residency training.

To alleviate these concerns, provide an explanation of the circumstances that led to the blemish. Was it a death or serious illness in the family? Were you sick at the time? Life presents everyone with challenges, and medical students are no exception. If a hardship of this sort caused academic difficulty during a short period of time, a brief explanation will generally suffice. Make sure you emphasize that you performed at a higher level outside of this time period. In other words, finish by pointing to your successes.

If poor grades or scores were the result of academic rather than nonacademic issues, you must take responsibility for your record. Acknowledge it. Don't make excuses and don't sound defensive. If you do, the interviewer may question your ability to handle criticism or your willingness to admit to mistakes. Apologizing is not a good idea because it may be viewed as an indicator of low self-confidence. Some candidates have tried to inject humor into their response, hoping to defuse a difficult situation. This is not a good approach. A serious question requires a serious answer.

Explain the situation, why it happened, what you learned, how you overcame it, and why it won't happen again. End by emphasizing that your performance since then is a far better indicator of your motivation and intellectual ability.

Addressing a disciplinary problem noted in the Dean's letter will be more challenging. Issues such as falsifying information, failure to respect patient confidentiality, failure to fulfill responsibilities, inappropriate interactions with team members, arrogance, inability to handle criticism, and inadequate personal commitment to patients are examples that will raise red flags. In fact, some studies have shown that these types of problems in medical school are predictive of future disciplinary action by state medical boards. You'll need to discuss these issues with your advisors, and formulate a response that emphasizes the lessons you learned and why you wouldn't repeat the behavior.

What type of people do you have difficulty working with?

"None. I get along well with everyone." This response will be viewed with skepticism. Few people can honestly make this claim, so avoid this answer.

The question, obviously, is asked to determine how well you work with others. One way to respond would be to state that you work well with all types of people, but you have found it challenging to work with people who "...." Examples would include people who don't fulfill their responsibilities, complete their share of the work, or who complain incessantly.

Do you prefer working as a member of a team or would you rather work alone?

While carrying out the duties of a resident requires the ability to work well with others as part of a team, it is also essential that you have the ability to perform individually. The best answer is one that demonstrates to the interviewer that you work well in both settings.

What do you perceive as the negatives about this program?

No program is perfect. In your research, you will undoubtedly come across some negatives. Some may be significant, while others may be minor. Should you be asked for your opinion about a program's negatives, tread carefully. The interviewer is hoping to hear that you don't see any major negatives, and therefore remain very interested in training at the program. Therefore, convey minor negatives, and always end your response with a positive spin.

What was your least favorite course or clerkship in medical school? Why?
What rotation was your most difficult?

Don't mention a course or clerkship that is related in any way to your chosen specialty. Stating that pharmacology was your least favorite course would be a poor answer for an applicant to anesthesiology. If asked why, avoid saying anything negative about those with whom you worked. For example, "I would have to say neurology. I had really looked forward to the rotation, but of all my rotations, it was the least hands-on."

Why did you attend your medical school?

Through this question, the interviewer is trying to learn about the way in which you make decisions. Provide a specific answer that demonstrates that your choice was not a random one. For example, you might comment on a particularly appealing aspect of the curriculum which was not available elsewhere. You can also use this opportunity to highlight the quality of your medical education.

How did you like your medical school?

Your answer should be positive. Your goal is to emphasize the strength of your medical education so that you are viewed as an individual who is well-prepared and ready for residency training.

What accomplishment are you most proud of?
What is the most distinct contribution you made to your medical school?

In preparing an answer to this question, consider those accomplishments that are unique or distinctive. Focus on those that would give your interviewer some insight into the type of contributions you would make as a resident in her program. Are you a leader of an organization? Are you a championship athlete? Are you an accomplished musician? Did you receive recognition for tutoring underclassmen? Did you publish an article in a leading journal?

A survey of emergency medicine residency program directors revealed that having a "distinctive factor" such as being a championship athlete or medical school officer was one of three factors most predictive of residency performance (Hayden). In a survey of plastic surgery residency program directors, leadership qualities were the most important subjective criterion used to evaluate applicants during the interview process (LaGrasso). In a study done to determine predictors of otolaryngology resident success using data available at the time of the interview, candidates having an exceptional trait such as leadership experience were found to be rated higher as residents (Daly).

Is there anything else you'd like to tell me before we conclude this interview?

This is the perfect opportunity to close the interview with a bang. Use this chance to give a brief summary of the skills and strengths you would bring to the residency program. End by restating your strong interest in the program and thanking the interviewer for her time. Since this is the last question, keep your response short.

What is your hospital's take on Obama Care
adequate ancillary staff.
ask about financially stability
what is your demographic.

contagious enthusiasm.
Bring to program: positivity, Innovative - contributing ideas,
resourceful, culturally aware/ness -
resilient/adaptable - make the best of every situation

Chapter 14

The Interview Day

Rule # 149 Your interview begins long before you meet your interviewer.

Your interview doesn't start when you sit down with your interviewer. It begins as soon as you enter the premises. Many applicants mistakenly assume they only need to "be on" during the interview. In reality, everything you say or do on the day of the interview may be noted and duly reported.

It's not unheard of for faculty to ask their secretaries and administrative staff for their opinions of the applicants. They may ask the secretary about a candidate's appearance or behavior. Our secretaries have commented on a host of negative behaviors. These range from the disinterested applicant leafing through the waiting room *Sports Illustrated* instead of program information, to the applicant with the arrogant, unfriendly demeanor, to the pesky applicant asking inappropriate questions, especially when the secretary is clearly busy.

Did you know ...

Dr. Lee, a professor in the department of ophthalmology at the University of Iowa, wrote that "many programs (including our own) use the informal feedback from the residency coordinator, the secretaries, and the other residents to obtain a more complete view of the applicant. Important sentinel behaviors both positive (e.g., politeness, altruism, helpfulness) and negative (e.g., condescension, arrogance, rudeness) may only manifest during applicant interactions with perceived subordinates (e.g., the appointment secretary)" (Lee).

Interviews often do not start on time. Applicants may wait as long as an hour or two. Since many interviewers are practicing physicians, patient care-related issues can arise at any point and require immediate tending. Some candidates lose their patience, and have been known to approach the secretary impatiently or rudely, demanding to know the reason for the delay. How you handle a situation of this type is very telling.

Tip # 102

Applicants should be on their best behavior, not just during the interview, but throughout the entire visit. Programs can gain much insight into your personal characteristics by observing your interactions with other applicants, program staff, residents, and others. The best rule of thumb is to conduct yourself as if there are hidden cameras watching your every move.

Tip # 103

Ask the receptionist where you can place your excess belongings (coat, umbrella, etc.). You don't want to walk into your interview bogged down with clutter.

Rule # 150 Be compulsive about bringing everything that you need for the interview.

Bring the following with you to your interview:

- Curriculum vitae (CV)
- Personal statement
- Application
- Board scores
- Medical school transcript
- Copies of any published articles
- Copies of submitted, accepted, or in press articles, with your advisors' permission
- All correspondence between you and the program
- Picture
- Notepad portfolio with pen
- Money
- Parking ticket
- Personal items (dental floss, mint, etc.)

While the program is likely to have your application (including CV, personal statement, board scores), you should be prepared with copies in the event that an interviewer asks for one of these items. You may have a closed file interview, or a patient emergency may result in an interviewer substitution. The pen that you use should be a nice one. Specifically, bring a pen that has not been provided by a drug rep.

Rule # 151 Arrive early for the interview.

Start your interview day properly by arriving early. Aim to reach the city on the day before the interview. Stay as close to the hospital as possible. If possible, make a trip to the hospital to gain familiarity with the interview destination. In the morning, plan to be at your destination an hour before the start time. This extra time will be useful when the unforeseen occurs—such as heavy traffic, inclement weather, or an accident. Running in at the last minute can affect your interview performance, as many applicants have learned the hard way.

Entering the designated interview location more than fifteen minutes before the start time can be just as bad. Arriving too early can make you seem anxious, and you may interrupt the staff as they set up for the interview day. When you do enter the reception area, introduce yourself to the residency program's secretary. "Good morning. My name is _____ and I have an interview today."

Even with meticulous planning, unforeseen circumstances may cause you to be late. Arriving late is one of the reasons that program directors cite for not ranking an applicant highly. It is possible to recover from this situation, but only if it is handled with great poise. If you will be late, call the program to apprise them of the situation. When speaking on the phone, be polite no matter how flustered you are. Once you have arrived, take time to compose yourself before entering the room. Apologize and explain, at an appropriate time, what detained you. Never rush in complaining about what happened.

Tip # 104

Make sure you have the phone number of the program readily accessible in the event that you are running late.

Tip # 105

If you are driving, determine in advance the route you will take. Having an alternate route in the event that you encounter heavy traffic is wise. If you're taking the train or bus, familiarize yourself with the bus or train line you will be riding, including the times. What will you do if service is interrupted for some reason? Always have a back-up plan.

Rule # 152 Project self-confidence, not anxiety.

It is common and completely natural to be nervous. However, you don't want to convey the message that you are an anxious, distracted, unqualified applicant. Your message should be that you're an extremely well qualified applicant, and therefore you are calm and confident. The first and best way to conquer anxiety is thorough preparation. Learning about the interview process, anticipating questions, preparing responses, rehearsing with friends, and performing a mock interview with an advisor are all important parts of interview preparation.

Despite extensive preparation, anxiety can remain a significant problem for some applicants. We have a few additional suggestions for the days before an interview:

- Utilize stress-reduction techniques. Many articles and books provide specifics on effective techniques utilized by actors, professional athletes, and public speakers. Such techniques include controlled breathing, progressive muscle relaxation, and visualization, among others.

- Channel your nervous energy into concrete, positive action. One example would be focusing on action items for interview preparation such as re-reading the program information or practicing some of your responses for anticipated interview questions.

- Direct your nervous energy into action that is unrelated to interview preparation. You've heard of the fight or flight response. Expend that extra adrenaline by heading to the gym or going for a run.

- Look over your CV to remind yourself of your accomplishments. The program would not be interviewing you if they weren't impressed with what you have to offer. You have a great deal to offer a residency program, and you should be specific when reminding yourself of what you can bring to a program.

- Your career does not ride on your performance at one interview. Remind yourself of this fact. Other interviews will follow.

Tip # 106

Although you will be nervous, you don't want to convey the impression of an anxious, nervous applicant. Residency is inherently stressful. As such, interviewers seek residents who are able to think clearly in the most stressful of situations. Avoid comments that convey anxiety.

Did you know ...

In evaluating interview performance, interviewers take note of both what you say and how you say it. High levels of anxiety have been shown to adversely affect a variety of factors, including eye contact, body language, voice level, and projected confidence (Freeman). In her article, "Anxiety patterns in employment interviews," Young wrote that "anxious individuals are less likely to be hired ... possibly because interviewers perceive highly anxious people to be less trustworthy, less task-oriented, ... than low anxiety interviewees" (Young).

Rule # 153 Shake hands properly.

You'll have the opportunity to shake hands when you first meet the interviewer and again when you complete the interview. You must be ready for a handshake at these two points. Not all interviewers will offer to shake hands. In general, the interviewee should follow the lead of the interviewer. If she doesn't extend her hand, don't offer yours.

The initial handshake is an important component of a first impression. Be prepared to shake hands by keeping your right hand free at your side, as opposed to clutching your portfolio. If you suffer from hyperhidrosis and are prone to sweaty palms, be prepared to subtly wipe your palm. Your goal is to convey self-confidence, not anxiety. Shake hands using a firm grip, conveying an impression of confidence. Avoid a weak, limp, or crushing grip. As it can be difficult to evaluate the quality of your own handshake, you may need to solicit input from friends or colleagues.

Did you know ...

In the *Lancet* article, "Getting a grip on handshakes," Larkin reported the results of a study by Chaplin in which the handshake characteristics of men and women were evaluated. Larkin wrote that "a strong correlation was found between a firm handshake— as evidenced by strength, vigor, duration, completeness of grip, and eye contact—and a good first impression... Given the power of first impressions, the researchers advise that women as well as men 'try to make that first handshake a firm one'" (Larkin) (Chaplin).

Rule # 154 The first few minutes of an interview can be critical.

As soon as you walk into the room, your interviewer will be sizing you up. Initial impressions may even dictate the course of the interview. A favorable first impression may lead to a more relaxed interview. An interviewer who perceives you to be disinterested or sloppy, though, may be more likely to grill you extensively to try to support or refute that impression.

Did you know ...

Dr. Ziegelstein, associate program director of the internal medicine residency at Johns Hopkins Bayview Medical Center, states that "individuals who interview and judge others for a living (e.g., program directors) often form very strong first impressions. Typically, those individuals are flexible and those impressions are changeable, but those first impressions are nevertheless important."

Below are key guidelines to promoting a favorable impression within the first few minutes of an interview:

- Dress well and be impeccably groomed.
- Stand up and greet the interviewer with a firm handshake ("Hello, Dr. Smith, I'm Evan Chen. It's a pleasure to meet you.")
- Smile when meeting the interviewer.
- Walk into the room with confidence.
- Make eye contact.
- Pronounce the interviewer's name early ("How do you do, Dr. Smith?")
- Make small talk easily.

You must have a polished entrance, introduction, and opening. In your mock interviews, practice even this early stage of the interview.

Tip # 107

After you are invited into the interviewing room, do not sit down until the interviewer offers you a seat. It's considered bad manners to be seated before the interviewer asks you to or does so herself.

Tip # 108

After introductions have been made, most interviewers will engage interviewees in some small talk. You may be asked the following:
   How was your trip here?
   Did you have any problems finding our office?
   What's the weather like in _____?
   In answering these questions, avoid long statements. The interviewer doesn't want to hear about the "terrible traffic," how much you "hate the snow," or the problems you had finding their office. To start off on the right foot, answer these questions with brief, positive answers.

Tip # 109

"How has your day with us been so far?" is a commonly asked question at the beginning of an interview. You can use this opportunity to say something positive about the program. Talk about how happy the residents looked, how much you enjoyed morning report, etc.

Rule # 155 Your nonverbal communication is a potent part of your message.

In all personal interactions, communication occurs in two fashions: verbal and nonverbal. So much focus is placed on what applicants should say during the interview that they often neglect to focus on how they say it. However, nonverbal communication can be as important, and in some cases more important, than verbal communication. Body language cues can overcome the content of your interview answers, especially if your body language conveys hesitation, uncertainty, or a lack of conviction.

Interviewers do analyze body language, although most of the time this is done on a subconscious level. Any inconsistency between verbal and nonverbal communication may raise red flags. We've interviewed applicants who can't send a consistent message. While their self-proclaimed greatest strength is passion and dedication, they're slouched in the chair, leaning on the armrest, and looking a little bored. Others say the right things, but seem to lack sincerity. In response to a question on why a resident is switching fields: "I found that my passion lay not in spending hours in the operating room, but in spending time in an outpatient setting speaking with patients." Although the content of the answer is fine, the poor eye contact suggests insincerity.

Tip # 110

Are you aware of how you communicate nonverbally? Most applicants are not. When preparing for an interview, applicants focus most of their attention on verbal communication. Much less emphasis is placed on nonverbal communication or body language. In fact, many applicants don't even think about nonverbal communication. However, it is estimated that 65 to 90% of every conversation is interpreted through body language (Cole). There are many qualified applicants who interview poorly because their nonverbal language is not congruent with the content of their interview answers. Participating in a mock interview is an excellent way of learning about how you communicate nonverbally.

It's difficult, and in some cases impossible, to evaluate your own body language. We've interviewed applicants who send strong, clear messages with their unconscious use of body language. The student who twirls her hair constantly. The applicant who rests his head on his hand during the interview. The other applicant who is slumped down in the chair. The student who can't seem to maintain eye contact, even when stating how much they love your program. The applicant who keeps smiling and laughing, even when discussing a sad patient case. The student who maintains such a blunted affect that it's difficult to tell if they're bored, tired, or just at baseline. You would be surprised how often such cues can lead an interviewer to make snap judgments about a candidate's qualifications.

Your own evaluation of this type of communication should include a conscious awareness of several items. What are you doing with your hands? How is your posture? Are you maintaining eye contact? While you can perform a self-evaluation, mock interviews are critical in evaluating your nonverbal cues. Mock interviews can be staged with colleagues, advisors, or interview coaches, and feedback should cover your nonverbal communication skills. Mock interviews can be videotaped as well. Reviewing your performance can prove uncomfortable but enlightening.

Successful nonverbal communication includes adhering to the following rules:

- Stand and walk with erect posture and shoulders back.
- Shake hands firmly. Avoid a limp or crushing handshake.
- Your facial expressions should be relaxed. Avoid indicators of excessive anxiety, such as the furrowed brow or tense jaw.
- Maintain appropriate eye contact. Don't stare down your interviewer.
- Hand gestures should be appropriate, and not overdone.

- Avoid excess. While you should smile and nod occasionally, some applicants exhibit nervous laughter or excessive head bobbing.

Did you know ...

Weiten, in his book *Psychology applied to Modern Life: Adjustment in the 21st Century,* wrote (citing the work of Riggio) "it has been found that interviewees who emit positive nonverbal cues—leaning forward, smiling, and nodding, are rated higher than those who do not" (Weiten).

Equally important is the avoidance of nervous and distracting habits. We could list endless examples, but here are a few of the most common:

- Looking down or glancing away
- Tapping the foot or drumming fingers on desk or chair
- Fiddling with jewelry or other accessories
- Twirling the hair
- Glancing often at the watch

Tip # 111

Failure to maintain eye contact while speaking may suggest a lack of confidence or even dishonesty. However, avoid prolonged eye contact. An interview is not a staring contest.

Body language 101

What should I do with my hands?

Rest your hands in your lap. It's acceptable to clasp your hands together, but don't clasp them too tightly or make a fist. Avoid folding your arms across your chest. This can create an impression of rigidity, unapproachability, or even dishonesty. Do not cover your mouth or touch your face while you speak. Avoid touching your tie, tugging at your collar, or straightening your clothing. We also recommend that you not hold your pen in your hand. Many applicants end up fiddling with it or tapping with it.

How should I sit?

Posture can weigh heavily in how others perceive you. Maintain an alert, straight posture while you sit, stand, and walk. Leaning forward slightly demonstrates interest. Applicants who slouch can appear lazy, unmotivated, or disinterested.

What should I do with my feet?

Keep your feet flat on the floor. You may cross your legs at your ankles. Do not rest your ankle on your opposite knee.

Tip # 112

With the mirroring technique, an individual makes subtle efforts to adopt the pose and position of those with whom they're speaking. It is based on the concept that people generally like those who are similar to them. Mirroring of body language may help to establish better rapport. In fact, in the book "Handbook of Cultural Psychology," Kitayama and Cohen reviewed the literature in this area and wrote that "people have more positive subjective experiences of rapport as a result of mirroring exhibited by interaction partners" (Kitayama).

Rule # 156 You need to know how well you're doing in an interview. Pay close attention to the nonverbal cues of the interviewer.

The interviewer's body language may be your only clue as to how well you're doing. Most interviewers won't interrupt you to tell you that you're rambling. They won't share with you that your last response came across as very defensive. Better than words, their posture, movements, facial expressions, and tone of voice can indicate their reactions. This type of indicator can be useful if you make it a point to notice these nonverbal cues. As we've stated before, interviews are stressful, and many applicants focus all of their attention on preparing their next response. In response to the simple "Tell me a little bit about yourself," one applicant went off on a five-minute monologue. She didn't notice the obvious impatience of my colleague and myself because she wasn't paying any attention to us. The interview is bilateral communication, and it is very important to monitor how well you are doing. In many cases, your only effective way to do so is by paying close attention to the nonverbal cues of the interviewer.

Rule # 157 Pay attention.

It is extremely stressful to be seated in front of an interviewer anticipating the next question. Most applicants nervously focus on what they're going to say. Instead of focusing on their next answer, they should be focused on the interviewer. Listening carefully doesn't mean waiting for the chance to speak. It means concentrating on what the interviewer is saying and making it clear that your entire attention is focused on the interviewer. Your goal is to create an impression of poise and confidence. We've sat in interviews where applicants were obviously nervous and distracted. They misunderstood the question or provided an answer that didn't address the question. Some asked questions that were answered earlier in the interview.

Rule # 158 Plan what you'll do when you don't know how to answer the question.

Among an applicant's greatest fears is that of being asked a question to which she doesn't know the answer. While practice is the best defense against the unexpected, we do think that some reassurances and suggestions here are necessary. Remember that one subpar interview response is unlikely to torpedo the entire interview. Most important is that you maintain your confidence and focus.

If you are asked a difficult question or one that you are not sure how to answer, avoid stammering, stuttering, apologizing, or making something up. Don't rush into a disjointed and hurried answer. Pause for a few seconds to gather your thoughts. Or you can say, "That's an interesting question. Let me think about it for a moment." If the question is ambiguous, you can also ask the interviewer for clarification. Remind yourself that with many questions, there are no simple right or wrong answers. If you still can't come up with anything other than "I don't know" or "I'm not sure how to answer that question," say so. Being able to say "I don't know" can take a great deal of confidence.

Don't view this as the end of the world. Your recovery is likely much more important than your response to a single question. Maintain your composure and focus on the next question. If, at the end of the interview, you come up with an answer, then volunteer it. "I've been thinking about one of the questions you asked me earlier. Would you mind if I expand on my answer?"

Rule # 159 Learn how to handle silence.

Silence during an interview can be a common occurrence. If inexperienced, the interviewer may not be able to come up with any more questions. At other times a savvy interviewer may purposefully become silent after you've answered a question. The interviewer may simply stare at you without saying a word. The natural response is to wonder what you did wrong. "Did I say something inappropriate?" "Did she not like my answer?" The other natural response is to reword your answer, repeat a comment you made earlier, or even retract your answer. Applicants may assume that the reason for silence is that the interviewer doesn't agree with your answer, or is searching for another one. However, the silent response is often used as a tactic to gauge an interviewee's confidence in their response.

The best course of action is simply to remain silent without fidgeting or displaying signs of anxiety. Look at the interviewer with interest as you wait for the next question. In time, the interviewer will break the silence with the next question.

How can you tell if your interviewer is testing you or just can't come up with anything else to say? If her attention is focused on you, it's more likely that she's utilizing this stress tactic. If, on the other hand, the interviewer appears nervous, is fidgeting, and isn't looking at you, she may be trying to come up with the next question. In this case, you could break the silence by asking some questions about the residency program.

Rule # 160 Convey enthusiasm.

Enthusiasm is contagious, even in the setting of an interview. It doesn't matter how well you've prepared the content of your interview answers. The manner in which that content is conveyed has a great deal to do with its reception. Your goal is to appear personable, sincere, and down-to-earth. You need to avoid appearing flat, blunted, tired, or robotic. It's easy to stiffen up, become too formal, or become so focused on what you're going to say that you fail to convey a personality. In all of these cases, you may fail to connect with your interviewer or even leave a frankly negative impression.

Your goal should be to appear enthusiastic about yourself, the specialty, and the residency program. As with any conversation, things go more smoothly if you can locate a topic that interests the other person. Ideally, you'd be able to find a topic in common that interests your interviewer. This rule is more applicable to interviews that occur late in the season. After your thirtieth conversation with an individual interviewer, you may find it difficult to muster the energy and enthusiasm that came so easily initially.

Did you know ...

In his advice to students at the University of Florida College of Medicine, Dr. Patrick Duff, Associate Dean for Student Affairs, recommends that applicants keep their "energy level up throughout the day. When I reviewed the interview performance of over 200 students who applied for our ob-gyn training program in the last 5 years, the single biggest reason for a low interview score was 'did not appear interested, no spark'" (www.med.ufl.edu/oea/osa/student_advice.shtml).

Rule # 161 Avoid phrases that suggest a lack of credibility.

Programs are on their guard against applicants who exaggerate their achievements, or outright lie. Therefore, you need to safeguard your own credibility. Avoid the following phrases:

- I'm going to be honest with you now ...
- To tell you the truth ...
- To be perfectly candid ...

Prefacing a statement with phrases such as these may raise a red flag in the interviewer's eyes. She may assume that what you're about to say will be a stretch of the truth or a flat out lie. The reason we specify these particular phrases is that many individuals who use them are unaware of their use, and are unaware of their connotations.

Rule # 162 You may be asked inappropriate or illegal questions. Plan in advance how to handle them.

Results of the 1996 AAMC Medical Student Graduation Questionnaire revealed that 45% of students were asked about marital status or family plans. Despite efforts to eradicate questionable interviewing practices, interviewers continue to ask applicants inappropriate, unethical, or outright illegal questions.

Federal and state civil rights acts make it unlawful for employers to discriminate on the basis of the following:

- Religion
- Age
- Race
- Gender
- Sexual preference
- Marital status/living situation
- Family planning
- Height
- Weight
- Military discharge status

Most of these questions are asked not out of malice, but out of simple ignorance. Naïve or less experienced interviewers may ask these questions simply to make conversation, not recognizing the inappropriateness of their queries.

Before you begin the interview process, develop an effective way to handle these types of questions. Some applicants, unprepared for such questions, have unfortunately reacted in an emotional manner. Some have refused to answer the question and some have even responded in a hostile manner: "That is a completely inappropriate question. I can't believe you would ask me that."

An outright refusal to answer an improper question is certainly your right. However, you will offend the interviewer and create a situation from which you may not be able to recover. It goes without saying that if the question is blatantly offensive, then you should choose this option.

If at all possible, however, you should try to answer the question as you would any other, with poise and confidence. There are several possible strategies to utilize. We describe two ways of handling these types of questions:

Answer the question directly

Some applicants will simply answer the question directly. If you're comfortable answering the question, then this may be the right approach for you. If the interviewer has asked the question just to make conversation, it's unlikely that your response would affect your chances of matching with that program. If the interviewer is deliberately asking the question, then your response may have a direct impact on your chances of matching.

"I see that you're a nontraditional student, already in your 30s. When do you plan on having children?"

Examples of direct responses:

My husband and I hope to have children in the next few years.

My spouse and I have discussed it, and we'd like to delay until after residency, since it would be so challenging during residency.

We really haven't come to any decision yet on that issue.

Answer the intent or concern behind the question

Using this approach, you won't directly answer the question. Your goal is to address the interviewer's concern. The key is to try to understand why the question is being asked.

"I see that you're a nontraditional student, already in your 30s. When do you plan on having children?"

This applicant assumes that the question is asked to determine if she would continue to be an effective resident in the event that she were to have a young child at home during residency:

"Dr. Lowell, I understand that the residents at Seymour Hospital deal with a very high patient volume when on call. I can assure you that I have a strong work ethic and sense of responsibility, along with the ability to deal with a demanding patient case load. You'll find that my transcript and letters of recommendation attest to this fact."

Did you know ...

In a survey of 230 urology residency applicants conducted in 1999, "being asked about marital status was recalled by 91% of male and 100% of female, if they had children by 25% of male and 62% of female, applicants, respectively" (Teichman).

Rule # 163 If the interviewer asks if you have any questions about the residency program, the correct answer is "Yes, ma'am, I do."

Most interviewers will set aside some time, usually at the end of the interview, for your questions. The advantage of asking questions is twofold:

- You can gather information about the program in order to make an informed decision about the program's place on your rank list.
- You can demonstrate to the interviewer your interest in the program.

When the interviewer asks, "Do you have any questions about the residency program?" the right answer is "Yes, I do." One of the worst answers you can give is "No, I don't have any questions." This is akin to saying, "I have no interest in your program," which may or may not be true.

Tip # 113

When the interviewer asks "Do you have any questions?" this generally signifies the closing phase of the interview. If you did not have the opportunity to communicate important points earlier, you can use this opportunity to do so. Simply say, "Before I ask my first question, I would like to take a moment to mention a few other points. Would you mind if I do so now?" Keep your comments concise, especially at this closing phase of the interview.

Often, applicants prepare a question or two, only to find that the questions are answered during the course of the interview. Then, when asked if they have any questions, they are forced to respond "No, I believe you've answered all my questions." To avoid this, prepare five or six questions. Although you need to prepare your questions in advance, don't read them off a piece of paper. Be careful not to ask a question that has already been answered. Doing so will prompt the interviewer to question your listening skills.

Even if a previous interviewer has answered all of your questions, there's no reason why you can't ask a different interviewer the same set of questions. It's better to repeat the same questions than to say, "I believe my questions were all answered by the other interviewer."

Did you know ...

In his article offering advice to dermatology applicants, Heymann encourages applicants to "ask questions that are stimulating and try to learn as much about us as we are trying to find out about you. There is a tremendous difference between the applicant who takes the time and effort to learn about our program and faculty's expertise compared with the person who only applies to be near his girlfriend in Philadelphia" (Heymann).

Did you know ...

Dr. Fitzgibbons, associate program director of the internal medicine residency program at Lehigh Valley Hospital, encourages applicants to "ask unique questions. Something that will make the interviewer remember you" (Kohli).

Rule # 164 The questions that you ask an interviewer send a message. Don't ask the wrong questions.

Don't ask questions to which you should already know the answers. If the answer is readily found in the program's brochure, the interviewers will assume that you didn't bother to read the brochure, and that you're clearly not all that interested in the program. Therefore, the first rule of asking the right questions is to research the program before you arrive. Read the brochure. Read the program information that is sent before the interview. Study the program's website. Read the profiles of the faculty members.

Also avoid asking faculty about issues pertaining to vacation, call schedule, salary, insurance, or benefits. The image you wish to portray is that of an individual who is hard working, even in the face of long, stressful hours. That's hard to do when you're focused on how much you'll be paid and how much time off you're going to get. This information should be available in the residency program information sent to you. If not, save these questions for the house staff.

There are other types of questions that may be perceived in a negative fashion:

- Don't get so personal that you make an interviewer uncomfortable. "Are you married?" "How many children do you have?"
- Do not reveal your biases. "Will I be working with a lot of HIV patients?"
- Do not exhibit a poor sense of taste or strange sense of humor.

- Don't ask questions that make you appear too aggressive. Be especially carefully with "why" questions. "Why doesn't the hospital have a liver transplant program?"

Tip # 114

Don't ask faculty about vacation, call schedule, salary, insurance, or benefits.

Did you know ...

On July 1, 2003, the Accreditation Council for Graduate Medical Education (ACGME) implemented common standards for resident work hours. The goals were to improve patient safety and resident well-being while maintaining the educational quality of the residency experience. Applicants are understandably interested in a program's compliance with work hour guidelines. However, you must realize that this is a sensitive area. In a 2004 survey of obstetric/gynecology residency program directors, many felt that the changes have negatively impacted resident education, the acquisition of key skills during residency, and work ethic (Nuthalapaty). In a survey of otolaryngology residency program directors, most program directors were opposed to work hour restrictions, with only 23.9% being in favor (Brunworth).

Your goal is to ask intelligent, thoughtful, and specific questions. Too often, applicants ask general questions that could be asked of any program. In phrasing your question, consider making a reference to the program's website, informational material, or a point that was raised earlier in the interview day (see example in Chapter 13: Interview Questions). When using this approach, though, don't go overboard. In some cases, it is clear that an applicant could care less about the answer, and in flaunting their research they only appear insincere. "I happened to notice that your residents last year published 14 original research articles, 20 case reports, and 10 book chapters."

Finally, ask your questions in an appropriate fashion. If you're not careful with your language usage or your tone of voice, your interviewers may feel that you are grilling, challenging, or confronting them. For example, rather than asking "What are your program's weaknesses?" Wiebe suggests modifying the question to "If you had unlimited resources as a program director, what would you improve in the program?" (Wiebe).

Tip # 115

While you are free to ask interviewers general questions about the program, specific questions that demonstrate that you have researched the program will have more of an impact.

Questions to ask interviewers (faculty)

General
What are the major strengths of the program?
What are the main differences between this program and others in the area?
If you could change one thing about your program, what would it be and why?
What changes in the residency program are likely in the next few years?
What qualities are you looking for in a residency applicant?

Education
How does your program demonstrate its commitment to the residents' education?
What percentage of attending or teaching rounds is spent at the bedside?
Is attendance at a national conference encouraged? Does the program offer any funding?
What resources are available to assist residents in the fellowship application process?
What resources are available to assist residents in locating an academic position following residency?
How does the program assist residents seeking private practice positions in the local area?
Is there flexibility to do rotations at other institutions?

Clinical duties/responsibilities
How autonomous would you say the residents are in the program?

Research opportunities
What research opportunities are available for residents?
Is protected time available for research during residency?
What type of research have the residents done in recent years?
What research projects are currently ongoing?

Teaching opportunities/responsibilities
What teaching responsibilities do residents have in regard to medical students?
Are there resources for improving resident teaching, such as workshops?

Advising/mentoring
Is there a formal advising/mentoring program for new residents? If so, how does this program work?
How often are advisors and advisees expected to meet?

Specialty board examination
How have your graduates performed on the specialty board exam?
Is there a didactic series to help residents prepare for the boards?

Graduates
Where are your graduates (private practice, academics, local area, etc.)?

What percentage of your graduates successfully place in fellowships? Which fellowships do they get into? Where?

What percentage pursues private practice? Where?

You will not have unlimited time to ask questions. Therefore, you must use your judgment to decide when to ask your last question. Keep track of the time and pay close attention to your interviewer's body language. If you sense that your time is up, proceed to your closing statement.

Rule # 165 You need to make a good first impression. You also need to leave the interviewer with a good final lasting impression.

Earlier we discussed the importance of making a good first impression. You also need to leave the interviewer with a good final lasting impression. You can do so by telling the interviewer you were glad to meet her. Thank her for this opportunity to meet, and for considering you for one of their positions. Leave with a smile, direct eye contact, and a firm handshake if the interviewer extends her hand to you.

Some applicants go a step further by expressing interest in the program:

> "Thank you very much for taking the time to interview me. I've really enjoyed my visit and have been quite impressed with your program. I would be very excited to be a resident here. Is there any other information I can provide for you?"

Tip # 116
Practice your closing statement so that you can deliver it smoothly.

Tip # 117
Although you will have feelings about how the interview went, do not reveal these emotions to your interviewer. We have seen candidates unfortunately end interviews with sighs of relief or disappointment. End your interview in a confident manner.

Rule # 166 Meet with the house staff on your interview day.

Some of the most valuable and forthright information about a residency program will come from the interns and residents currently in training. They will usually be honest about their experience and are usually willing to answer any questions.

As we've mentioned, certain types of questions are best asked of residents. Questions regarding call schedule, salary, vacation, and moonlighting are examples. However, even when speaking to residents, be very careful about what you ask, how you ask, and when you ask. Program directors frequently ask the current residents for their impressions of the candidates. Your interactions with the residents are all up for later discussion. Meeting a resident for the first time, and then immediately jumping in with questions about benefits or salary, could lead one to wonder about your priorities and values. Save these questions for later in the discussion.

Since questions about programs often arise after the interview day, ask several residents for their e-mail address. Follow up later if necessary.

Questions to ask house officers

General
What are the major strengths of the program?
What are the major weaknesses of the program?
Do you feel that you have received good training?
Are the residents happy?
Are you happy?
What do residents like the most?
What do residents like the least?
What is an average day like?
What are the main differences between this program and others in the area?
What is the morale of residents? Faculty?
If you could change one thing about your program, what would it be and why?
What changes in the residency program are likely in the next few years?
What has changed since you came to the program?
Is the program responsive to suggestions for change?
Knowing what you now know, would you still train here?

Inpatient clinical duties/responsibilities
What is the patient load like? How does it vary from service to service?
Do you feel the patient load is too much, too few, or just right?
How many residents/interns are present on each service?
What is the call schedule like? What is the experience like?
When you are on call, which patients are you responsible for?
What are your on-call responsibilities?
What rotations are required during the first year of residency?
What rotations are required during the second and third years of residency?
How are the clinics organized? Are attending physicians present?
Do you feel that you have enough faculty supervision on the floors? What about the clinics?
Do you feel that you have enough autonomy?
What kind of attending backup support is available while on call?
What type of ancillary support (phlebotomy, physical therapy, respiratory therapy, social workers/discharge planning) is available at each of the affiliated-hospitals? How is it different on weekends?

How much time do you spend in the operating room?
When in the residency do you begin to operate?
What are the total number and variety of procedures/surgeries per resident?

Outpatient clinical duties/responsibilities

How much time is spent in the clinics? What about subspecialty clinics?
Are residents able to follow patients whom they have discharged from the
    hospital?
What is the teaching like in the clinics?

Patients

What is the nature of the patient population?
Are residents involved in the care of patients followed by private physicians? If so,
    what percentage of my patients will be private? With regards to private patients,
    who writes the patient orders?
Do private physicians take the time to discuss patient-related issues with
    residents?

Resident education

Can you fill me in on the conference schedule (lectures, grand rounds, morbidity
    and mortality, morning report, journal club, board review course)?
How many of the resident conferences are required?
Do you have time to attend conferences?
What is the quality of the conferences?
Who runs these conferences—faculty or residents?
Is there an appropriate balance between service obligations and the educational
    program?
Are there opportunities for research? Is research required?

Medical student teaching

Are there medical students on the team? If so, how many patients do they follow?
What are the expectations for residents as teachers?

Radiology

Does the program offer any formal training in the reading of films, CT scans, etc.?
Is a radiologist available 24 hours a day?
Are there formal radiology rounds every day?
How difficult is it to schedule radiology tests and procedures after the regular work
    day?

Faculty

What is the relationship between residents and faculty?
How responsive and committed to the residents are the faculty?
How much teaching do they do?
How much supervision do you have?
Are there any known upcoming faculty changes?
Is the department stable?
How approachable is the faculty?
Are the program director and faculty open to suggestions about the program?
Is there a particular subspecialty lacking in either quality or quantity?

Residents

What do residents do in their free time?
Is it a collegial environment?
What is the level of camaraderie among the residents?
Have any residents left the program in the past few years? If so, why?

What is the function of the upper level residents on the team?
How well do senior residents relate to their junior colleagues?

Specialty board examination
Do you feel that the program prepares you well for boards?
Do you have enough time to read?

Graduates
Do residents have any difficulty finding jobs in private practice?
Do residents have any difficulty securing fellowship positions?
How does the program support residents who plan to pursue subspecialty training?
How many people get the fellowships they want?
How many people were unable to land a fellowship position last year?
Do any of the residents stay on as faculty?

Employment benefits
What is the starting salary?
What are the basic resident benefits?
Does the program pay for parking? Is it easily available?
Are meals paid for? What about on call?
How late does the cafeteria stay open?
Are coats/scrubs free of charge to the residents? Is there a charge for laundry?
How is the health/life insurance?
Is there a stipend for travel to conferences? If so, how much?
Can you moonlight during residency? If so, what are the rules? What opportunities are available locally?
Is there a resident union or association? Is membership mandatory? Does it cost anything to be a member?
What is the program's family leave policy? Do you have maternity/paternity leave?

Vacation/time off/sick leave
What is the vacation schedule?
Do you have any days off during a rotation?
Is the program in compliance with ACGME work hour guidelines?
Do you ever exceed the maximum work hours?

City
What is it like to live in this city?
Where do most of the residents live? What is the housing situation? What is the cost of housing?
What is the cost of living?
Is the area safe?

During most interview days, applicants typically have an hour or so, perhaps at lunch, to meet with the house staff. This may not be enough time, especially if the ratio of applicants to residents is high. In your interactions with the residents, strive to find answers to the important basic questions:

- Are the residents happy?
- Would I fit in with the current group of house staff?
- Would I be happy as a resident in this program?

> **Did you know ...**
>
> In survey after survey, among the most important factors affecting medical student ranking of programs was the perceived happiness of the current residents.

If you aren't offered an opportunity to meet with the residents, consider this a red flag. It is quite possible that the program is shielding you from their residents because they want to discourage a free exchange of candid information. If the program remains one in which you are seriously interested, be aggressive about contacting the residents at a later date.

> **Tip # 118**
>
> Because there is often insufficient time to spend with residents on the interview day, make it a point to attend all pre-interview dinners. Also, don't be afraid to contact residents to follow up on issues after your interview day.

> **Tip # 119**
>
> Don't just focus on the first year of residency, as many applicants do. Learn and ask questions about each year.

Rule # 167 During your interview visit, meet with faculty or house staff from your own institution.

During your interview visit, try to meet with faculty or house staff who trained at your own medical school. Seek out these individuals. They can be a valuable source of information. Because you share a common bond, they may be forthright with you about the strengths and weaknesses of the residency program you are considering. In addition, they can compare and contrast the program with the residency program you know best, the one at your medical school.

Not sure how to locate these individuals? Start with your student affairs office. Ask to see a list of senior medical students who have graduated over the past three to five years. Make a note of those who are now training at the institutions you will be visiting. Call or e-mail them to schedule a time to talk over the phone. If you can't locate their e-mail address, write to them using the program's address. See if you can meet with them on the interview day.

Tip # 120

While on the interview trail, you'll meet students from a variety of schools. Discussions with these applicants can be informative, especially if they attend schools affiliated with programs to which you've applied.

Rule # 168   Grade the residency program immediately after your visit.

As soon as you have a chance, write down your impressions of the program. What did you like? What didn't you like? Do this as soon as possible while the program is fresh in your mind. Be as specific as possible. After just a few interviews, it will be difficult to keep track of each program's particulars. Before you know it, you will forget what happened and where. Similarities and differences between programs will blur.

Prior to your first interview, make a list of characteristics that are important to you in a residency program. For an example, see the "Residency Program Evaluation Guide" in the publication Strolling Through the Match (available at www.aafp.org). After the interview, grade each program on a scale of 1 to 5 according to each criterion. After your last interview compare the grades, notes, and information from the various programs. This will help you create your rank list for the final decision process.

Tip # 121

As soon as you can, jot down some points discussed during the interview. This will help you personalize your thank-you notes.

Did you know ...

In their article "Impact of the interview in pediatric residency selection," Swanson and colleagues offered some insight into what happens following an interview at their institution (Swanson). At the conclusion of the interview, the interviewer completes a score form. The candidate is given a score from 1 to 6 with a 1 indicating "outstanding: a must have" and a 6 indicating "poor fit." The candidate is presented to the selection committee by the interviewer at a meeting that takes place the day following the interview.

Did you know ...

In a survey of radiology residency program directors, it was learned that 76.5% of programs use residents and fellows as interviewers (Otero). All members of the interviewing body vote in the ranking of candidates in 88.1% of the programs; 6.5% of the programs use panel interviews, and 15 directors stated that the "fit" of the candidates in the program and a "gut feeling" were the most important criteria for deciding admission. The interviewing body is responsible for making the final ranking in 62.9% of the programs, while the program director has the final word in 33.8%.

Rule # 169 Grade yourself after the interview.

Some candidates leave an interview thinking that they "aced it" while others feel like they "blew it." Such impressions are based on opinions that students form from the interviewer's disposition and bearing during the interview. Because interviewers will not usually share their thoughts about your performance, this type of thinking is not productive. In fact, there are many students who match into a residency program despite feeling as if they "blew it" during the interview. There are many examples of the opposite as well—interviewees who were sure that they "aced" the interview but didn't match.

There are many more interviews to come. It is more productive to ask the following questions after every interview:

- Did I make a good first impression?
- Did I answer each question appropriately and effectively? Was my answer concise?
- Were my answers supported by evidence whenever possible?
- Could I have answered some questions better?
- Did any of the questions surprise me? If so, which ones? Why did they surprise me?
- Was I able to establish rapport with the interviewer?
- Did I make a good final impression?
- How can I use this experience to better prepare for my next interview?

Chapter 15

After the Interview

Rule # 170 Communicating with a residency program after the interview is an important aspect of the application process.

Applicants can initiate post-interview communications in several ways. Most communicate with programs by sending letters, handwritten notes, or e-mail. Some candidates will even phone program directors or revisit institutions. There are many reasons that applicants communicate with programs following an interview:

- Common courtesy
- To thank the program
- To help the program remember them
- To demonstrate interest in the program
- To communicate their intent to rank the program highly
- To ask questions that come up after the interview day
- To request a "second look"
- For fear that not communicating will lower their place on the rank list

We review in more detail the three cornerstones of post-interview communication:

1. Plan to thank every program for the opportunity to interview.
2. Plan how to communicate and what to say to the top programs on your rank list.
3. Plan how to respond to programs that initiate contact with you following the interview.

Rule # 171 You should communicate with every program at which you interviewed.

Unless a program specifically makes it known that it does not wish to be contacted, you must at the very least send a thank-you note. Not only is this common courtesy, but at *some* programs post-interview communication may serve as a selection factor, as we more fully describe below.

Note we specified "some" programs. We've talked to some faculty who don't care if they never received any notes from applicants, and in fact find the flood of mail after an interview to be a hassle.

However, the opposite is true for many faculty members. "This applicant didn't even bother to send a thank you note. They must not be interested in our program. If they're not interested in coming here, they wouldn't be a good fit for us."

While some applicants recognize these facts and are diligent about communicating with programs following the interview, not enough applicants do so. In one study, only 39% of applicants sent follow-up communication to every program with whom they interviewed. 55% communicated only with select programs (Anderson).

Rule # 172 Your expressed interest in a program can impact their interest in you.

Is there a chance that your communication with a program following the interview can influence your ranking? Absolutely. Not for every faculty member, and not for every program, but there is a chance that at some programs your expressed interest in the program may influence your ranking.

How would your interest in a program affect their interest in you? Your negative interest can provide a negative influence. For some faculty, the fact that an applicant didn't even bother to send a thank-you note sends the message that they're not interested in a particular program. Programs don't wish to rank applicants who have no interest in the program, because lack of interest can be an indicator of a poor fit.

A positive interest can have a positive influence. An applicant who ranks a program highly is likely to feel that the program would be a good fit for their interests and abilities, which is what a program seeks. An applicant who plans to rank a program highly would be thrilled to match there, and that hopefully translates to an enthusiastic, hard-working resident. It is also a point of pride for many programs to match those applicants at the top of their own rank list. In a study examining communication between programs and applicants, the authors wrote that "some program directors appear to construct their match lists with the goal of 'matching well' i.e., not having to go too far down their lists. To achieve this, knowing where applicants plan to rank them is a high priority" (Miller).

However, programs do differ widely in their beliefs on the value of post-interview communication. For some programs, what you say following the interview will have no effect whatsoever on the program's decision-making process. In a study of general surgery program directors, the authors found that they "were very skeptical of student ranking assurances, and were seldom influenced by such information" (Anderson). In another study looking at recruitment behavior, the authors wrote that "program directors were very skeptical of student ranking assurances" (Carek).

However, the authors did feel that such assurances had an effect on ranking decisions at some programs. They felt that the impact of the rank order list was "limited to one third of programs" (Carek). Such information is clearly important to some programs.

Surveys of applicants support this belief. When Miller and colleagues surveyed graduating students at ten U.S. medical schools with respect to post-interview communication from programs to applicants, they found that 23% were asked how they planned to rank the program, and 21.7% were told that their level of interest would have bearing on their ranking (Miller).

Surveys of program directors support this belief as well. In one study, emergency medicine residency program directors were asked to rate the importance of 20 items in the resident selection process. An applicant's expressed interest in the program was found to be a moderately important selection factor, although the standard deviation was noticeably high. In this study, it ranked of higher importance than the USMLE Step 1 score. The large standard deviation, however, indicates that there were significant differences in how program directors viewed this factor (Crane). Other surveys indicate that programs commonly tell applicants to keep in touch if they have an interest in matching with their program, as outlined below.

Post-interview communication: does it help?	
Study	**What was found**
Survey of emergency medicine residency program directors (Crane)	Respondents were asked to rate the importance of 20 items in the resident selection process on a scale of 1 to 5, with five being most important. An applicant's expressed interest in the program was found to be a moderately important selection factor with a mean score of 3.30 and a standard deviation of 1.19. Of note, it was ranked of higher importance than the USMLE Step 1 score and nearly as high as the USMLE Step 2 score. The authors commented on the large standard deviation, emphasizing considerable differences between programs in the way they viewed post-interview communication.
Survey of fourth-year students at three medical schools (Anderson)	Following the interview 57% were told by programs to keep in touch if they had an interest in matching there; 21.4% of program directors said that confirmatory rank-order statements from applicants had some positive effect; 2% of directors stated that such statements had a significant positive effect.
Survey of family practice program directors (Carek)	82% of programs told at least some of their applicants to keep in touch if they had an interest in matching with their program.
Survey of urology residency program directors (Teichman)	67% of programs told applicants to keep in touch if they had an interest in matching in their program.

Rule # 173 The top programs on your rank list should be informed of this fact.

As detailed previously, your expressed interest in a program can, in some situations, impact their interest in you. Therefore, we recommend that you inform the top programs on your rank list of this fact. However, this can be a difficult area in which to proceed. *You must never lie*. We can't state it any more clearly than that. However, if you are certain that a program is your number one choice, and you rank that program number one on your rank list, you may legally and ethically let them know that fact. There is no NRMP rule against stating your interest in a program. The NRMP states that "the Match Participation Agreement does not prohibit either an applicant or a program from volunteering how one plans to rank the other" (www.nrmp.org). What is prohibited is asking for that information.

While such ranking statements are not binding, we all know of applicants who have made such statements, only to be proven as liars after the match results are available. Medicine can be a surprisingly small world, and your reputation is one of your most important assets. There are too many opportunities to lose your moral compass during the residency application process. Maintain the highest ethical and moral standards now and throughout your career, and your reputation will reflect that fact. Proven a liar now, and that reputation will follow you.

There is a potential negative in informing the top programs on your rank list of that fact. The world of program directors can be a small one, and there is a small chance that your strong interest in a particular program may be conveyed to another program.

A more important consideration is that you may not be able to inform the top programs on your rank list, because you may not have identified those programs. One small study of 21 anesthesiology residents found that 76% made their final ranking choices within a week prior to the final submission date (Lewis). There is no point in informing programs at that late date, because most have submitted their own rank lists by that point. In order to take advantage of this rule, you would have to confirm your choices earlier in the process.

Tip # 122

If you have any reason to believe that you won't be ranked high enough to match at one of your top programs, there are concrete steps that you can take following the interview that may improve your chances. First, communicate with the program following the interview to remind them of your interest in and enthusiasm for the program. Second, consider updating your file with new course/clerkship grades, USMLE Step 2 CK score, an additional letter of recommendation, or a recently received award (e.g., election to AOA). Third, consider a "second look" visit to programs. Finally, talk to one of your letter writers to see if she might call the program to rave about you. If you have a compelling reason to match at a certain program, you can let the program know that as well.

Rule # 174 The thank-you letter serves as another chance to emphasize your overall message, so don't send a generic one. Send a compelling and memorable thank you.

The most effective thank you letters contain the following information:

- Statement of appreciation for the opportunity to interview, and for the interviewer's time
- Statement indicating that you enjoyed meeting the interviewer
- Expression of appreciation for information shared with you
- Expression of interest/enthusiasm for the position
- Brief statement why you are a good fit for the program (i.e., highlighting your ability to make a contribution to the program)
- Reference to a point raised or topic discussed during the interview (i.e., personalizing the note)
- Intent to rank program highly (optional, as this must be truthful)
- Final statement of thanks

It is particularly important to emphasize how your qualities, skills, or strengths match the program's needs. What did you learn about the program that can help you explain more effectively why you are a good fit for the program? Few applicants take this additional step. Those that do so distinguish themselves from other candidates. The sample thank you letter we've included in this chapter demonstrates how to emphasize your fit with a program.

Tip # 123

If the interviewer raised a concern about your application and you feel that you did not address it to the best of your ability, you may consider addressing it further in the thank you letter.

Rule # 175 Thank you letters may be sent in the form of a handwritten note, a typed letter, or an e-mail.

All forms of thank you correspondence are acceptable. While individual faculty members may have their own preference, it would be impossible for you to know that preference. The handwritten note implies a great deal of time and care in its production, and immediately sends a more personal message. However, the production of multiple handwritten notes is difficult, especially if you follow the norms of sending one to every single interviewer, and include sufficient information to personalize the note. While the typed letter can easily be expanded to include more information, it can give an impression of mass production, and therefore may not be as memorable. However, you can include sufficient detail to create a memorable letter and overcome this negative. The e-mail thank you may be seen as too informal and suggestive of a shortcut, particularly for more traditional faculty, but has the benefit of speed.

Our suggestion is to immediately send an e-mail thank you letter to every interviewer, preferably within one day. This should be followed by either a typed letter or handwritten note. Either type should include specific details that refer back to the interview, and should include specific information that substantiates your fit for the program.

Note that these are not necessarily the norms of post-interview correspondence. Hardly any students send immediate thank you e-mails, and few of the thank you letters we receive include the type of specific details that we suggest. Therefore, your utilization of these suggestions will aid in your goal of creating a memorable impression.

Rule # 176 As a general rule, thank you letters should follow the norms of a business letter.

A typewritten thank you letter that is to be mailed should follow the proper format. It should be considered a form of business correspondence and should follow the norms of a business letter. It should convey a professional message, and should be sent on professional stationery.

Proper format of the typewritten thank-you letter

Return address (your full name and address)

Date

Inside address (full name, including title/position, of interviewer and address)

Salutation ("Dear Dr. Smith:")

Body of letter

Closing ("Sincerely," or "Yours truly,")

Signature line (your signature above your typewritten full name)

AAMC ID #

Note that the above format is for typewritten letters that will be mailed. If you are planning on sending your letter by e-mail, the format will differ to some extent. Your e-mail message will begin with the salutation. You will then proceed to word the letter in the same way. Below your signature line, you should include your AAMC ID # so that your correspondence makes its way to your file. Before sending the e-mail, double check your subject line to make sure it is clear and concise. A subject line with "Thank you—residency interview" will ensure that your e-mail is not ignored or deleted as junk.

Rule # 177   A thank you letter should be personalized.

Some applicants send a thank you letter to each interviewer, but fail to personalize their letters. A thank you letter that is tailored to the individual faculty member is more effective and more memorable. If every applicant sends a generic thank you letter, the impact of your generic letter can easily be lost. Unfortunately, after reading the fifth "Thank you for the opportunity to interview at Baylor. The strength of your faculty and the diversity of clinical experience were very impressive. I would be honored to train at such a program," the letters tend to blur into one. Use the thank you letter to further emphasize your message, and use it to help your interviewer remember you as an individual, not as one of many candidates. This can easily be done by mentioning items that were discussed in the interview. "I enjoyed hearing about your favorite restaurants in Chicago." This should be followed by a reminder of why you as a candidate are a perfect fit for the program, as we demonstrate later in this chapter.

Rule # 178   Send a thank you letter to each individual with whom you interviewed.

To whom should you send a thank you letter? Our recommendation is to send a letter to each individual with whom you interviewed. Many applicants choose to send a letter only to the program director. These applicants fail to realize that the residency selection process varies markedly from program to program. While the program director may make ranking decisions at one program, at another ranking decisions may be made by all residency selection committee members. For example, at the general surgery residency program at the Medical

University of South Carolina, Brothers wrote that "... all surgical faculty are given equal input, with individual members providing insight into applicants whom they interviewed" (Brothers). Therefore, you should send a letter to each interviewer. We also recommend sending a letter to the program coordinator who has worked diligently and tirelessly to make sure your interview visit goes smoothly. They often don't get the credit they deserve.

Rule # 179 Send notes early.

Post-interview communication should be sent early. By early, we mean sending a thank you e-mail or delivering a thank-you letter within hours after your interview. Why? To be most effective, your thank you message should reach your interviewer before she completes her interview evaluation form or meets with the residency selection committee to discuss your candidacy. Therefore, time is of the essence. At some programs, interviewers are even asked to complete their evaluation form at the end of the interview day.

In our years of experience, a few applicants have sent an e-mail within hours of an interview. A few have prepared notes or letters that are delivered to the clinic mailboxes the same day. However, the more common scenario is to receive an e-mail a few days later. For postal mail, the thank you letter may take many days to arrive. In the university or hospital setting, there are often additional delays as mail is routed within the institution. As we mentioned, if you choose to send an immediate e-mail thank you, we recommend that you follow it with a more traditional, formal form of correspondence.

Rule # 180 A poorly written thank you can damage your candidacy.

Not bothering to send a thank you note can affect your chances of matching at a particular program. However, sending a poorly written note can prove more damaging. Avoid the following indicators of a poorly written thank you letter.

● **Poor readability**

It is acceptable to send handwritten letters, but only if your handwriting is legible. If your penmanship leaves a lot to be desired, send a typewritten letter instead.

● **Informal**

Your letter should be written in a formal manner, even if it is sent by e-mail. Throughout your letter, your goal is to maintain the image of a professional and polished individual. Avoid "cutesy" stationery. Avoid the use of informal language, smiley faces and other emoticons, as well as internet lingo such as lol.

- **Misspelled words/poor grammar/improper punctuation**

  Your letter must be flawless. This means that it cannot contain any misspelled words, grammatical errors, or improper punctuation. Failure to correct these errors suggests a lack of attention to detail on your part and will significantly detract from your candidacy.

- **Making manual corrections to the letter**

  If you catch a mistake, don't make manual corrections to your typewritten letter. This may seem obvious, but we have received such letters.

- **Bragging or overassertive**

  While you must feel comfortable writing about your strengths, take care with the words you use and the tone in which you write. You never want to appear as if you are bragging or over-assertive.

- **Focusing entirely on yourself**

  Too often, thank you letters focus entirely on what the program can do for the applicant, rather than what the applicant can do for the program. Think about how you can make valuable contributions to the program and include specifics in your letter.

- **Too much information**

  To be effective, your thank you letter must be concise. Often, applicants write and write, cramming as much information as they can into the letter. Faculty members don't have the time to read through such letters.

Sample Thank you letter
456 Stuyvesant Circle
Le Blanc, Wisconsin 60322
December 16, 2008

Dr. Josephine Brooks
Assistant Professor of Pediatrics
Department of Pediatrics
General Hospital
456 Huron Drive
Muskegon, MI 43567

Dear Dr. Brooks:

Thank you for the opportunity to interview for a position in the pediatrics residency program at General Hospital. I really enjoyed our conversation and appreciated the time you spent getting to know me.

I particularly enjoyed our discussion of how personal digital assistants can improve the quality of care we deliver to our patients. As a medical student, I had the opportunity to contribute to a PDA drug database. During residency training, I plan to continue my work in developing user-friendly PDA resources for clinicians. I know that there are faculty members at General Hospital who are involved in this area, and I would welcome the opportunity to work with them.

I was thoroughly impressed with all aspects of your pediatrics residency program, and I would be thrilled to be one of your residents. I plan to rank your program at the top of my rank order list.

Thank you again for the opportunity to meet with you and I hope that we have the chance to work together in the future. If you have any additional questions, please contact me.

Yours truly,

Candace Liu
AAMC ID 22222

Rule # 181   Plan what you'll do and say when you are contacted by a program following the interview.

Post-interview communication from programs to applicants occurs much more often than applicants would suspect. Not only is it a common practice, but it can be a stressful one for applicants. Programs may contact you via e-mail, postal mail, or phone. The chairman, program director, or faculty member may send a simple e-mail stating how much they enjoyed meeting you during the interview. They may ask you to keep in touch if you are interested in their program. They may go further and make informal commitments to you. They may even ask how you plan to rank their program. They may even ask which program will be first on your rank list. Every applicant must plan well ahead of time how to handle these situations.

Did you know ...

In a survey of graduating students at ten U.S. medical schools, the following was found with respect to post-interview communication from programs to applicants (Miller):

41.7% of applicants received guarantees of the program's intent to rank them highly
23% were asked how they planned to rank the program
21.7% were told that their level of interest would have bearing on their ranking
17% were asked which program would be first on their rank list

As a result of this communication, many applicants felt pressured to offer assurances to programs. Nearly 30% of respondents felt either very or moderately pressured. Communication by phone posed the most pressure.

Your strategy to handle these situations must be established well before you need it. A phone call from a program director calling to say how highly the program feels about your potential as a resident is a highly stressful situation, and is not the ideal time to be formulating a response. Your response must be one that does not jeopardize your chances of matching into the program, and must be one that in no way compromises your ethics.

The easiest response is when you know the program will be first on your rank list. There is no legal or ethical injunction against volunteering that the program will be first on your rank list. If the program won't be first on your list, or you're not sure, you can still honestly convey your interest in the program and admiration for it.

As we've emphasized throughout the book, always include specifics. When you're speaking to a program director, these specifics add credibility and emphasize that you're interested enough in the program to have done your research. The use of specifics also emphasizes that the program made a significant impression. You should have already created summary sheets for each of the programs at which you interviewed. These sheets, listing the strengths and weaknesses of each program, should be kept easily accessible. In the event of an e-mail or phone call, you'll be able to honestly convey your impressions of the program.

> "It would be a privilege to train at your program, especially because of my interest in … and the opportunities in…provided by Pickens University."

> "I haven't finished interviewing yet, but I was very impressed by the program at Dow University. I'm most interested in obtaining strong clinical training, and the quality of the faculty, the subspecialty interests, and the strong didactic program all support that."

> "I'm so honored that you took the time to contact me and am excited about the opportunity to train at Berkshire University. The …. of the program, the … of the faculty, and the …are all reasons that I was so impressed with the residency training."

Tip # 124

Be prepared for a phone call, e-mail, or letter from a program informing you of their intent to rank you highly. Are you prepared to handle such a situation? Have your strategy in place before this occurs.

Did you know …

In a survey of students graduating from three medical schools, 13% of applicants were contacted by one or more programs, stating their intent to rank them number one (Anderson).

Rule # 182 Don't lie.

"Although truthfulness and honesty have long been considered fundamental values within the medical profession, lying and deception have become standard practices within medicine's residency selection process" (Young).

These were the words of Tara Young in her article, "Teaching medical students to lie." She also wrote that candidates must "lead their interviewers to believe that they are interested in the program they are being interviewed for, even if they have no intention of ranking it anywhere near the top of their list of choices." Although written after her experiences with the residency selection process in Canada, her discussion of the potential negative effects of the process is pertinent to both the NRMP and San Francisco matches.

We've touched upon this subject elsewhere, and yet feel compelled to review this rule in more depth. Lying and unethical practices are rampant in the residency application and residency selection process. These practices are shockingly common, as the literature demonstrates. In one survey of graduating medical students, 12.4% of respondents reported making misleading statements or assurances to programs (Miller). Recognize that these were the students who actually admitted to such a practice. A review of residency program directors suggests that the numbers may be much higher. A survey of emergency medicine residency program directors found that 42% frequently felt that applicants had lied to them, while another 42% sometimes felt lied to by applicants (Wolford).

Many applicants believe that they must be dishonest with programs to avoid an unfavorable match outcome. They fear that being completely honest about their level of interest will harm their candidacy at programs. While some applicants report feeling uncomfortable, most would describe it as just playing along with "the game." Consider the results of the following studies:

- In a survey of urology residency program directors following the 1999 match, 20% of program directors reported receiving informal commitments from applicants (Teichman). However, over 50% of these commitments failed to result in actual matches.

- In a survey of general surgery residency program directors following the 1998 match, nearly 40% felt that they had received informal commitments from applicants (Anderson). However, half of these commitments failed to lead to actual matches.

- In a survey of family practice residency program directors after the 1999 match, about half felt that they had received informal commitments from applicants (Carek). However, two thirds of these commitments did not lead to actual matches.

- In a survey of emergency medicine residency program directors, 42% reported receiving informal commitments by applicants (Wolford). Forty-two percent frequently felt lied to by applicants. Another 42% sometimes felt lied to by applicants.

- In a survey of graduating medical students from ten U.S. medical schools, 12.4% of respondents reported making misleading statements or assurances to programs (Miller).

Such unethical practices are not limited to applicants. In Rule #188, we describe how program directors may also make misleading statements or assurances to applicants. The bottom line is this:

you must proactively plan how to navigate the complex application process, while being completely honest and without ever compromising your ethics.

Did you know ...

Dr. Ziegelstein, associate director of the internal medicine residency program at Johns Hopkins Bayview Medical Center, wrote that you should not "tell a program director that you are ranking that program # 1 on your list if it is not true. The statement is not binding, but you do not want someone to develop bad feelings about you that could count against you later. Most physicians have good memories or they would not have passed anatomy" (Ziegelstein).

Rule # 183 You do have the option of visiting a program again.

After completing your interviews, you will review in detail the information that you have gathered. You will use this information to create your rank list. As you may suspect, this is not an easy process. You will be spending three or more years at the program where you match, and it can be difficult to make such an important decision based on a few hours spent at a program.

Although it isn't usually necessary, you do have the option of visiting a residency program after your interview. You would simply call the program and ask if you can arrange for another visit, known as a "second look." Some programs are receptive to such requests, and in fact may view your request as a sign of your interest in their program. Second look visits are not routine and should be used only when you truly feel the need to obtain more information about a program. Some students may view the second look as a technique to strengthen their application, but when used for this reason the visit just typically reinforces their insincerity.

Before your repeat visit, review all program information. Since the reason for your visit is to collect more information about the program, start by formulating new questions to ask. During this second visit, you may be able to spend a full day observing a resident as she fulfills her responsibilities. You should take note of the interactions between faculty and residents, evaluate the hospital and program resources, participate in the didactic sessions, and ask your additional questions. You may gain valuable insight about the program, information that can help you assess whether the program is a good fit for you. An experience such as this can often put to rest any lingering doubts you may have about the program.

Your visit will essentially be an extended interview. While you are more fully evaluating the program, the program is evaluating you as well. If you perform well, this second visit may have the potential to improve your chances of matching with the program.

Tip # 125
Some programs are receptive to applicants who wish to take a "second look" at their program. Some programs, however, do not recommend it, making it clear to applicants that second look opportunities are not available. Other programs may not be so explicit. Try to gain some insight into how a program views a "second look" on your interview day. Avoid making such a request to any program that you feel might view it is an inconvenience. Dr. Amorosa of the radiology department at UMDNJ/Robert Wood Johnson Medical School states that "a second look should be a sincere effort to clarify a specific aspect of the residency, not just one more hurdle the student thinks he needs to jump over to get higher on the match list."

Tip # 126
If you are unable to arrange a "second look" visit, you can still call or e-mail the program with questions. In fact, follow-up questions may demonstrate your continued interest in and enthusiasm for the program.

Chapter 16

Ranking Residency Programs

The last step in the residency application process is the creation and submission of your rank order list. On the official rank list, you list those programs, in order of preference, which you would be willing to attend. Programs also submit their own rank lists, in the order in which they would extend offers. Sometime in February, the Match takes place. A computer matches each applicant to the highest ranking program on the applicant's list which has offered him a position. The results are announced throughout the country in mid-March on "Match Day."

For many, Match Day is the happy culmination of a very long, hard application process. Other applicants experience bitter disappointment. There are a whole host of reasons as to why match results may not be favorable. However, we've seen some students who do everything right, only to make crucial errors when it comes time to create and submit their rank list. Errors at this final step in the process can undo all of your previous efforts.

Rule # 184 Always rank according to your own criteria.

After the interview season ends, the process of finalizing your rank list begins in earnest. The rank list is a list of the residency programs at which you interviewed, placed in your order of preference. This involves sorting through a great deal of data. Some students are tempted to rank based on reputation alone. "I'd like to attend the most prestigious program I can get into." Ranking programs is rarely that simple. You will be spending a minimum of three years of your life at this program, and you need to take into account a whole host of other factors. A useful checklist for evaluating residency programs can be found in Strolling Through the Match, a publication produced by the American Academy of Family Physicians. It is accessible free to applicants at www.aafp.org. Consider also the following questions:

- Will the residency program provide me with strong clinical training?
- Will that training be broad-based, with exposure to all facets of the field?
- Will it provide some subspecialty training in my areas of interest?

- Will it provide training in additional areas important to me, such as research training?
- How did I feel when I visited the program?
- Would I be able to work with the people there?
- Could I live and work in this city for the next several years?
- What are the strengths and weaknesses of the program relative to the others?
- Does the program offer an environment that will allow me to reach my full potential?

Tip # 127

Don't ignore your gut feeling about a program. A program may look outstanding on paper, but if your visit left you feeling that you would be miserable there, consider that an important data point. While objective information is obviously important in the ranking process, emotions can, and should, play an important role.

Rule # 185 Never rank a program that you wouldn't want to attend.

If you have serious doubts about a program, *do not* put that program on your rank list. If you place it on the rank list and you match, you are bound to accept it. In fact, in registering for the Match, the NRMP has applicants affix their passwords to the Match Participation Agreement. This agreement states that a "match between an applicant and a program creates a binding commitment to accept or offer a position. A decision not to honor that commitment is a breach of the Agreement and will be investigated by the NRMP ..." (www.nrmp.org)

While applicants can be granted a waiver from their Match commitment, only the NRMP can grant this waiver. Programs are not allowed to grant waivers and must report all waiver requests to the NRMP. If the NRMP denies the waiver request, you will be expected to honor your commitment to the program. Failure to accept the position may lead the NRMP to prohibit you from gaining entrance into another NRMP-participating program for a period of one year following the decision.

While the NRMP has approved some waiver requests, others have been denied. Overall, it would be better to not match at all than to match at a program you have no desire to attend. In the event that you don't match, you still have additional opportunities to strengthen your application and apply again.

Tip # 128

Think long and hard before you rank any program where you feel you would be unhappy. You may ultimately match there.

Rule # 186 Rank every single program that you would consider attending.

You should place every program you would consider attending on your rank list. Submitting a longer list will not affect your chances of matching with those programs that are higher on your rank list. This is clearly explained in the information the NRMP provides to applicants regarding the Match.

Some students, for various and often misguided reasons, do not wish to rank every program that they would consider attending. Before you leave any programs off your list, factor in the following:

- Competitiveness of the specialty
- Your qualifications
- Competition for the specific programs being ranked

We do encounter students who create too short of a rank list because they feel confident of matching into one of their top choices. These students are devastated when they don't match at all. Don't let overconfidence ruin your chances.

Did you know ...

Per the words of the San Francisco Matching Program:

"Pay attention to the bottom of your list! Each year some applicants tell us that they omitted a lower choice because they overestimated their chances elsewhere. They ended up unmatched because the omitted program turned out to be their only offer. The only reason not to list a program is that you would rather remain unmatched to explore other options after the match" (www.sfmatch.org).

This is echoed by the American Urological Association:

"Maximize your chances! Previous years' matches have demonstrated the need for applicants to include on their preference lists all of the programs they would be willing to attend. Some applicants who were not matched at all received offers from programs they did not list. If the applicants had listed all programs preferable, some of these 'misses' might have been avoided" (www.auanet.org/residents/resmatch.cfm).

Rule # 187 Don't wait until the last minute to certify your rank order list.

Candidates are allowed to modify their rank order lists as often as necessary until the posted deadline, which is usually in the middle of

February. Before the deadline, you must certify your list; otherwise, the NRMP will not receive it.

The following advice is offered by the NRMP:

"Participants are advised not to wait until the last minute to enter their Rank Order Lists so as to avoid any problems at the deadline.

"If you make a change to your Rank Order List by moving or deleting a program, the change is saved and the previous rankings are deleted, and your old Rank Order List is NOT certified if previously certified. You must then certify your ROL again for it to be used in the match" (www.nrmp.org).

Tip # 129

You are free to modify your list as often as necessary. However, several days before the posted deadline, you must certify your list. The NRMP will not act on your list until you certify it.

Rule # 188 **You cannot believe everything that you hear. Not only are misunderstandings common, but some programs do engage in questionable ethical practices.**

Although the first match was run in 1952, it did not become known as the National Resident Matching Program (NRMP) until 1978. The system was designed to allow students and applicants to confidentially rank one another and make selection decisions without pressure.

However, every year both parties try to influence selection decisions in their favor. While the NRMP expects that all match participants will conduct themselves in an above-board and ethical manner, in reality this may be compromised.

Programs may engage in questionable ethical practices, and this may be more common than one would think. Misunderstandings are also common. These practices include the following:

- Making informal commitments

  In a survey of fourth-year students at three schools, 43% felt that they had received informal commitments from at least one program (Anderson). A similar result was found in a survey of urology residency applicants (Teichman). In this study, 40% of applicants felt that they had received informal commitments.

- Dishonesty with applicants

  A survey of urology residency applicants found that over 50% of the informal commitments failed to result in an actual match. In this same survey, only about half of the program directors felt uncomfortable being dishonest with applicants. Another study surveyed family practice residency program directors and learned that 94% felt pressured to be dishonest with applicants in an attempt to recruit coveted applicants (Carek). In the previously cited survey of graduating fourth year medical students, 33% of students felt that programs had lied to them at some point during the Match process (Anderson).

- Asking applicants how they planned to rank the program

Clearly, programs want to match well. In an effort to do so, some programs may act in an unethical manner. Misunderstandings are also common. Recognize that this may occur, and recognize as well that you cannot believe everything that you hear.

Did you know ...

In their Statement on Professionalism, the NRMP states that "although the Match Participation Agreement does not prohibit either an applicant or a program from volunteering how one plans to rank the other, it is a violation of the Match Participation Agreement to request such information" (www.nrmp.org).

Tip # 130

You stand the best chance of matching into the residency program that you want if you rank it as your top choice. Do not create your rank list based upon where you think you will be accepted.

Rule # 189 You cannot naively believe comments made by program directors.

After interviewing at a program, you may receive a follow-up e-mail, letter or telephone call from the program director stating that the program plans on ranking you at the top of their list. You may be thrilled to hear such great news. Beware. Such a statement made by a program in no way serves as a guarantee that they will rank you highly. You cannot allow comments such as these to affect the order of your rank list.

Surveys have shown that students for the most part are skeptical about any assurances made by programs regarding their place on the program's rank list. They generally report that these assurances, including informal commitments, have little effect on their rank order list.

However, some applicants are in fact influenced by these types of statements. They may let a program's expression of interest change the way in which they rank programs on their list. They may even create too short of a rank list believing that they are an "in" or a "lock" at a certain program because they were told so. These students have been devastated when they learn they didn't match into any residency program.

At the NRMP website, it is clearly stated that applicants should not rely on statements made by programs when creating their rank order lists. As thrilling as it may be to hear "Our program plans to rank you high on our list," this isn't binding in any way. We know of multiple cases in which students have been given such assurances, only to subsequently not match at those programs.

Did you know ...

In their Statement on Professionalism, the NRMP writes that each year it is "contacted by applicants who believe that an error has occurred in the Match because they did not match to programs whose directors had promised them positions (i.e., had promised to rank them high enough to ensure a match.) In every case, the NRMP has determined that the applicant did not match to the desired program because, contrary to the applicant's expectation, the program did not rank the applicant high enough on the program's rank order list for the applicant to match there" (www.nrmp.org).

Tip # 131

While some programs will remain in contact with all applicants, some will only communicate with selected applicants. Other programs have a policy not to communicate whatsoever with any applicant. Don't let the lack of communication alter the position of the program on your rank list.

Rule # 190 Know what constitutes a match violation.

Applicants often seek an understanding of the Match policy, including what might constitute a violation, from their peers. This practice often leads to misinformation. In one study, nearly half of students perceived a violation that did not meet the NRMP definition for a violation (Phillips).

Myth or fact?

1) Programs that tell you where they're ranking you on their list are in violation of the NRMP guidelines.

   Myth. Programs and applicants can volunteer how they plan to rank one another. However, the NRMP prohibits either party from asking one another of their plans.

2) It is against the rules for a program director who participates in the NRMP Main Match to offer a contract to a U.S. allopathic medical student senior before Match Day.

   Fact.

3) Programs are prohibited from asking applicants if they are applying to another specialty.

   Myth. Programs are free to ask you if you are interviewing in more than one specialty.

4) It is permissible for a program director to ask me where else I am applying.

   Fact.

5) Programs are not allowed to contact you following the interview.

   Myth. Programs are free to contact applicants following the interview, but they are not allowed to ask applicants how they plan to rank their program.

To gain a solid understanding of the Match policy, attend all orientation and information sessions about the process at your school. Read carefully the rules of the Match, which are often given to students by their schools and are also available at the NRMP website (www.nrmp.org).

Tip # 132
Feel free to turn to your peers for information, but realize that they're not the ideal source of information. Always verify what you hear.

Did you know...

A study found that 12.1% of general surgery program directors felt it was ethically wrong to interview in more than one specialty (Anderson). In the same study 75.4% of directors reported that an applicant's forthright admission to multispecialty interviewing would have a negative effect on the applicant's rank order.

Chapter 17

International Medical Graduates

There are over 900,000 physicians in the United States, a substantial number of which are international medical graduates (IMGs). According to the AMA, 228,665 of these doctors are IMG physicians, representing 25.3% of the total physician population (http://www.ama-assn.org/ama1/pub/upload/mm/18/img-workforce-paper.pdf).

Since most are involved in direct patient care, IMGs have had a vital role in meeting the medical manpower needs of the United States. IMGs have also made valuable contributions to medical education, furthered biomedical and health services research, and held leadership positions in academic medicine. In fact, 17% and 10% of department chairs in the basic sciences and clinical sciences at U.S. medical schools, respectively, are IMGs (Alexander).

The Educational Commission for Foreign Medical Graduates (ECFMG) is responsible for certifying the readiness of IMG physicians for entry into U.S. residency training. As you can see from the following table, the ECFMG has certified hundreds of thousands of IMGs from a number of countries in its 50 plus years of existence.

Top countries by country of origin ECFMG certificates issued, 1958 - 2005					
Citizenship at time of entry to medical school	Issued 1958-2005: No. (%)		Issued 1996-2005: No. (%)		Issued 2001-2005: No. (%)
India	54,292	(18.9)	17,378	(20.8)	8,710	(22.8)
United States	40,051	(13.9)	13,476	(16.1)	7,919	(20.8)
Philippines	19,870	(6.9)	2,519	(3.0)	1,081	(2.8)
Pakistan	13,706	(4.8)	4,930	(5.9)	2,394	(6.3)
United Kingdom	7,534	(2.6)	1,183	(1.4)	467	(1.2)
China	7,072	(2.5)	3,791	(4.5)	1,214	(3.2)
Germany	6,863	(2.4)	1,862	(2.2)	539	(1.4)
USSR	6,171	(2.2)	3,282	(3.9)	1,201	(3.2)
Iran	6,169	(2.2)	1,956	(2.3)	870	(2.3)
Egypt	6,006	(2.1)	1,883	(2.3)	516	(1.4)
Korea	5,955	(2.1)	820	(1.0)	415	(1.1)
Syria	4,292	(1.5)	1,473	(1.8)	677	(1.8)

Top countries by country of origin ECFMG certificates issued, 1958 - 2005						
Nigeria	4,016	(1.4)	1,858	(2.2)	812	(2.1)
Australia	3,819	(1.3)	666	(0.8)	182	(0.5)
Taiwan	3,763	(1.3)	240	(0.3)	55	(0.1)
Lebanon	3,481	(1.2)	1,269	(1.5)	588	(1.5)
Total certificates issued	287,382	(100)	83,476	(100)	38,142	(100)

From Hallock JA, Kostis JB. Celebrating 50 years of experience: an ECFMG perspective. *Acad Med* 2006; 81(12): S7-S16.

Although the sheer number of IMGs receiving ECFMG certification is impressive, these numbers tell you nothing of the difficulties these IMGs have experienced in their efforts to secure a position in a U.S. residency program. While gaining a desired residency position is difficult for U.S. medical students, it is more so for IMGs.

IMGs also have to deal with adapting to a new culture in a foreign land, often without friends or family close by for support. For many IMGs, the lack of understanding of the criteria which programs find important makes the residency application process extremely stressful and difficult. In working with IMGs, we have come to realize that misperceptions abound, with IMGs frequently overestimating or underestimating certain residency application criteria. These misperceptions may result in a failure to match.

In this chapter, our goal is to provide you with evidence-based advice from the literature on resident selection as it pertains to IMGs. In addition, we seek to deliver information from those individuals who are directly involved in the residency selection process—namely program directors and other members of the residency selection committee. What do programs value the most? How important are letters of recommendation? Why do programs prefer applicants with U.S. medical experience? These are among some of the questions we answer in our effort to help you develop an application strategy that will lead to match success.

Rule # 191 Research the competitiveness of your chosen specialty.

Certain specialties are far more competitive than others. Specialties such as ophthalmology, otolaryngology, radiation oncology, dermatology, urology, plastic surgery, and orthopedic surgery are highly competitive. There are many more U.S. applicants who wish to enter these fields than positions available. Consequently, a significant number of U.S. applicants fail to match every year.

As you might expect, IMGs find these specialties the most difficult to enter. For example, 93.1% of available orthopedic surgery residency positions in the 2008 Match were filled by U.S. seniors (www.nrmp.org). Of the 3187 resident physicians in orthopedic surgery, only 73, or 2.3%, were IMGs (Brotherton). Contrast this with family medicine, internal medicine, and psychiatry. In these specialties, IMGs account for over 30% of all resident physicians.

PERCENTAGE OF RESIDENT PHYSICIANS WHO ARE IMGS BY SPECIALTY

	Total number of residents*	Number of IMG residents	Percentage
Anesthesiology	4,970	735	14.8%
Dermatology	1,069	32	3.0%
Emergency medicine	4,379	234	5.3%
Family medicine	9,456	3,708	39.2%
Internal medicine	22,099	9,737	44.1%
Neurological surgery	881	92	10.4%
Neurology	1,507	550	36.5%
Obstetrics and gynecology	4,739	1,004	21.2%
Ophthalmology	1,225	98	8.0%
Orthopedic surgery	3,187	73	2.3%
Otolaryngology	1,292	36	2.8%
Pathology	2,310	690	29.9%
Pediatrics	7,964	1,903	23.9%
Physical medicine and rehabilitation	1167	195	16.7%
Plastic surgery	609	40	6.6%
Psychiatry	4,613	1,411	30.6%
Radiation oncology	556	16	2.9%
Diagnostic radiology	4,368	283	6.5%
General Surgery	7,651	1,462	19.1%
Urology	992	36	3.6%

*Includes resident physicians on duty as of December 1, 2006

From Brotherton SE, Etzel SI. Graduate Medical Education, 2006-2007. *JAMA* 2007; 298 (9): 1081-1096.

While IMG applicants have successfully matched into highly competitive specialties, it requires a well thought out application strategy. Because of the large numbers of IMG applicants matching into less competitive specialties such as internal medicine and family medicine, IMGs often believe that it is easy to match into these fields. Statistics from the 2007 and 2008 Match results shown below debunk this common misconception.

Key statistics from the 2008 Match results...

10,304 IMGs participated in the 2008 Match. 5,565, or 54.9%, failed to match.

7,335 IMG participants were not U.S. citizens. Of this group, 4,227, or 57.6%, failed to match.

2,969 IMG participants were U.S. citizens. Of this group, 1,541, or 41.9%, failed to match.

Key statistics from the 2007 Match results ...

2,342 independent applicants, most of whom were IMGs, failed to match into internal medicine.

1,012 independent applicants, most of whom were IMGs, failed to match into family medicine.

Information from www.nrmp.org.

. As you can see from this data, thousands of IMGs fail to match every year. Failure to match can be distressing. Those who fail to match often report feeling shocked, depressed or embarrassed. "I couldn't believe it," said one applicant. "I've never failed anything before."

Not to be minimized are the financial effects of not matching. The financial cost of the residency application process for IMGs is substantial. IMG applicants incur significant costs every step of the way. Leon and Aranha described these costs in more detail (Leon):

"Economic constraints impede many competitive FMGs from applying because of the prohibitive fees requested, when analyzed in the context of average foreign wages. To begin with, international medical schools charge very high fees to issue all documents necessary to apply, including medical school transcripts...Several educational courses are available to FMGs to prepare for the USMLE tests. These courses often have prohibitive costs...For a 4-month period, some courses charge about U.S. $9000...Testing costs by themselves are equivalent to average annual gross income in many countries."

These costs are just the start. Another area of high expense is that of travel, including travel to the United States and the costs incurred during the interviewing process. In one survey, the median expense per interview was $330 (Kerfoot).

Regardless of your chosen specialty, the key to a successful match hinges on the development of a well thought-out strategy. Such an approach will significantly increase your chances of a successful match.

Rule # 192 Becoming ECFMG certified is key.

To secure a position in an accredited U.S. residency program, IMGs must first be certified by the Educational Commission for Foreign Medical Graduates (ECFMG). The ECFMG, which came into existence in 1956, is responsible for certifying the readiness of IMGs for entry into U.S. residency training.

Did you know ...

ECFMG certification is required before an IMG can take the USMLE Step 3 examination or obtain an unrestricted license to practice medicine in the U.S.

To be eligible for ECFMG certification, you must meet the following criteria:

- Take and pass the USMLE Step 1, Step 2 Clinical Knowledge (CK), and Step 2 Clinical Skills (CS) exams

- Fulfill medical education credential requirements

- Your medical school and graduation year must be listed in the International Medical Education Directory (IMED) which is available at http://imed.ecfmg.org.

- You must have had at least four credit years in attendance at the medical school.

- You must submit copies of your medical school diploma. The ECFMG will verify your diploma with your medical school and request your school to provide ECFMG with your final medical school transcript.

Tip # 133

Start the process of obtaining an ECFMG certificate as early as you can. As those before you have learned, this process can take considerable time. Note that several steps in this process are beyond your control. For example, you may have no control over the length of time it takes your medical school to verify your medical school diploma and provide the ECFMG with an official copy of your final medical school transcript.

Did you know ...

Some residency programs will consider IMG applicants who are not ECFMG certified, as long as the results of one or more USMLE exams are available at the time of application review. However, all programs will require you to provide them with documentation of your ECFMG certification prior to the deadline for ranking applicants. In other words, programs at which you have interviewed will not place you on their rank list unless you show them you are ECFMG certified.

Rule # 193   Learn the selection criteria that are most important to residency program directors.

In a survey of 102 internal medicine residency program directors, directors were asked to rate the importance of 22 selection criteria that best predicted the performances of foreign-born medical graduates during internal medicine residencies (Gayed). Criteria rated highest included performance on the NBME (precursor to the USMLE), interview performance, and postgraduate clinical experience in the U.S.

Importance of 22 residency selection criteria for IMG applicants	
Criteria	Rating*
Score on NBME II#	4.34
Fluency in English as determined during interview	4.30
Number of attempts on NBME II#	4.30
Postgraduate clinical experience in U.S.	4.20
Number of attempts on NBME I#	4.10
Score on NBME I#	4.07
Interview performance on nonmedical issues (e.g., personality)	4.02
Medical school (if known to program director)	3.98
Year of graduation (recent graduates perform better)	3.84
Performance during interview with medical questions (e.g., quiz, case presentation)	3.65
Country of medical education	3.64
Score on FLEX	3.54
Rank order in medical school class	3.35
Age (younger graduates performing better respective to graduation date)	3.33
Letter of recommendation from the U.S.	3.27
Postgraduate clinical experience in foreign country	3.12
Passing FLEX before applying for residency	3.12
Duration of living in U.S.	3.03

Importance of 22 residency selection criteria for IMG applicants	
Criteria	Rating*
Medical school grades (transcript)	2.94
Nonclinical graduate work in the U.S. (e.g. basic science graduate studies, research)	2.74
Dean's letter	2.32
Other letters of recommendations from foreign country	1.93

*Directors were asked to rate the importance of each criterion on a scale of 1 (least important) to 5 (most important).
#NBME I and II exams were the immediate precursors of the USMLE Step 1 and 2 CK exams, respectively.
From Gayed NM, Residency directors' assessments of which selection criteria best predict the performances of foreign-born medical graduates during internal med residencies. *Acad Med* 1991; 66(11): 699-701.

Did you know ...

Your year of graduation is important to programs. Some programs prefer recent graduates because they believe these applicants will do better during residency training. These programs may even screen out applications from IMGs who have graduated "too far in the past." Others evaluate such applicants on a case by case basis. As Rao stated, these applicants "may have gained valuable life and career experiences through professional work since graduation from medical school. They may have obtained additional postgraduate medical qualifications and administrative or research experience or may have worked in various cultures" (Rao). In Gayed's survey, while 27% of program directors agreed that "IMGs straight out of medical school performed better than those who had done clinical work in a foreign country," 33% disagreed and 40% were neutral (Gayed).

Rule # 194 The USMLE is important. Very important.

As discussed, to become certified by the ECFMG, you must take and pass the United States Medical Licensing Examinations (USMLE). These include the USMLE Step 1, USMLE Step 2 Clinical Knowledge (CK), and USMLE Step 2 Clinical Skills (CS) exams. The USMLE Step 1 and 2 CK exams were developed to assess medical knowledge. The Step 2 CS exam was designed to evaluate communication and interpersonal skills.

While the USMLE exams were not developed to be used as residency selection tools, scores have taken on significant importance in the residency selection process. This is true for both U.S. and IMG applicants, but even more so for the latter. According to 2006 data supplied by the ECFMG, nearly 300,000 IMGs from over 200 countries had received certification since the organization's inception. It is difficult for U.S. residency programs to accurately assess the quality of medical education in 200 plus countries, let alone the quality of each of the 1500 plus medical schools operating throughout the world.

While you may have been a "star medical student" or physician in your native country, your past performance will have little bearing on your chances of securing a residency position in the U.S. Program directors will simply not be familiar with the quality of your medical education. Instead, programs will place considerable emphasis on a tool they are intimately familiar with—the USMLE exams. These exams have made it easier for programs to assess the medical knowledge of IMG applicants. Since all applicants are required to take these exams, programs are readily able to compare scores of one applicant with another.

The reality of the situation is this: the higher your USMLE scores, the better your chances of matching with a program in your chosen specialty. The following points deserve emphasis:

- With the exception of the USMLE Step 2 CS exam, the USMLE exams are not pass/fail exams. However, if you pass, you cannot take the exam again, and you cannot try to get a better score. In other words, once you pass, the score that you achieve will be the score used by residency programs in their decision-making process.

- The USMLE Step 1 and 2 CK exams are difficult. In 2006, Boulet and colleagues reported the USMLE first attempt pass rates (i.e. what percent of test-takers passed the exam on their first try) for IMGs who sought ECFMG certification between 1995 and 2004.

USMLE First Attempt Pass Rates for International Medical Graduates		
	First attempt pass rate for U.S. IMGs*	First attempt pass rate for non-U.S. IMGs#
USMLE Step 1	60.5%	64.3%
USMLE Step 2 CK	70.4%	66.1%
USMLE Step 2 CS	91.6%	84.2%

*U.S. IMGs = IMGs who are citizens of the U.S.
#Non-U.S. IMGs = IMGs who are not citizens of the U.S.

From Boulet JR, Swanson DB, Cooper RA, Norcini JJ, McKinley DW. A comparison of the characteristics and examination performances of U.S. and non-U.S. citizen international medical graduates who sought Educational Commission for Foreign Medical Graduates certification: 1995 - 2004. *Acad Med* 2006; 81 (10 Suppl): S116-119.

Since that study, first attempt pass rates have improved to some extent. In 2007, 70% of the 15,762 IMGs who took the USMLE Step 1 exam passed on their first attempt. The percentage was even better for first time takers of the USMLE Step 2 CK exam. 79% of the 12,584 IMGs passed. (www.usmle.org/Scores_Transcripts/performance/2007.html).

Many programs will not consider applications from IMGs who do not pass on the first attempt. Given the importance of these exams in the residency selection process, and the relatively high first-time fail rates, you must prepare properly for these exams.

- Some residency programs will not consider applications from IMGs until the results of USMLE Step 1, 2 CK, and 2 CS exams are all available. Other programs will extend interview invitations to IMG applicants who have completed either the USMLE Step 1 or Step 2 CK exam.

- Many programs have score cutoffs for IMG applicants. Applicants who are at or above this threshold will be considered for an interview. Those with scores below this threshold will not be considered further. At times, this information is made available to applicants at program websites.

- IMG applicants are not required to take the USMLE Step 1 exam prior to taking the USMLE Step 2 CK exam. In other words, you are free to choose the order in which you would like to take these exams. The Step 1 exam is essentially a basic science exam, while the focus of the Step 2 CK exam is on the clinical sciences. If you are closer to the latter, consider taking the Step 2 CK exam first.

- The USMLE Step 3 exam is not a major factor used by programs in the residency selection process. Many IMG applicants, however, take the exam since it is not possible to secure a H1-B visa without passing the Step 3 exam. In 2007, of the 9,384 IMGs who took the exam, 21% failed (http://www.usmle.org/Scores_Transcripts/performance/2007.html).

While low USMLE scores or a failed attempt will not eliminate you from securing a residency position in the U.S., the road you must travel to realize your professional goals becomes much more difficult. To overcome low scores, you will need to strengthen every aspect of the residency application.

While high USMLE scores increase the likelihood of a successful match, every year IMGs with high scores fail to match. In the 2007 Match, 277 of the 828 independent applicants with Step 1 scores > 230 failed to match to an internal medicine residency program.

Clearly, attention needs to be given to every aspect of the application in order to maximize your chances of a successful match, even for applicants with competitive scores.

Did you know ...

In a study done to determine application criteria predictive of IMG residency success, researchers examined the performance of 46 IMGs in the internal medicine residency program at Wright State University between 1985 and 1991 (Part). They found that NBME Part 1 scores (precursor of the USMLE exam) were one of only two factors that related significantly to subsequent performance in residency.

Did you know ...

With completion of residency training, physicians are eligible to take the specialty board exam. Passing this exam makes the physician "board certified." Having the ability to pass the specialty board examination is important to programs because "specialty board certification has a demonstrated relationship with clinical outcomes and other measures of physician competence" (Norcini). Failing the specialty board exam may also impact the program's ability to recruit residents, since some specialties require programs to make public the average pass rate. For these reasons, programs try to identify applicants who might be at higher risk of failing these exams. In several studies, USMLE test scores have been found to predict board passage (Sosenko, Case, Fish). Yet another reason why USMLE scores are an important factor in the residency selection process.

Rule # 195 Understand the concerns of program directors with respect to IMG applicants.

Residency programs seek to select applicants who will be successful residents. However, performance as a resident can be difficult to predict. While this holds true for both U.S. MGs and IMGs, program directors have a more difficult time assessing the potential of IMG applicants.

A major goal for program directors is to avoid selecting applicants who may become problem residents. The problem resident is defined as a "trainee who demonstrates a significant enough problem that requires intervention by someone of authority, usually the program director or chief resident" (American Board of Internal Medicine. Association of Program Directors in Internal Medicine (APDIM) Chief Residents' Workshop on Problem Residents; 1999).

In a survey of 298 internal medicine residency program directors, Yao and Wright found that the mean point prevalence of problem residents was 6.9% for the academic year 1998 - 1999 (Yao). According to the American Board of Internal Medicine, 8% to 15% of residents have significant areas of learner difficulty, and 94% of internal medicine residency programs reported having one or more problem residents during the academic year 1998 - 1999 (Yao). While U.S. medical graduates and IMGs can become problem residents, in this study program directors felt that IMGs were more likely to be identified as problem residents.

Problem residents can negatively impact a program by compromising patient care and increasing the workload of their resident colleagues. In addition, to remediate the problem, considerable time, support, and guidance is required from the faculty. When a disproportionate amount of a program's resources are spent on one or two problem residents, less time my be available for the rest of the residents. The end result of this is often a lowering of the entire residency program's morale.

Also of concern to programs is whether a resident, once selected, will complete residency training. Several studies have examined resident attrition rates:

- In a study examining resident attrition rates from family practice residencies, a significantly higher attrition rate (18.5% vs. 7.8%) was found for IMGs than for U.S. medical graduates (Laufenburg).

- In another study, while the overall rates were found to be lower, the attrition rate of IMGs (3.7% vs. 1.4%) was higher than U.S. medical graduates (Baldwin).

- A higher attrition rate (3.6% vs. 2.5%) for IMGs was also found in another study (van Zanten).

From these studies, it is apparent that IMGs are less likely to complete residency training. While the attrition rate in the latter two studies seems small, the loss of even a single resident has significant effects on a residency program. Therefore, programs make it a priority to accurately identify applicants at higher risk of becoming problem residents, as well as those that are less likely to complete training.

In a study by Yao and Wright, apparent deficiencies in problem residents were identified and are shown in the following table:

Frequency of apparent deficiencies and underlying causes in problem residents	
Apparent deficiency	Half of the time or more frequently
Insufficient medical knowledge	48%
Poor clinical judgment	44%
Inefficient use of time	44%
Inappropriate interaction with colleagues or staff	39%
Provision of poor or inadequate medical care to patients	36%
Unsatisfactory clinical skills	31%
Unsatisfactory humanistic behavior with patients	23%
Excessive and unexplained tardiness or absences	21%
Unacceptable moral or ethical behaviors	15%
Taken from Yao DC, Wright SM. National survey of internal medicine residency program directors regarding problem residents. *JAMA* 2000; 284: 1099-1104.	

Insufficient medical knowledge is at the top of this list. As discussed earlier, programs assess knowledge attainment mainly from an applicant's performance on the USMLE exams. To determine if an applicant is likely to become a problem resident for other reasons, such as inefficient use of time or inappropriate interaction with colleagues or staff, residency programs will rely on other components of the application. These other components include letters of recommendation and U.S. medical experience.

Rule # 196 Don't underestimate the importance of letters of recommendation.

While you may have been a highly competent physician in your home country, will you be one in the United States? How strong are your clinical skills? How readily and easily will you adapt to medicine as it is practiced in the U.S? How will you relate to U.S. patients? How well do you work with others? Do you have the written and oral communication skills needed to succeed? These are among the many questions that residency programs are trying to answer as they consider your application.

Programs wish to determine if you have both the professional and personal qualities to succeed as a resident and, later, as a practicing physician. To make this determination, programs rely heavily on letters of recommendation. In contrast to your USMLE scores, recommendation letters supply programs with qualitative, rather than quantitative information, about your cognitive and non-cognitive characteristics. A number of studies have shown that behavior, attitude, and other non-cognitive skills are important predictors of resident success. As such, programs place great importance on these letters in evaluating your application.

IMGs often underestimate the importance of these letters, but these letters are crucial. We are often asked if it is acceptable to submit recommendation letters written by non-U.S. faculty members or physicians. While it is possible to match without having a single letter written by a U.S. faculty member, you will significantly strengthen your application and improve the chances of a favorable match outcome if you are able to submit letters from a U.S. faculty member. In a survey of 102 directors of internal medicine residency programs, directors were asked to rate the importance of 22 selection criteria (Gayed). Rated lowest were letters of recommendation from a foreign country. "Only 7% of the program directors disagreed with the statement that such letters are useless." In other words, 93% of program directors felt that letters of recommendation from a foreign country were useless.

In further support of this were the results of a survey of psychiatry residency program directors (Rao). Less importance was attached to letters of recommendation written by foreign faculty. The authors wrote that "letters from abroad may be superficial and filled with generalities, addressing qualities that are more important in the applicant's culture of origin. For example, many reference letters from India mention loyalty, good behavior, and the devotion of an applicant as contrasted with articulateness, assertiveness, clinical competence, and ability to think independently. "

The following points deserve emphasis:

- Letters of recommendation written by non-U.S. faculty members or physicians carry very little weight in the residency selection process. In contrast, letters written by U.S. faculty members are highly valued because these physicians are familiar with the cognitive and non-cognitive skills and traits essential for success during residency.

- Can IMGs match without any U.S. letters of recommendation? Yes, but it is much more difficult. Many IMGs contact us after failing to match, wondering what went wrong. In many cases, these applicants had strong applications, including high USMLE scores, but were lacking letters of recommendation written by U.S. faculty members. We encourage these applicants to obtain these letters and reapply. The effects of doing so can be dramatic. Following submission of these letters, we have seen many of these applicants receive significantly more interview invitations. As you interview at more programs, you increase your chances of matching.

- When considering IMG applicants of the same caliber, programs will offer an interview invitation to the applicant having letters of recommendation written by U.S. faculty members.
- Aim to obtain three or four recommendation letters from U.S. faculty. If this is not possible, then obviously one letter is better than no letter.
- IMGs often ask their friends or family members for letters of recommendation. However, these letters are useless, even if the writer is in the medical field. Letters of recommendation should be written by physicians who have worked with you in a clinical capacity. Chapter 7: Letters of Recommendation outlines in comprehensive detail what factors make for a powerful letter of recommendation. Letters written by medical friends or family members who have not worked with you in a clinical capacity will be filled with generalities and superficial information. These types of letters can actually work to weaken your application.

Did you know ...

In 2007, the ECFMG posted an announcement on their website regarding fraudulent letters of recommendation after investigating a dozen cases in which applicants had fabricated their letters. These letters were brought to ECFMG attention mainly by program directors after attempts to verify their authenticity raised suspicion. In this announcement, the ECFMG reminded applicants that submission of these letters was considered a form of irregular behavior, the consequences of which can be devastating. If irregular behavior is confirmed, the ECFMG may place a permanent annotation in the applicant's ECFMG Status Report. The behavior may also be reported to directors of graduate medical education programs, the Federation of State Medical Boards, and state medical licensing authorities. In 11/12 cases, the ECFMG revoked the applicant's standard ECFMG certificate (http://www.ecfmg.org/reporter/2007/iss116.html).

Did you know ...

We have heard of some services, and even physicians, offering to write IMGs letters of recommendation for a fee, sometimes as high as $500. While such offers may be tempting, you should never have to pay for a letter of recommendation, and you should never do so. Services or individuals that charge for writing letters are displaying questionable ethics, and you should question the quality of their letter as well. Furthermore, such actions may be considered irregular behavior by the ECFMG. As we've discussed, the consequences of irregular behavior can be very severe.

Your next step...

See chapter 7 of this book and visit www.ImgAssist.com for further information about letters of recommendation.

Rule # 197 To secure strong letters of recommendation, you must perform well, and you must do so during rotations in the United States.

As we've emphasized, letters of recommendation from U.S. faculty members can significantly strengthen your application. To secure a strong letter of recommendation from a U.S. faculty member, you must work with that physician in a capacity that allows him or her to evaluate you in the same way that they would evaluate a third or fourth year U.S. medical student.

During the third year of U.S. medical school, students generally rotate through their core rotations in internal medicine, family medicine, psychiatry, general surgery, pediatrics, and obstetrics/gynecology. These rotations typically offer students a "hands-on experience" taking care of patients. Students learn how to take histories, perform physical exams, analyze test results, make diagnoses from the available information, formulate a treatment plan, and follow their patients throughout the hospitalization until discharge. Students are also asked to write progress notes and present their patients daily to the rest of the team, which typically consists of the faculty preceptor, resident, and intern. Through these interactions, faculty preceptors are able to assess students' medical knowledge, clinical judgment, initiative, work ethic, ability to receive constructive feedback, quality of medical care given, clinical skills, interpersonal skills, punctuality, and professionalism. Letters written by faculty preceptors often comment on these skills and traits.

For IMGs, participating in rotations allows preceptors the chance to evaluate their skills and qualities in the same manner. This can result in a letter containing the type of information that program directors seek. Rotations also offer IMGs a chance to gain familiarity with the U.S. medical system. Because most IMGs have never worked in a U.S. hospital or medical center, gaining such experience will help ease the transition from foreign training to U.S. residency training, leading to fewer professional adjustment problems. Programs seek to avoid these types of adjustment problems, as they can lead to poor residency performance.

Following are some important points about U.S. medical experience:

- International medical graduates often underestimate the importance of U.S. medical experience to residency programs.

- Some programs will not consider you as a candidate unless you have U.S medical experience.

- Programs that do not have U.S. medical experience requirements per se will still often favor applicants who have such experience. When two applicants with similar credentials and qualifications are compared, programs will most certainly favor the applicant who has U.S. medical experience.

- Is it possible to match without any U.S. medical experience? It can and does happen, but you should realize that many IMG applicants have failed to match despite having competitive USMLE scores. Gaining such experience can make you a more desirable candidate.

- The duration of the experience required varies from program to program. Some programs will require at least one year of experience, while others may simply state that several months is sufficient. We are often asked whether a few days or weeks are sufficient. However, since one of your goals is to secure a strong letter of recommendation from the faculty member with whom you work, a short duration of experience may not result in the type of letter you truly need to strengthen your application. However, if your time is limited, some experience is better than none.

- Ideally, the rotation should be in your chosen specialty. Letters written by faculty in your field are valued more highly. However, at some programs, gaining U.S. medical experience in other fields may meet their application requirements.

- IMGs often participate in observerships. The American Medical Association (AMA) defines an observership as a "structured opportunity for an IMG to observe clinical practice in a variety of health care settings under the guidance of a physician mentor and to learn about the general structure, characteristics, and financing of health care delivery in the U.S." (http://www.ama-assn.org/ama1/pub/upload/mm/471/cme12.doc). While this type of rotation might satisfy some programs, others require "hands-on" experience. Rotations that offer hands-on experience are commonly referred to as externships.

- Obtaining a position as an observer or extern is difficult. In a survey of 33 IMG residents in an internal medicine residency program, 18 voiced frustration over the difficulties they experienced in finding such positions (Woods).

- Opportunities to do externships are limited, especially for IMGs who have graduated from medical school. It is considerably easier to arrange an externship while still in medical school, because you remain eligible to qualify for student group malpractice insurance rates.

- In the survey by Woods, one respondent stated that "a lot of programs request clinical experience in the U.S. from IMGs. This is even more difficult because a lot of residency programs do not give IMGs the opportunity for an externship." Another commented that "no one would give me an opportunity to prove myself." For those that were successful in arranging these rotations, some reported that without the assistance of family or friends, it would have been much more difficult to secure a position.

- Externships are more highly valued because faculty preceptors are able to assess your skills while you are involved in hands-on care of patients. Since no clinical contact is allowed during observerships, these rotations do not allow preceptors to accurately gauge key skills. Letters of recommendation written by observership preceptors are limited in what they can say about your skills.

- One advantage of these rotations is that you have the chance to make a strong impression on those with whom you work. This can be particularly helpful in gaining an interview at that particular program.

- Many IMGs have found rotation experience valuable in their preparation for the USMLE Step 2 CS exam.

- Impressing faculty preceptors during these rotations can be difficult for IMGs. Most IMGs are unfamiliar with the U.S. medical education system, usual expectations of U.S. physician supervisors, and the qualities which these supervisors value most. Bates wrote that "the usual style of North American Medical Education is a Socratic method in which trainees attempt to support their decisions to their supervising physicians and defend their actions. However, many IMGs come from cultures and training programs where deference to authority is the norm and questioning a professor's opinion is unthinkable. Unfortunately, in North

America, the IMG's silence may be interpreted as lack of knowledge, lack of interest, or lack of confidence" (Bates).

To make the most of your rotation experiences, you need to be well informed of the qualities, skills, and behaviors that are highly valued. We have written or edited a series of books guiding U.S. medical students through their rotations. Feedback we have received from IMGs has informed us that these books have also been useful for observerships and externships. These resources are listed in the following table.

Observership or externship	Recommended reading
Before your first rotation (either observership or externship)...	250 Biggest Mistakes 3ʳᵈ Year Medical Students Make And How To Avoid Them
Before your internal medicine observership or externship....	Internal Medicine Clerkship: 150 Biggest Mistakes And How To Avoid Them
Before your surgery observership or externship...	Surgery Clerkship: 150 Biggest Mistakes And How To Avoid Them
Before your pediatrics observership or externship...	Pediatrics Clerkship: 101 Biggest Mistakes And How To Avoid Them
Before your psychiatry observership or externship...	Psychiatry Clerkship: 150 Biggest Mistakes And How To Avoid Them

Your Next Step

Visit www.ImgAssist.com for further information, including answers to the following questions:

1) How do I find an observership/externship?
2) How do I find the right observership/externship?
3) When should I do an observership/externship?
4) Should I do a research elective instead?
5) Does it matter who I work with?
6) Should I work in an office or hospital setting?
7) Does it matter at which hospital I do the rotation?
8) What is expected of me during the rotation?
9) How can I impress my preceptor/attending/supervisor?
10) How can I obtain a strong letter of recommendation?

Rule # 198   Create a powerful personal statement.

While individual specialties, residency programs, and application reviewers assign varying degrees of importance to the personal statement, there is data showing that the personal statement is of major importance to the specialties that IMGs are most likely to pursue.

A 1993 study of family practice residency program directors found that the personal statement ranked second only to the Dean's letter for making decisions about whom to interview (Taylor). With regard to the ranking of applicants, it was third in importance, following only the interview and the Dean's letter.

Psychiatry residency programs also place considerable emphasis on the personal statement. Dr. Rao, chair of the department of psychiatry and behavioral sciences at Nassau University Medical Center, wrote that the personal statement "has proven to be a very useful method of assessing IMG applicants at the preinterview stage" (Rao). IMGs should also heed the words of the department of psychiatry at Stonybrook University School of Medicine:

> "Writing skills are an essential component of medical record keeping, particularly in psychiatry...The Selection Committee will evaluate the preparation of the application and in particular the Personal Statement for evidence of writing skills...Applicants with poorly written essays, e.g., multiple spelling and grammatical errors will not be invited for an interview" (http:// www.hsc.stonybrook.edu/som/psychiatry/ selection_procecess.cfm).

Your next step...

See chapter 8 of this book and visit www.ImgAssist.com for further information about the personal statement.

Rule # 199   The interview is extremely important.

In Gayed's survey of internal medicine residency program directors, the interview was found to be of major importance in the residency selection process. Most important in the interview process were fluency in the English language, personality, and medical knowledge.

- Determination of the candidate's fluency in the English language

  Having the ability to understand and communicate with English-speaking patients is essential to delivering quality medical care and understandably important to program directors. For IMGs coming from English-speaking countries, this may pose little difficulty. However, for those who have practiced medicine in their native country using their mother tongue, this can be extremely challenging. Poor command of the English language can make it difficult for physicians to interview patients effectively, establish rapport, and interact with other healthcare professionals.

  Difficulties exist even for IMGs who are trained in English. Husain wrote that "variations in pronunciation, rhythm, and voice inflection may combine to produce a foreign accent that interferes with efficient transmission of the desired message, and this problem may occur despite excellent grammar and vocabulary use" (Husain).

To determine your level of English language proficiency, programs will initially rely on the results of your USMLE Step 2 CS test. While passage of this exam is a measure of your communication skills, the interview will be the chief means by which your overall proficiency is assessed. Rao stated that "of primary importance for the interviewer is an assessment of the applicant's communication skills with respect to pronunciation, grammar, grasp of idiom, and vocabulary...In listening to the applicant's responses to questions, the interviewer can assess the applicant's ability to express and understand abstract thought" (Rao).

- Assessment of personality

During the interview, your interviewer will learn more about your noncognitive traits, including your communication skills, your interpersonal skills, your strengths, and your drive. Interview questions are also asked to determine "fit" with the program.

An interviewer can't learn about your interpersonal skills from your application alone. He can't learn about your strengths or weaknesses. He can't find out what drives or motivates you. He can't discover how well you handle pressure. Do you have the qualities that make someone a valued team member? Will you fit in and work well with others in the department? The only way an interviewer can learn any of these things is by speaking with you and asking questions. While the personal statement and letters of recommendation provide some information, the interview is the chief means by which programs can directly assess these noncognitive factors.

- Assessment of medical knowledge

In contrast to U.S. applicants, IMGs are more likely to be asked questions that gauge their medical knowledge. One IMG commented on his experience. They "would ask you medical questions and give you patient scenarios and...they made me examine and talk to a patient...it was awful. They asked all kinds of questions and gave you labs...it's like an exam. It was horrible" (Woods).

> ### Your next step…
> See chapters 12-14 of this book and visit www.ImgAssist.com for further information about the residency interview.

Rule # 200 Understand immigration and visa issues as they relate to residency training.

Without obtaining the legal authority to work in the U.S., you will be unable to begin residency training. For foreign-born IMGs who are naturalized U.S. citizens or holders of a permanent resident (immigrant) visa, this poses no difficulty. For IMGs who do not fit into these two groups, options generally include obtaining either a J-1 Exchange visitor visa or a H-1 B Temporary Professional Worker visa.

The ECFMG is authorized to sponsor IMGs for J-1 visas. To qualify for this visa, the IMG must show proof of acceptance into an accredited residency training program. In addition, a statement of need is also necessary. This statement is essentially a letter from the ministry of health of the country of nationality or last legal permanent residence, stating that a need exists in that country for physicians with the skills that IMGs are hoping to acquire through residency training.

The J-1 visa is an "exchange visitor" program that allows an IMG to reside in the U.S. while completing residency training. After completing training, the IMG must return to his or her country for a minimum of two years. After this period of time, the IMG becomes eligible for a change in visa status, permitting him or her to return to the U.S.

Since most IMGs prefer to stay in the U.S. permanently following completion of residency training, this requirement of the J-1 visa makes this visa unattractive. To avoid returning home, IMGs often explore ways to avoid fulfilling this requirement. One option is the receipt of the J-1 waiver from the U.S. government. IMGs who receive a waiver have to practice in a medically underserved area for at least three years.

Because there is no "2-year home requirement," many IMGs prefer to train on a H-1 B visa. However, the H-1 B visa has traditionally been harder to obtain. To be eligible for this visa, you must pass the USMLE Step 3 exam, which can be challenging. In 2007, of the 9,384 IMGs who took the exam, 21% failed (http://www.usmle.org/Scores_Transcripts/performance/2007.html).

In addition, the process is more involved, sometimes requiring the assistance and efforts of an attorney. Furthermore, the H-1 B visa is not sponsored by the ECFMG but rather by the residency training program. Because of the effort and expense involved, fewer programs have traditionally offered the H-1 B visa. Recent data, however, suggests that this is changing. In 2006, 15.1% of IMG resident physicians were found to be on H visas (which include H1B), a significant rise over the 6.5% reported in 2000 (Brotherton).

Citizenship/visa status of IMG resident physicians in ACGME-accredited programs as of December 1, 2006		
Citizenship/visa status	Number	Percentage
Native U.S. citizen	4,066	14.4%
Naturalized U.S. citizen	2,812	9.9%
Permanent resident	6,589	23.4%
H-1, H-1B, H-2, H-3 temporary worker	4,242	15.1%
J-1, J-2 exchange visitor	3,960	14.1%
Other/unknown	6,507	23.1%

Adapted from Brotherton SE, Etzel SI. Graduate medical education, 2006-2007. *JAMA* 2007; 298 (9): 1081-1096.

Did you know...

In 2003, according to the ECFMG, 18% of J-1 physicians arrived 31 days or more after their residency program start date because of delays in the processing of visas (http://www.ama-assn.org/ama/pub/category/11928.html).

References

Aagaard EM, Hauer KE. A cross-sectional descriptive study of mentoring relationships formed by medical students. *J Gen Intern Med* 2003; 18: 298-302.

Adams LJ, Brandenburg S, Blake M. Factors influencing internal medicine program directors decisions about applicants. *Acad Med* 2000; 75: 542-3.

Alexander H, Lang J. Full-time faculty at U.S. medical schools with MD or equivalent degree: IMGs compared to U.S./Canadian graduates. Research Brief RB06-5. Washington, DC: Assoc of American medical colleges; April 2006.

Altmaier EM, Smith WL, O'Halloran CM, Franken EA. The predictive utility of behavior-based interviewing compared with traditional interviewing in the selection of radiology residents. *Invest Radiol* 1992; 27 (5); 385-389.

Amorosa JK. How do I mentor medical students interested in radiology. *Acad Radiol* 2003; 10: 527-535.

Amos DE, Massagli TL. Medical school achievements as predictors of performance in a physical medicine and rehabilitation residency. *Acad Med* 1996; 71: 678-680.

Ances, BM. The away neurology rotation: is the grass greener on the other side? *Neurology* 2006; 66(9): E35-36.

Anderson KD, Jacobs. General surgery program directors' perceptions of the match. *Curr Surg* 2000; 57(5): 460-465.

Armstrong WB. Residency selection handbook: otolaryngology. From www.ucihs.uci.edu.

Bajaj G, Carmichael KD. What attributes are necessary to be selected for an orthopedic surgery residency position: perceptions of faculty and residents. *South Med J* 2004; 97 (12): 1179-1185.

Bak MK, Louie AK, Tong LD, Coverdale J, Roberts LW. Applying to Psychiatry Residency. *Acad Psychiatry* 2006; 30(3): 239-247.

Baker DR, Jackson VP. Misrepresentation of publications by radiology residency applicants. *Acad Radiol* 2000; 7(9): 727-729.

Baldwin D, Roley B, Daughterty S, Bay C. Withdrawal and extended leave during residency training: results of a national survey. *Acad Med* 1995; 70: 1117-24.

Balentine J, Gaeta T, Spevack T. Evaluating Applicants to Emergency Medicine Residency Programs. *J Emerg Med* 1999; 17:131-134.

Bandiera G, Regehr G. Reliability of a structured interview scoring instrument for a Canadian postgraduate emergency medicine training program. *Acad Emerg Med* 2004; 11 (1): 27-32.

Bates BP, Bates CK, Tolstrup K. Selection criteria in postgraduate osteopathic medical education. *J Am Osteopath Assoc* 1988; 88: 391-395.

Bates BP. Selection criteria for applicants in primary care osteopathic graduate medical education. *J Am Osteopath Assoc* 2002; 102 (11): 621- 626.

Bates J, Andrew R. Untangling the roots of some IMGs' poor academic performance. *Acad Med* 2001; 76(1): 43-46.

Bell JG, Kanellitsas I, Shaffer L. Selection of obstetrics and gynecology residents on the basis of medical school performance. *Am J Obstet Gynecol* 2002; 186(5): 1091-1094.

Bellini LM. Printing brochures for residency training programs: is it worth the expense any longer? SGIM Forum. 1998; 21(9): 5. Accessed from http://www.sgim.org/userfiles/file/Forum/forum9809.pdf.

Bernstein AD, Jazrawi LM, Elbeshbeshy B, Della Valle CJ, Zuckerman JD. Orthopaedic resident-selection criteria. *J Bone Joint Surg Am* 2002; 84-A (11): 2090-2096.

Bilge A, Shugerman RP, Robertson WO. Misrepresentation of authorship by applicants to pediatric training programs. *Acad Med* 1998; 73 (5): 532-33.

Biros M, Adams J. Medical students and research: getting started in emergency medicine research. Available at www.saem.org.

Blanchard A, Gilmore-Bradford E. Pritzker residency process guide: obstetrics and gynecology. Available at http://pritzker.uchicago.edu/current/students/ResidencyProcessGuide.pdf.

Blumstein HA, Cone DC. Medical Student Career Advice Related to Emergency Medicine. *Acad Emerg Med.* 1998; 5:69-72.

Boor M, Wartman SA, Reuben DB. Relationship of physical appearance and professional demeanor to interview evaluations and rankings of medical residency applicants. *J Psychol* 1983; 113: 61-65.

Boulet, JR, Swanson DB, Cooper RA, Norcini JJ, McKinley DW. A comparison of the characteristics and examination performances of U.S. and non-U.S. citizen international medical graduates who sought Educational Commission for Foreign Medical Graduates Certification: 1995-2004. *Acad Med* 2006; 81 (10 Suppl): S116-119.

Boyd AS, Hook M, King LE Jr., An evaluation of the accuracy of residency applicants' curricula vitae: Are the claims of publication erroneous? *J Am Acad Dermatol* 1996; 35 (4):606-608.

Boyse TD, Patterson SK, Cohan RH, Korobkin M, Fitzgerald JT, Oh MS, Gross BH, Quint DJ. Does medical school performance predict radiology resident performance? *Acad Radiol* 2002; 9(4): 437-445.

Brandenburg, S, Kruzick T, LinCT, Robinson A, Adams LJ. Residency selection criteria: what medical students perceive as important. *Med Educ Online* 2005; 10: 1-6 (www.med-ed-online.org).

Britt, LD. How to interview for a residency position. From http://www.facs.org/medicalstudents/britt.pdf.

Brothers TE, Wetherholt S. Importance of the faculty interview during the resident application process. *J Surg Educ* 2007; 64(6): 378-385.

Brotherton SE, Etzel SI. Graduate medical education, 2006-2007. *JAMA* 2007; 298 (9): 1081-1096.

Brunworth JD, Sindwani R. Impact of duty hour restrictions on otolaryngology training: divergent resident and faculty perspectives. *Laryngoscope* 2006; 116: 1127-1130.

Caplan JP, Borus JF, Chang G, Greenberg WE. Poor intentions or poor attention: misrepresentation by applicants to psychiatry residency. *Acad Psychiatry* 2008; 32(3): 225-229.

Carek PJ, Anderson KD, Blue AV, Mavis BE. Recruitment behavior and program directors: how ethical are their perspectives about the match process? *Fam Med* 2000; 32(4): 258-260.

Carson KD, Carson PP, Fontenot G, Burdin JJ Jr. Structured interview questions for selecting productive emotionally mature, and helpful employees. *Health Care Manag* 2005; 24(3): 209-215.

Case SM, Swanson DB. Validity of NBME part I and part II scores for selection of residents in orthopaedic surgery, dermatology and preventive medicine, *Acad Med* 1993; 68 (suppl): S51-S56.

Chaplin WF, Phillips JB, Brown JD, Clanton NR, Stein JL. Handshaking, gender, personality, and first impressions. *Journal of Pers Soc Psychol* 2000; 79: 110-117.

Chew FS, Ochoa ER, Relyea-Chew A. Spreadsheet application for radiology resident match rank list. *Acad Radiol* 2005; 12: 379-384.

Clarke JT, Miller JJ, Sceppa J, Goldsmith LA, Long E. Success in the dermatology resident match in 2003: perceptions and importance of home institutions and away rotations. *Arch Derm* 2006; 142: 930-932.

Cohen BL, Friedman E, Zier K. Publications by students doing a year of full-time research: what are realistic expectations? *Am J Med* 2008; 121: 545-548.

Cohen-Gadol AA, Koch CA, Raffel C, Spinner RJ. Confirmation of research publications reported by neurological surgery residency applicants. *Surg Neurol* 2003; 60(4): 280-283.

Cohen JJ. The role and contributions of IMGS: a U.S. perspective. *Acad Med* 2006; 81(12): S17-S21.

Cole AF. Plagiarism in graduate medical education. *Fam Med* 2007; 39(6): 436-8.

Cole K. *The Complete Idiot's Guide to Clear Communication*. Published by Alpha books in 2002.

Connell P. Pritzker residency process guide: radiation oncology. Available at http://pritzker.uchicago.edu/current/students/ResidencyProcessGuide.pdf.

Counselman FL, Griffey RT. Fourth-year Elective Recommendations for Medical Students Interested in Emergency Medicine. *Am Emerg Med* 1999; 17:745-746.

Coupe K. Career counseling: orthopedic surgery. Available at http://www.uth.tmc.edu/med/administration/student/ms4/2003CCC.htm.

Crane JT, Ferraro CM. Selection criteria for emergency medicine residency applicants. *Acad Emerg Med* 2000; 7 (1): 54-60.

Cruz PD. Residency selection: the Southwestern experience. *Arch Dermatol* 2001; 137 (6): 808-811.

Curtis DJ, Riordan DD, Cruess DF, Brower AC. Selecting radiology resident candidates. *Invest Radiol* 1989; 24 (4): 324-330.

Dale JA, Schmitt CM, Crosby LA. Misrepresentation of research criteria by orthopedic surgery applicants.

Daly KA, Levine SC, Adams, GL. Predictors for resident success in otolaryngology. *J Am Coll Surg* 2006; 202(4): 649-654.

DaRosa DA, Folse R, McCarthy MC, Sharp K. *Am J Surg* 1989; 157(2): 245-249.

DeBlieux P, Keim S, Chisholm C. Taming the Residency Application Process. Medical Student Emergency Medicine Symposium, May 22, 2000. Society for Academic Emergency Medicine Website.

DeLisa JA, Jain SS, Campagnolo DI. Factors used by physical medicine and rehabilitation residency training directors to select their residents. *Am J Phys Med Rehabil* 1994; 73: 152-156.

DeLisa JA, Leonard JA Jr, Smith BS, Kirshblum S. Common questions asked by medical students about physiatry. Brief report. *Am J Phys Med Rehabil* 1995; 74(2): 145-154.

DeLisa, Leonard JA Jr, Meier RH III, et al. Educational survey: common questions asked by medical students about physiatry. *Am J Phys Med Rehabil* 1990; 69: 259-265.

Delorio NM, Yarris LM, Kalbfleisch ND. Early invitations for residency interviews: the exception or the norm. *J Emerg Med* 2007; 33(1): 77-79.

DeSantis M, Marco CA. Emergency medicine residency selection: factors influencing candidate decisions. *Acad Emerg Med* 2005; 12 (6): 559-561.

Dumas, C. Career counseling: family practice. Available at http://www.uth.tmc.edu/med/administration/student/ms4/2003CCC.htm.

Easdown LJ, Castro PL, Shinkle EP, Small L, Algren J. The behavioral interview, a method to evaluate ACGME competencies in resident selection: a pilot project. *JEPM* 2005; 7 (1); 1-10.

Edmond M, Roberson M, Hasan N. The dishonest dean's letter: an analysis of 532 dean's letters from 99 U.S. medical schools. *Acad Med* 1999; 74(9): 1033-1035.

Embi PJ, Desai S, Cooney TG. Use and utility of Web-based residency program information: a survey of residency applicants. *J Med Internet Res* 2003; 5(3): e22.

Englander R, Carraccio C, Zalneraitis E, Sarkin R, Morgenstern B. Guiding medical students through the match: perspectives from recent graduates. *Pediatrics* 2003; 112(3): 502-505.

Ertel NW, Gunderman RB. Helping medical students to prepare for radiology residency interviews. *Acad Radiol* 2006; 13 (9): 1168-1171.

Espey E, Ogburn T. Guidelines for pursuing a residency in obstetrics and gynecology: 2005-2006. From (http://obgyn.unm.edu/clerkship).

Fabri PJ, Powell DL, Cupps NB. Is there value in audition extramurals? *Am J Surg* 1995; 169(3): 338-340.

Farnie, MA. Career counseling: internal medicine. Available at http://www.uth.tmc.edu/med/administration/student/ms4/2003CCC.htm.

Fish DE, Radfar-Baublitz LS, Choi H, Felsenthal G. Correlation of standardized testing results with success on the 2001 American board of physical medicine and rehabilitation part 1 board certificate examination, *Am J Phys Med Rehabil* 2003; 82: 686-691.

Fling M. A guide to the perplexed: residency guide. From www.ucdmc.ucdavis.edu.

Frim D, Rice H. Pritzker residency process guide: neurological surgery. Available at http://pritzker.uchicago.edu/current/students/ResidencyProcessGuide.pdf.

Fortune JB. The content and value of letters of recommendation in the resident candidate evaluative process. *Curr Surg* 2002; 59 (1): 79-83.

Freeman T, Sawyer CE, Behnke RR. Behavioral inhibition and the attribution of public speaking anxiety. *Communication Education* 1997; 46: 175-187.

Galazka SS, Kikano GE, Zyzanski S. Methods of recruiting and selecting residents for U.S. family practice residencies. *Acad Med* 1994; 69 (4): 304-306.

Gallin EK, Le Blancq SM. Clinical Research Fellowship Program Leaders. Launching a new fellowship for medical students: The first years of the Doris Duke Clinical Research Fellowship Program. *J Investig Med* 2005; 53: 73-81.

Garden FH, Smith BS. Criteria for selection of physical medicine and rehabilitation residents. A survey of current practices and suggested changes. *Am J Phys Med Rehabil* 1989; 68(3): 123-127.

Garmel GM. Letters of Recommendation: What Does "Good" Really Mean? *Acad Emerg Med* 1997; 4:833-834.

Gayed NM. Residency directors' assessments of which selection criteria best predict the performances of foreign-born foreign medical graduates during internal medicine residencies. *Acad Med* 1991; 66 (11): 699-701.

Gimenez, K. Residency selection handbook: anesthesiology. From www.ucihs.uci.edu.

Girzadas DV, Harwood RC, Dearie J, Garrett S. A comparison of standardized and narrative letters of recommendation. *Acad Emerg Med* 2000; 7(8): 963.

Girzadas DV, Harwood RC, Delis SN, Stevison K, Keng G, Cipparrone N, Carlson A, Tsonis GD. Emergency medicine standardized letter of recommendation: predictors of guaranteed match. *Acad Emerg Med* 2001; 8(6): 648-653.

Gong H, Parker NH, Apgar FA, Shank C. Influence of the interview on ranking in the residency selection process. *Med Educ* 1984; 18(5): 366-9.

Greenburg AG, Doyle J, McClure DK. Letters of Recommendation for surgical residencies: what they say and what they mean. *J Surg Res* 1994; 56 (2): 192-8.

Grover M, Dharamshi F, Goveia C. Deception by applicants to family practice residencies. *Fam Med* 2001; 33: 441-446.

Gurudevan SV, Mower WR. Misrepresentation of research publications among emergency medicine residency applicants. *Ann Emerg Med* 1996; 27 (3): 327-330.

Hallock JA, Kostis JB. Celebrating 50 years of experience: an ECFMG perspective. *Acad Med* 2006; 81(12): S7-S16.

Harwood RC, Girzadas DV, Carlson A, Delis S, Stevison K, Tsonis G, Keng G. Characteristics of the emergency medicine standardized letter of recommendation. *Acad Emerg Med* 2000; 7(4); 409-410.

Hauer KE, Teherani A, Dechet A, Aagaard EM. Medical students' perceptions of mentoring: a focus-group analysis. *Med Teach* 2005; 27(8): 732-734.

Hauge LS, Stroessner SJ, Chowdhry S, Wool NL. Evaluating resident candidates: does closed file review impact faculty ratings? *Am J Surg* 2007; 193: 761-765.

Hayden SR, Hayden M, Gamst A. What characteristics of applicants to emergency medicine residency programs predict future success as an emergency medicine resident. *Acad Emerg Med* 2005 Mar;12(3):206-10.

Hebert A. Career counseling: dermatology. Available at http://www.uth.tmc.edu/med/administration/student/ms4/2003CCC.htm.

Hebert RS, Smith CG, Wright SM. Minimal prevalence of authorship misrepresentation among internal medicine residency applicants: Do previous estimates of "misrepresentation" represent insufficient case finding? *Ann Intern Med* 2003; 138(5): 390-392.

Henderson M. A guide to the perplexed: residency guide. From www.ucdmc.ucdavis.edu.

Hern T, Hickner J, Ewigman B. Pritzker residency process guide: family medicine. Available at http://pritzker.uchicago.edu/current/students/ResidencyProcessGuide.pdf,

Heymann WR. Advice to the dermatology residency applicant. *Arch Dermatol* 2000; 136: 123-124.

Hunt DD, MacLaren C, Scott C, Marshall SG, Braddock CH, Sarfaty S. A follow-up study of the characteristics of dean's letters. *Acad Med* 2001; 76(7): 727-733.

Hunt DD, MacLaren CF, Scott CS, Chu J, Leiden LI. Characteristics of dean's letters in 1981 and 1992. *Acad Med* 1993; 68(12): 905-911.

Husain S, Munoz R, Balon R. International medical graduates in psychiatry in the United States: challenges and opportunities. *American Psychiatric Press* 1997.

Jackson VA, Palepu A, Szalacha L, Caswell C, Carr PL, Inui, T. "Having the right chemistry: a qualitative study of mentoring in academic medicine." *Acad Med* 2003; 78(3): 328-334.

Kahana M, Fromme B, Schwab. Pritzker residency process guide: pediatrics. Available at http://pritzker.uchicago.edu/current/students/ResidencyProcessGuide.pdf.

Kassebaum DG, Szenas PL. Medical students' career indecision and specialty rejection: roads not taken. *Acad Med* 1995; 70(10): 937-943.

Katta R, Bogle MA, Levy ML. Primary cutaneous opportunistic mold infections in a pediatric population. *J Am Acad Dermatol* 2005; 53(2): 213-219.

Katz ED, Shockley L, Kass L, Howes D, Tupesis JP, Weaver E, Sayan OR, Hogan V, Begue J, Vrocher D, Frazer J, Evans T, Hern G, Riviello R, Rivera A, Kinoshita K, Ferguson E. Identifying inaccuracies on emergency medicine residency applications. BMC Med Educ 2005; 5: 30.Keim SM, Rein JA, Chisholm C, et al. A Standardized Letter of Recommendation for Residency Application. *Acad Emerg Med.* 1999;6:1141-1146.

Kellaway J. Career counseling: ophthalmology. Available at http://www.uth.tmc.edu/administration/student/ms4/2003CCC.htm.

Kerfoot BP, Asher KP, McCullough DL. Financial and educational costs of the residency interview process for urology applicants. *Urology* 2008; epub 990-994.

Kia KF, Gielczyk RA, Ellis CN. Academia is the life for me, I'm sure. *Arch Dermatol* 2006; 142: 911-913.

Kitayama S, Cohen D. *Handbook of Cultural Psychology.* Guildford Press; 2007.

Kohli N. 411 on acing the residency interview. *ACP Impact;* 2004; 10 (4).

Konstantakos EK, Laughlin RT, Markert RJ, Crosby LA. Follow-up on misrepresentation of research activity by orthopedic residency applicants: has anything changed? *J Bone Joint Surg Am* 2007; 89: 2084 - 8.

Koscove EM. An Applicant's Evaluation of an Emergency Medicine Internship and Residency. *Ann Emerg Med.* 1990;19:774-780.

Ksiazek S. Taylor TL. Pritzker residency process guide: ophthalmology. Available at http://pritzker.uchicago.edu/current/students/ResidencyProcessGuide.pdf.

Kuo, J. Residency selection handbook: radiation oncology. From www.ucihs.uci.edu.

LaGrasso JR, Kennedy DA, Hoehn JG, Ashruf S, Pryzbyla AM. Selection criteria for the integrated model of plastic surgery residency. *Plast Reconstr Surg* 2008; 121 (3): 121e-125e.

Lamke N, Watson AB, Fisher RG. Radiology resident selection: objective restructured interview to assess five essential attributes. *SQU Journal for Scientific Research: Medical Sciences* 2003; 5(1-2): 27-30.

Landau C, Hall S, Wartman SA, Macko MB. Stress in social and family relationships during the medical residency. *J Med Educ* 1986; 61(8): 654-660.

Larkin GL, Marco CA. Ethics seminars: beyond authorship requirements - ethical considerations in writing letters of recommendation. *Acad Emerg Med* 2001; 8 (1): 70-3.

Larkin M. Getting a grip on handshakes. *Lancet* 2000; 356: 227.

Laufenburg HF, Turkal NW, Baumgardner DJ. Resident attrition from family practice residencies: United States versus international medical graduates. *Fam Med* 1994;26:614-617.

Lee AG, Gonik KC, Oetting TA, Beaver HA, Boldt HC, Olson R, Greenless E, Abramoff MD, Johnson AT, Carter K. Re-engineering the resident applicant selection process in ophthalmology: a literature review and recommendations for improvement. *Surv Ophthalmol* 2008; 53 (2): 164-176.

Lehrmann JA, Walaszek A. Assessing the quality of residency applicants in psychiatry. *Acad Psychiatry* 2008; 32(3): 180-182.

Leon LR, Aranha G. The journey of a foreign-trained physician to a United States residency. *J Am Coll Surg* 2006; 204(3): 486-494.

Leonard A, Harris I. An approach for defining selection criteria of applicants for medical residency training. *J Med Educ* 1980; 55: 57-59.

Leuhr S. Career counseling: anesthesiology. Available at http://www.uth.tmc.edu/med/administration/student/ms4/2003CCC.htm.

Levine MS. The art of clinical research with medical students. *Acad Radiol* 2003; 10: 527-535.

Lewis MC, Banks S, Dollar B, Cobas M, Katz J. The residency selection process: The when and how of the match order list. *Anesthesiology* 2007; 107: A409.

Loftipour S, Luu R, Hayden SR, Vaca F, Hoonpongsimanont W, Langdorf M. Becoming an emergency medicine resident: a practical guide for medical students. *J Emerg Med* 2008; Jun 10 (epub 339-344).

Low R. A guide to the perplexed: residency guide. From www.ucdmc.ucdavis.edu.

Lubavin B, Phelps M. Pearls of Wisdom for Your Emergency Medicine Rotation. *J Emerg Med.* 2001; 20:211-212.

Lurie SJ, Lambert DR, Grady-Weliky TA. Relationship between Dean's letter rankings and later evaluations by residency program directors. *Teach Learn Med* 2007; 19(3): 251-256.

Mahadaven SV, Garmel GM. The Outstanding Medical Student in Emergency Medicine. *Acad Emerg Med.* 2001; 8(4): 402-403.

Martin-Lee L, Park H, Overton DT. Does interview date affect match list position in the emergency medicine national residency matching program match? *Acad Emerg Med* 2000; 7 (9): 1022-1026.

Mavis BE, Shafer CL, Magallanes BM. The intentions of letter writers for applicants to a baccalaureate-M.D. program: self-report and content analyses of letters of reference. Med Educ Online [serial online] 2006; 11:6 (available from http://www.med-ed-online.org).

McDade W. Residency programs: an inside look. From www.ama-assn.org.

McDaniel MA, Whetzel D, Schmidt FL, Maurer SD. The validity of employment interviews: a comprehensive review and meta-analysis. *J Appl Psychol* 1994; 79 (4): 599-616,

McGarry KA, Tammaro D, Cyr MG. Crafting a Great Personal Statement. ACP IMpact September 2006.

McMahon GT. Coming to America - international medical graduates in the United States. *N Engl J Med* 2004; 350 (24): 2435 - 2437.

Melendez MM, Xu X, Sexton TR, Shapiro MJ, Mohan EP. The importance of basic science and clinical research as a selection criterion for general surgery residency programs. *J Surg* 2008; 65: 151-154.

Messner AH, Shimahara E. Letters of recommendation to an otolaryngology/head and neck surgery residency program: their function and the role of gender. *Laryngoscope* 2008; 118: 1-10 (epub).

Metro DG, Talarico JF, Patel RM, Wetmore AL. The Resident Application Process and its correlation to future performance as a resident. *Anesth Analg* 2005; 100: 502-505.

Miller JB, Schaad DC, Crittenden RA, Oriol NE, MacLaren C. Communication between programs and applicants during residency selection: effects of the match on medical students' professional development. *Acad Med* 2003; 78(4): 403-411.

Miller JB, Schaad DC, Crittenden RA, Oriol NE. The departmental advisor's effect on medical students' confidence when the advisor evaluates or recruits for their own program during the match. *Teach Learn Med* 2004; 16(3): 290-295.

Miller J, Miller OF, Freedberg I. Dear dermatology applicant. *Arch Derm* 2004; 140: 884.

Molidor JB, Barber KR. I can't believe you asked that! *Acad Med* 1998; 73 (7): 731-733.

Monga M, Yoemans E. Career counseling: obstetrics and gynecology. Available at http://www.uth.tmc.edu/med/administration/student/ms4/2003CCC.htm.

Moore P. A guide to the perplexed: residency guide. From www.ucdmc.ucdavis.edu.

Morgenstern BZ, Zalneraitis E, Slavin S. Improving the letter of recommendation for pediatric residency applicants: an idea whose time has come? *J Pediatr* 2003; 2: 143-144.

Motowidlo SJ, Carter GW, Dunnette MD et al. Studies of the structured behavioral interview. *J Appl Psychol* 1992; 77 (5): 571-587.

Muizelaar JP. A guide to the perplexed: residency guide. From www.ucdmc.ucdavis.edu.

Nawotniak R, Gray E. General surgery resident applicants perception of program coordinators. *Curr Surg* 2006; 63(6): 473-475.

Nelsen K. A guide to the perplexed: residency guide. From www.ucdmc.ucdavis.edu.

Newton DA, Grayson MA, Thompson LF. The variable influence of lifestyle and income on medical students' career specialty choices: data from two U.S. medical schools, 1998 - 2004. *Acad Med* 2005; 80(9): 809-814.

Norcini JJ, Boulet JR, Whelan GP, McKinley DW. Specialty board-certification among U.S. Citizen and non-U.S. citizen graduates of international medical schools. *Acad Med* 2005; 80(10): S42-S45.

Nuthalapaty FS, Carver AR, Nuthalapaty ES, Ramsey PS. The perceived impact of duty hour restrictions on the residency environment: a survey of residency program directors. *Am J Obstet Gynecol* 2006; 194 (6): 1556-62.

Nuthalapaty FS, Jackson JR, Owen J. The influence of quality-of-life, academic, and workplace factors on residency program selection. *Acad Med* 2004; 79 (5): 417-425.

O'Halloran CM, Altmaier EM, Smith WL, Franken EA. Evaluation of resident applicants by letters of recommendation: a comparison of traditional and behavioral-based formats. *Invest Radiol* 1993; 28: 274-7.

Ogle AA, Garrison SJ, Kaelin DL, Atchison JW, Park YI, Currie DM. Roadmap to physical medicine and rehabilitation: answers to medical students' questions about the field. *Am J Phys Med Rehabil* 2001; 80(3): 218-224.

Oldham S. Career counseling: radiology. Available at http://www.uth.tmc.edu/med/administration/student/ms4/2003CCC.htm.

Oman J. Residency selection handbook: emergency medicine. From www.ucihs.uci.edu.

Opel D, Shugerman R, McPhillips H, Swanson W, Archibald S, Diekema D. Professionalism and the match: a pediatric residency program's postinterview no-call policy and its impact on applicants. *Pediatrics* 2007; 120: e826 - e831.

Otero HJ, Erturk SM, Ondategui-Parra S, Ros PR. Key criteria for selection of radiology residents: results of a national survey by. *Acad Radiol* 2006; 13: 1155-1164.

Paik C. A guide to the perplexed: residency guide. From www.ucdmc.ucdavis.edu.

Part HM, Markert RJ. Predicting the first-year performances of international medical graduates in an internal medicine residency. *Acad Med* 1993 ; 68(11): 856-858.

Peabody T, Manning D. Pritzker residency process guide: orthopedic surgery. Available at http://pritzker.uchicago.edu/current/students/ResidencyProcessGuide.pdf.

Pereira K. Career counseling: otolaryngology. Available at http://www.uth.tmc.edu/med/administration/student/ms4/2003CCC.htm/

Phipps GJ. Residency selection handbook: orthopedic surgery. From www.ucihs.uci.edu.

Potts JR. Career counseling: general surgery. Available at http://www.uth.tmc.edu/med/administration/student/ms4/2003CCC.htm.

Provan JL, Cuttress L. Preferences of program directors for evaluation of candidates for postgraduate training. *CMAJ* 1995; 153 (7): 919-923.

Pulito AR, Donnelly MB, Plymale M, Mentzer RM Jr. What do faculty observe of medical students' clinical performance? *Teach Learn Med* 2006; 18(2): 99-104.

Raff MJ, Schwartz IS. An applicant's evaluation of a medical house officership. *NEJM* 1974; 291(12) : 601-605.

Rao NR, Meinzer AE, Primavera LH, Augustine A. Psychiatry residency selection criteria for American and foreign medical graduates. *Acad Psychiatry* 1991; 15(2): 69-79.

Rao NR, Meinzer AE, Berman SS. Perspectives on screening and interviewing international medical graduates for psychiatric residency training programs. *Acad Psychiatry* 1994; 18(4): 178-188.

Reilly EF, Leibrandt TJ, Zonno AJ, Simpson MC, Morris JB. General surgery residency program websites: usefulness and usability for resident applicants. *Curr Surg* 2004; 61(2): 236-240.

Reilly E. Career counseling: psychiatry. Available at http://www.uth.tmc.edu/med/administration/student/ms4/2003CCC.htm.

Ritchey M. Career counseling: urology. Available at http://www.uth.tmc.edu/med/administration/student/ms4/2003CCC.htm.

Robin AP, Bombeck CT, Pollak R, Nyhus LM. Introduction of bias in residency-candidate interviews. *Surgery* 1991; 110 (2): 253-8.

Roellig MS, Katz ED. Inaccuracies on applications for emergency medicine residency training. *Acad Emerg Med* 2004; 11(9): 992-994.

Rosen P, Hamilton GC. *Pro vs Con: Four vs Three.* Society for Academic Emergency Medicine Website.

Rosenblum J. Pritzker residency process guide: radiology. Available at http://pritzker.uchicago.edu/current/students/ResidencyProcessGuide.pdf.

Ross CA, Leichner P. Criteria for selecting residents: a reassessment. *Can J Psychiatry* 1984; 29: 681-686.

Ryu J. A guide to the perplexed: residency guide. From ww.ucdmc.ucdavis.edu

Scheiss M. Career counseling: neurology. Available at http://www.uth.tmc.edu/med/administration/student/ms4/2003CCC.htm.

Scherer L. A guide to the perplexed: residency guide. From www.ucdmc.ucdavis.edu.

Schwartz RA. Medical student publications: a faculty mentor's perspective. *J Am Acad Dermatol* 1997; 37 (4): 667-668.

Servis M. A guide to the perplexed: residency guide. From www.ucdmc.ucdavis.edu.

Shalhav AL. Pritzker residency process guide: urology. Available at http://pritzker.uchicago.edu/current/students/ResidencyProcessGuide.pdf.

Shaver EG. Neurosurgery. From www.womensurgeons.org (Association of Women Surgeons).

Shea CR. Pritzker residency process guide: dermatology. Available at http://pritzker.uchicago.edu/current/students/ResidencyProcessGuide.pdf.

Simmonds AC, Robbins JM, Brinker MR, Rice JC, Kerstein MD. Factors important to students in selecting a residency program. *Acad Med* 1990; 65(10): 640-643.

Simpson J. Residency selection handbook: ophthalmology. From www.ucihs.uci.edu.

Singhal K, Ramakrishnan K. Training needs of international medical graduates seeking residency training: evaluation of medical training in India and the United States. The Internet Journal of Family Practice 2004; 3(1).

Smilen SW, Funai EF, Bianco AT. Residency selection: should interviewers be given applicant's board scores. Am J Obstet Gynecol 2001; 184 (3): 508-513.

Smith EA, Weyhing B, Mody Y, Smith WL. A critical analysis of personal statements submitted by radiology residency applicants. Acad Radiol 2005; 12: 1024-1028.

Sosenko J, Stekel KW, Soto R, Gelbard M. NBME examination part 1 as a predictor of clinical and ABIM certifying examination performance, J Gen Intern Med 1993; 8: 86-88.

Speer A, Khilnani N. Applying for Residency: Providing Advice to Medical Students. Academic Internal Medicine Insight 2005; Volume 2 Issue 4; 10 (www.im.org/AAIM/Pubs/Insight/Winter2005/page10.htm).

Spitz D,Penna N. Pritzker residency process guide: psychiatry. Available at http://pritzker.uchicago.edu/current/students/ResidencyProcessGuide.pdf.

Suskind D. Pritzker residency process guide: otolaryngology. Available at http://pritzker.uchicago.edu/current/students/ResidencyProcessGuide.pdf.

Swanson WS, Harris MC, Master C, Gallagher PR, Maruo AE, Ludwig S. The impact of the interview in pediatric residency selection. Amb Pediatr 2005; 5 (4): 216-220.

Taber's Cyclopedic Medical Dictionary (edition 17). F.A.Davis Company; Philadelphia 1993.

Taylor CA, Weinstein L, Mayhew HE. The process of resident selection: a view from the residency director's desk. Obstet Gynecol 1995; 85 (2): 299-303.

Teichman JM, Anderson KD, Dorough MM, Stein CR, Optenberg SA, Thompson IM. The urology residency matching program in practice. J Urol 2000; 163(6): 1878-1887.

Travis C, Taylor CA, Mayhew HE. Evaluating residency applicants: stable values in a changing market. Fam Med 1999; 31 (4): 252-256.

Tsarnas CD, Fessenden J. Audition electives during surgical residency and selection for post-residency fellowship positions. Curr Surg 2002; 59(4): 412-415.

Twede JV. Being a visual person. Arch Dermatol 2006; 242: 1357-1358.

UAB guidelines for pursuing a residency in obstetrics and gynecology. Taken from www.obgyn.uab.edu.

Uthman MO. Career counseling: pathology. Available at http://www.uth.tmc.edu/med/administration/student/ms4/2003CCC.htm.

van Zanten M, Boulet JR, McKinley D, Whelan GP. Attrition rates of residents in postgraduate training programs. Teach Learn Med 2002; 14(3): 175-177.

Villanueva AM, Kaye D, Abdelhak SS, Morahan PS. Comparing selection criteria for residency directors and physicians' employers. Acad Med 1995; 70(4): 261-271.

Vogt HB, Thanel FH, Hearns VL. The audition elective and its relation to success in the National Resident Matching Program. Teach Learn Med 2000; 12(2): 78-80.

Wagner PJ, Moseley GC, Grant MM, Gore JR, Owens C. Physicians' emotional intelligence and patient satisfaction. Fam Med 2002; 34(10): 750-754.

Wagoner NE, Gray GT. Report on a survey of program directors regarding selection factors in graduate medical education. J Med Educ 1979; 74: 51-58.

Wagoner NE, Suriano JR, Stoner JA. Factors used by program directors to select residents. J Med Educ 1986; 61 (1): 10-21.

Wagoner NE, Suriano JR. Program directors' responses to a survey on variables used to select residents in a time of change. Acad Med 1999; 74: 51-8.

Wajda MC, O'Neill D, Tepfenhardt L, Yook I, Kim J. Timing of applicants residency interview can not predict if they will match your residency program. *Anesthesiology* 2006; 105: A167.

Weiten W, Lloyd MA. *Pscyhology applied to modern life: adjustment in the 21st century.* Thomas Wadsworth 2005.

West D. A guide to the perplexed: residency guide. From www.ucdmc.ucdavis.edu.

Wiebe C. Face-to-face value. *New Physician* 1994; 43: 15-17.

Wilhelm G. Career counseling: emergency medicine. Available at http://www.uth.tmc.edu/med/administration/student/ms4/2003CCC.htm.

Wolford RW, Anderson KD. Emergency medicine residency director perceptions of the resident selection process. *Acad Emerg Med* 2000; 7(10): 1170-1171.

Wood PS, Smith WL, Altmaier EM, Tarico VS, Franken EA. A prospective study of cognitive and noncognitive selection criteria as predictors of resident performance. *Invest Radiol* 1990; 25 (7): 761-2

Woods SE, Harju A, Rao S, Koo J, Kini D. Perceived biases and prejudices experienced by international medical graduates in the U.S. post-graduate medical education system. *Med Educ Online* 2006; 11: 20.

Yang GY, Schoenwetter MF, Wagner TD, Donohue KA, Kuettel MR. Misrepresentation of publications among radiation oncology residency applicants. *J Am Coll Radiol* 2006; 3(4): 259-264.

Yao DC, Wright SM. The challenge of problem residents. *J Gen Intern Med* 2001; 16(7): 486-492.

Yao DC, Wright SM. National survey of internal medicine residency program directors regarding problem residents. *JAMA* 2000; 284(9): 1099-1104.

Young MJ, Behnke RR, Mann YM. Anxiety patterns in employment interviews. *Communication Reports* 2004; 17(1): 49-57.

Young T. Teaching medical students to lie—the disturbing contradiction: medical ideals and the resident-selection process. *CMAJ* 1997; 156(2): 2219-2222.

Zagumny MJ, Rudolph J. Comparing medical students' and residency directors' ratings of criteria used to select residents. *Acad Med* 1992; 67(9): 613.

Ziegelstein RC. "Rocking the match": applying and getting into residency. *J Natl Med Assoc* 2007; 99(9): 994-999.

Index

A

academic criteria
  erroneous focus on 118
  in residency selection 83
Academic Emergency Medicine 269
Accreditation Council for Graduate
  Medical Education (ACGME) 95, 335
action verbs, list 129
advance planning for research 271
advisor 87, 88, 90, 95, 103, 259, 269
After the Interview 344–358
Alpha Omega Alpha Honor Medical
  Society (AOA) 2, 81, 102, 103
American Medical Association
  Fellowship and Resiency Electronic
  Interactive Database Access (AMA-
  FREIDA) 93
anesthesiology 21–25
  AOA 24
  letters of recommendation (LOR) 24
  positions filled 2004-08 (table) 21
  program rankings of academic criteria
    used (table) 22
  research 24
  selection goals 107
  USMLE Step 1 score 24
applicant characteristics 280
application timeline (table) 92
Association of American Medical
  Colleges (AAMC) 246
Association of Program Directors in
  Radiology (APDR) 72
audition elective 9, 109, 248
  benefits and drawbacks 244–245
  evaluating programs 245
  for competitive programs 137
  importance by specialty 238–239
  impressing program 251
  in less competitive specialites 239
  opportunities 247
  power of 243
  strong letter of recommendation 251
away elective 243, 246, 250, 252, 257
  how to apply 249–250
  steps in applying for 249

B

behavioral interviews 287
behavioral questions
  examples 287–288
block of time for research 271
body language 17, 293, 323, 326, 327,
  328

C

case reports 256, 259
  classic case 260
  clinical features in 261
  in Postgraduate Medicine 255
  leads to more projects 254
  types 254
  working with faculty 257
  writing an outstanding 258–259
case series 256
case study
  needs a "hook" 259
common application form (CAF) 9
compatibility 110, 280, 292
competitive edge 11, 253–274
  recommendations 253
control over interview 288
conversational interview 291
curriculum vitae (CV) 8, 123–157
  characteristics of (table) 136
  correct format 124
  education 126
  ERAS format for 124
  importance of 123
  language style 128
  length 133
  order of elements 126
  personal interests 128
  professional membership 128
  research experience 129
  review 131
  review form 132
  sample 151, 153, 156
  standard sections of (table) 126
  work experience 131

250 Biggest Mistakes 3rd Year Medical Students Make And How To Avoid Them

By Samir P. Desai, MD, and Rajani Katta, MD
ISBN # 9780972556163

How important is the third year of medical school?

One survey of residency program directors found that grades in third year clerkships were the most important academic criteria used to select residents. Some students excel in their clerkships, while others remain average.

What sets apart these top students? Compiled from discussions with hundreds of faculty, residents, and students, along with extensive review of the literature, this evidence-based guide was written with the express intent of answering that question. This book will provide you with a specific strategy for success during the most important year of medical school.

"Does a thorough job demystifying the elements and culture of the clerkships."
> —The Journal, *Teaching and Learning in Medicine*

"House staff and attending physicians with teaching responsibilities may also benefit from the text."
> —The journal, *Mayo Clinic Proceedings*

"This book is a useful resource to avoid both common and not-so-obvious pitfalls, and serves as an excellent introduction to performing well on the wards. I would highly recommend this book for a beginning 3rd year student."
> —J. Reddy, M.D., Physician Preceptor for University of Illinois pediatric rotation (review posted on Amazon.com)